current procedural terminology

# *cpt*®

# 2013

# Changes

## An Insider's View

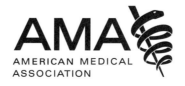

AMA

AMERICAN MEDICAL
ASSOCIATION

For information regarding the reprinting or licensing of CPT® Changes 2013: An Insider's View, please contact:

CPT Intellectual Property Services
American Medical Association
515 N. State St. Chicago, IL 60654
312 464-5022

Additional copies of this book may be ordered by calling: 800 621-8335 or from the secure AMA Web site at www.amabookstore.com. Refer to product number OP512913.

This book is intended for information purposes only. It is not intended to constitute legal advice. If legal advice is desired or needed, a licensed attorney should be consulted.

ISBN: 978-1-60359-685-5
AC34: 12-P-004:11/12

# Contents

Foreword. . . . . . . . . . . . . . . . . . . . . . . . . . . . . . . . . . . . . . . . . . . . . . . . . . . . . . . . . . . . . . vii

Using This Book . . . . . . . . . . . . . . . . . . . . . . . . . . . . . . . . . . . . . . . . . . . . . . . . . . . . . . . . ix

    The Symbols . . . . . . . . . . . . . . . . . . . . . . . . . . . . . . . . . . . . . . . . . . . . . . . . . . . . . . . . ix

    The Rationale . . . . . . . . . . . . . . . . . . . . . . . . . . . . . . . . . . . . . . . . . . . . . . . . . . . . . . . . ix

    Reading the Clinical Examples . . . . . . . . . . . . . . . . . . . . . . . . . . . . . . . . . . . . . . . . . . . . . x

    The Tabular Review of the Changes. . . . . . . . . . . . . . . . . . . . . . . . . . . . . . . . . . . . . . . . . x

    CPT Codebook Text and Guidelines . . . . . . . . . . . . . . . . . . . . . . . . . . . . . . . . . . . . . . . . x

CPT Nomenclature Reporting Neutrality . . . . . . . . . . . . . . . . . . . . . . . . . . . . . . . . . . . 1

Explicit Code Ranges . . . . . . . . . . . . . . . . . . . . . . . . . . . . . . . . . . . . . . . . . . . . . . . . . . 45

Evaluation and Management . . . . . . . . . . . . . . . . . . . . . . . . . . . . . . . . . . . . . . . . . . . 53

    Definitions of Commonly Used Terms . . . . . . . . . . . . . . . . . . . . . . . . . . . . . . . . . . . . . . 55

    Hospital Inpatient Services. . . . . . . . . . . . . . . . . . . . . . . . . . . . . . . . . . . . . . . . . . . . . . 56

    Domiciliary, Rest Home (eg, Assisted Living Facility), or Home Care Plan Oversight Services . . . . 57

    Prolonged Services . . . . . . . . . . . . . . . . . . . . . . . . . . . . . . . . . . . . . . . . . . . . . . . . . . . 58

    Case Management Services. . . . . . . . . . . . . . . . . . . . . . . . . . . . . . . . . . . . . . . . . . . . . . 60

    Care Plan Oversight Services . . . . . . . . . . . . . . . . . . . . . . . . . . . . . . . . . . . . . . . . . . . . 61

    Non-Face-to-Face Services. . . . . . . . . . . . . . . . . . . . . . . . . . . . . . . . . . . . . . . . . . . . . . 62

    Inpatient Neonatal Intensive Care Services and
Pediatric and Neonatal Critical Care Services. . . . . . . . . . . . . . . . . . . . . . . . . . . . . . . . . 63

    Complex Chronic Care Coordination Services . . . . . . . . . . . . . . . . . . . . . . . . . . . . . . . . 71

    Transitional Care Management Services . . . . . . . . . . . . . . . . . . . . . . . . . . . . . . . . . . . . 73

Surgery . . . . . . . . . . . . . . . . . . . . . . . . . . . . . . . . . . . . . . . . . . . . . . . . . . . . . . . . . . . . 81

    Services. . . . . . . . . . . . . . . . . . . . . . . . . . . . . . . . . . . . . . . . . . . . . . . . . . . . . . . . . . . 83

    CPT Surgical Package Definition . . . . . . . . . . . . . . . . . . . . . . . . . . . . . . . . . . . . . . . . . . 83

    Supplied Materials . . . . . . . . . . . . . . . . . . . . . . . . . . . . . . . . . . . . . . . . . . . . . . . . . . . 83

    Reporting More Than One Procedure/Service . . . . . . . . . . . . . . . . . . . . . . . . . . . . . . . . 83

    Integumentary System . . . . . . . . . . . . . . . . . . . . . . . . . . . . . . . . . . . . . . . . . . . . . . . . 84

    Musculoskeletal System. . . . . . . . . . . . . . . . . . . . . . . . . . . . . . . . . . . . . . . . . . . . . . . 85

    Respiratory System. . . . . . . . . . . . . . . . . . . . . . . . . . . . . . . . . . . . . . . . . . . . . . . . . . . 95

    Cardiovascular System . . . . . . . . . . . . . . . . . . . . . . . . . . . . . . . . . . . . . . . . . . . . . . . 105

    Hemic and Lymphatic Systems. . . . . . . . . . . . . . . . . . . . . . . . . . . . . . . . . . . . . . . . . . 145

    Digestive System . . . . . . . . . . . . . . . . . . . . . . . . . . . . . . . . . . . . . . . . . . . . . . . . . . 148

    Urinary System . . . . . . . . . . . . . . . . . . . . . . . . . . . . . . . . . . . . . . . . . . . . . . . . . . . . 153

Nervous System . . . . . . . . . . . . . . . . . . . . . . . . . . . . . . . . . . . . . . . . 155

Eye and Ocular Adnexa . . . . . . . . . . . . . . . . . . . . . . . . . . . . . . . . . . . . 158

Operating Microscope . . . . . . . . . . . . . . . . . . . . . . . . . . . . . . . . . . . . . 161

**Radiology** . . . . . . . . . . . . . . . . . . . . . . . . . . . . . . . . . . . . . . . . . . . . . . **163**

Diagnostic Radiology (Diagnostic Imaging) . . . . . . . . . . . . . . . . . . . . . . 165

Diagnostic Ultrasound . . . . . . . . . . . . . . . . . . . . . . . . . . . . . . . . . . . . . 170

Radiologic Guidance . . . . . . . . . . . . . . . . . . . . . . . . . . . . . . . . . . . . . . 171

Radiation Oncology . . . . . . . . . . . . . . . . . . . . . . . . . . . . . . . . . . . . . . . 173

Nuclear Medicine . . . . . . . . . . . . . . . . . . . . . . . . . . . . . . . . . . . . . . . . 174

**Pathology and Laboratory** . . . . . . . . . . . . . . . . . . . . . . . . . . . . . . . . . **181**

Evocative/Suppression Testing . . . . . . . . . . . . . . . . . . . . . . . . . . . . . . 183

Molecular Pathology . . . . . . . . . . . . . . . . . . . . . . . . . . . . . . . . . . . . . . 183

Multianalyte Assays with Algorithmic Analyses . . . . . . . . . . . . . . . . . . 203

Chemistry . . . . . . . . . . . . . . . . . . . . . . . . . . . . . . . . . . . . . . . . . . . . . . 209

Immunology . . . . . . . . . . . . . . . . . . . . . . . . . . . . . . . . . . . . . . . . . . . . 211

Transfusion Medicine . . . . . . . . . . . . . . . . . . . . . . . . . . . . . . . . . . . . . 218

Microbiology . . . . . . . . . . . . . . . . . . . . . . . . . . . . . . . . . . . . . . . . . . . . 218

Cytopathology . . . . . . . . . . . . . . . . . . . . . . . . . . . . . . . . . . . . . . . . . . . 223

Cytogenetic Studies . . . . . . . . . . . . . . . . . . . . . . . . . . . . . . . . . . . . . . 223

Surgical Pathology . . . . . . . . . . . . . . . . . . . . . . . . . . . . . . . . . . . . . . . 224

Reproductive Medicine Procedures . . . . . . . . . . . . . . . . . . . . . . . . . . . 225

**Medicine** . . . . . . . . . . . . . . . . . . . . . . . . . . . . . . . . . . . . . . . . . . . . . . **227**

Immunization Administration for Vaccines/Toxoids . . . . . . . . . . . . . . . . 229

Vaccines, Toxoids . . . . . . . . . . . . . . . . . . . . . . . . . . . . . . . . . . . . . . . . 229

Psychiatry . . . . . . . . . . . . . . . . . . . . . . . . . . . . . . . . . . . . . . . . . . . . . . 232

Gastroenterology . . . . . . . . . . . . . . . . . . . . . . . . . . . . . . . . . . . . . . . . . 247

Ophthalmology . . . . . . . . . . . . . . . . . . . . . . . . . . . . . . . . . . . . . . . . . . 248

Cardiovascular . . . . . . . . . . . . . . . . . . . . . . . . . . . . . . . . . . . . . . . . . . 249

Pulmonary . . . . . . . . . . . . . . . . . . . . . . . . . . . . . . . . . . . . . . . . . . . . . . 296

Allergy and Clinical Immunology . . . . . . . . . . . . . . . . . . . . . . . . . . . . . 296

Neurology and Neuromuscular Procedures . . . . . . . . . . . . . . . . . . . . . . 300

Hydration, Therapeutic, Prophylactic, Diagnostic Injections and Infusions,
and Chemotherapy and Other Highly Complex Drug or Highly Complex
Biologic Agent Administration . . . . . . . . . . . . . . . . . . . . . . . . . . . . . . . 319

Physical Medicine and Rehabilitation . . . . . . . . . . . . . . . . . . . . . . . . . . . . . . . . . . . . . . . . . . . . . . . 321

Non-Face-to-Face Nonphysician Services . . . . . . . . . . . . . . . . . . . . . . . . . . . . . . . . . . . . . . . . . . . . 321

Other Services and Procedures . . . . . . . . . . . . . . . . . . . . . . . . . . . . . . . . . . . . . . . . . . . . . . . . . . . . 323

**Category II Codes** . . . . . . . . . . . . . . . . . . . . . . . . . . . . . . . . . . . . . . . . . . . . . . . . . . . . . . . . . **325**

Footnotes. . . . . . . . . . . . . . . . . . . . . . . . . . . . . . . . . . . . . . . . . . . . . . . . . . . . . . . . . . . . . . . . . . . . 327

Patient History . . . . . . . . . . . . . . . . . . . . . . . . . . . . . . . . . . . . . . . . . . . . . . . . . . . . . . . . . . . . . . . . 327

Diagnostic/Screening Processes or Results. . . . . . . . . . . . . . . . . . . . . . . . . . . . . . . . . . . . . . . . . . . 328

Therapeutic, Preventive, or Other Interventions . . . . . . . . . . . . . . . . . . . . . . . . . . . . . . . . . . . . . . . 330

Patient Safety . . . . . . . . . . . . . . . . . . . . . . . . . . . . . . . . . . . . . . . . . . . . . . . . . . . . . . . . . . . . . . . . . 332

**Category III Codes** . . . . . . . . . . . . . . . . . . . . . . . . . . . . . . . . . . . . . . . . . . . . . . . . . . . . . . . . . . **333**

**Appendixes** . . . . . . . . . . . . . . . . . . . . . . . . . . . . . . . . . . . . . . . . . . . . . . . . . . . . . . . . . . . . . . . . **369**

Appendix A . . . . . . . . . . . . . . . . . . . . . . . . . . . . . . . . . . . . . . . . . . . . . . . . . . . . . . . . . . . . . . . . . . . 371

Appendix I. . . . . . . . . . . . . . . . . . . . . . . . . . . . . . . . . . . . . . . . . . . . . . . . . . . . . . . . . . . . . . . . . . . . 371

Appendix J . . . . . . . . . . . . . . . . . . . . . . . . . . . . . . . . . . . . . . . . . . . . . . . . . . . . . . . . . . . . . . . . . . . 371

Appendix O . . . . . . . . . . . . . . . . . . . . . . . . . . . . . . . . . . . . . . . . . . . . . . . . . . . . . . . . . . . . . . . . . . . 373

**Tabular Review of the Changes** . . . . . . . . . . . . . . . . . . . . . . . . . . . . . . . . . . . . . . . . . . . . . . . . . **375**

# Foreword

The American Medical Association is pleased to offer *CPT® Changes 2013: An Insider's View*. Since this book was first published in 2000, it has served as the definitive text on additions, revisions, and deletions to the CPT code set.

In developing this book, it was our intention to provide CPT users with a glimpse of the logic, rationale, and proposed function of CPT changes that resulted from the decisions of the CPT Editorial Panel and the yearly update process. American Medical Association (AMA) staff members have the unique perspective of being both participants in the CPT editorial process and users of the CPT code set. *CPT Changes* is intended to bridge understanding between clinical decisions made at the CPT Editorial Panel regarding appropriate service or procedure descriptions with functional interpretations of coding guidelines, code intent, and code combinations necessary for users of the CPT code set. A new edition of this book, like the codebook, is published annually.

To assist CPT users in applying new and revised CPT codes, this book includes clinical examples that describe the typical patient who might receive the procedure and detailed descriptions of the procedure. Both of these are required as a part of the CPT code change proposal process and are used by the CPT Editorial Panel in crafting language, guidelines, and parenthetical notes associated with the new or revised codes. In addition, many of the clinical examples and descriptions of the procedures are used in the AMA/Specialty Society RVS Update process for conducting surveys on physician work and in developing work relative value recommendations to the Centers for Medicare and Medicaid Services (CMS) as part of the Medicare Physician Fee Schedule (MPFS).

We are confident that the information contained in *CPT Changes* each year will prove to be a valuable resource to CPT users not only as they apply changes for the year of publication, but also as a resource for frequent reference as they continue their education in CPT coding. The AMA makes every effort to be a voice of clarity and consistency in an otherwise confusing system of health care claims and payment, and *CPT Changes 2013: An Insider's View* demonstrates our continued commitment to assist users of the CPT code set.

# Using This Book

This book is designed to serve as a reference guide to understanding the changes contained in *Current Procedural Terminology (CPT®) 2013* and is not intended to replace the CPT codebook. Every effort is made to ensure accuracy, however, if differences exist, you should always defer to the information contained in the *CPT 2013* codebook.

## The Symbols

This book uses the same coding conventions that appear in the CPT nomenclature.

● Indicates that a new procedure number was added to the CPT nomenclature

▲ Indicates that a code revision has resulted in a substantially altered procedure descriptor

✚ Indicates a CPT add-on code

⊘ Indicates a code that is exempt from the use of modifier 51 but is not designated as a CPT add-on procedure/service

►◄ Indicates revised guidelines, cross-references, and/or explanatory text

⊙ Indicates a code that typically includes moderate sedation

⁄ Indicates a code for a vaccine that is pending FDA approval

\# Indicates a resequenced code

○ Indicates a reinstated or recycled code

Whenever possible, complete segments of text from the CPT codebook are provided, however, in some cases the text has been abbreviated.

## The Rationale

After each change or series of changes is a rationale. The rationale is intended to provide a brief explanation as to why changes occurred, but note that it may not answer every question that may arise as a result of the changes.

## Reading the Clinical Examples

The clinical examples and their procedural descriptions included in this text with many of the codes provide practical situations for which the new and/or revised codes in the *CPT 2013* codebook would be appropriately reported. It is important to note that these examples do not suggest limiting the use of a code but only represent the typical patient and service or procedure. They do not describe the universe of patients for whom the service or procedure would be appropriate. In addition, third-party payer reporting policies may differ.

## The Tabular Review of the Changes

The table beginning on page 377 allows you to see all of the code changes at a glance. By reviewing the table you can easily determine the level to which your particular field of interest has been affected by the changes in the *CPT 2013* codebook.

## CPT Codebook Text and Guidelines

In *CPT Changes 2013*, guideline and revised CPT codebook text appears in brown indented type. Any revised text, guidelines, and/or headings are indicated with the ►◄ symbols. This convention matches the style used in the codebook, ie, symbols are placed at the beginning and end of a paragraph that contains a revision or revisions.

The CPT code set is a work of medical nomenclature consisting of a set of codes, descriptions, and guidelines that describe procedures and services performed by physicians and other qualified health care professionals. Any procedure or service in any section of the CPT code set may be used to designate the services rendered by any qualified physician or other qualified health care professional or entity (eg, hospital, clinical laboratory, home health agency). To provide consistency with this statement, the following is a list of those CPT codes, guidelines, and/or parenthetical instructions whose terminology has been revised with the intent of reporting neutrality in the CPT code set.

# CPT® Nomenclature Reporting Neutrality

The CPT Editorial Panel is required to adhere to the policy of neutrality with respect to indentifying who may perform a procedure or service that is described in the CPT® code set. Therefore, the CPT code set avoids statements about who is or is not qualified to perform the services and procedures described in the CPT code set, other than to state that he or she must be qualified. The introductory section of the CPT codebook describes the reporting neutrality aspect of CPT code sets in the **Instructions for Use of the CPT Codebook:**

> Select the name of the procedure or service…. It is important to recognize that the listing of a service or procedure and its code number in a specific section of this book does not restrict its use to a specific specialty group. Any procedure or service in any section of this book may be used to designate the services rendered by any qualified physician or other qualified health care professional or entity (eg, hospital, clinical laboratory, home health agency).

> A "physician or other qualified healthcare professional" is an individual who is qualified by education, training, licensure/regulation (when applicable), and facility privileging (when applicable) who performs a professional service within his/her scope of practice and independently reports that professional service. These professionals are distinct from "clinical staff." A clinical staff member is a person who works under the supervision of a physician or other qualified healthcare professional and who is allowed by law, regulation and facility policy to perform or assist in the performance of a specified professional service, but who does not individually report that professional service. Other policies may also affect who may report specific services.

Therefore, it would be inconsistent with the guidance cited above to include in any CPT descriptor accompanying guidance, or any explicit or implicit direction as to who is or is not qualified to perform any service or procedure.

In the following revisions, it should be noted that a limited number of code series have been created or modified to distinguish between physicians and other qualified health care professionals performing essentially the same service. These distinctions were created to better align CPT codes with the reporting and payment policies of the Centers for Medicare and Medicaid Services (CMS) and/or private payers. These distinctions are not inconsistent with the statement of reporting neutrality stated previously. Other revisions are denoted in a more comprehensive revision of a section or subsection of this publication (eg, Inpatient Neonatal Intensive Care Services and Pediatric and Neonatal Critical Care Services/Inpatient Neonatal and Pediatric Critical Care, Psychiatry, Allergy and Clinical Immunology, Neurology and Neuromuscular Procedures).

Because of the number of refinements, reference is only made to revised code number, section, or subsection language. Therefore, complete guidelines, code families, and all applicable parenthetical instructions are not represented in the following table. For complete information, refer to the CPT 2013 code set. The following code revisions include long descriptors. In instances in which a code revision has occured, the revised code symbol (▲) is placed before the code number. Underlined text indicates new language, while stricken text indicates deleted language. (For complete information, refer to the *CPT 2013* codebook.)

| CPT Code/Section/Subsection | Revision/Addition/Deletion |
|---|---|
| **Introduction** | *Current Procedural Terminology* (CPT®), Fourth Edition, is a set of codes, descriptions, and guidelines intended to describe procedures and services performed by physicians and other health care <u>professionals</u> ~~providers~~. <u>The CPT code set is also used by other entities to report outpatient services</u>......<br><br>Inclusion of a descriptor and its associated five-digit code number in the CPT codebook is based on whether the procedure is consistent with contemporary medical practice and is performed by many <u>individuals</u> ~~practitioners~~ in clinical practice in multiple locations.....<br><br>..... The interval between the release of the update and the effective date is considered the implementation period and is intended to allow physicians and other ~~qualified health care professionals~~ <u>providers</u>, payers, and vendors to incorporate CPT changes into their systems. |
| **Instructions for Use of the CPT Codebook** | *Select the name of the procedure or service that accurately identifies the service performed.....*<br><br>*It is important to recognize that the listing of a service or procedure and its code number...*<br><br><u>Throughout CPT code set the use of terms such as "physician," "qualified health care professional," or "individual" is not intended to indicate that other entities may not report the service. In selected instances, specific instructions may define a service as limited to professionals or limited to other entities (eg, hospital or home health agency).</u> |
| **Place of Service and Facility Reporting** | <u>Throughout CPT code set the use of terms such as "physician," "qualified health care professional," or "individual" is not intended to indicate that other entities may not report the service. In selected instances, specific instructions may define a service as limited to professionals or limited to other entities (eg, hospital or home health agency).</u><br><br>~~Facilities are entities that may also report the same services listed in CPT. For example, a physician may report a procedure performed in the outpatient department of the hospital and the hospital may report the same procedure (confusing because a "hospital" cannot perform a service but rather an employee of the hospital can perform the service and the hospital may report it  or the hospital may report the technical component of some services and the provider may report the professional component~~ . The CPT code set uses the term *facility* to describe such ~~circumstances~~ <u>providers</u> and the term *nonfacility* to describe services <u>settings, or circumstances</u> in which no facility reporting may occur. Services provided in the home by an agency are facility services. Services provided in the home by a physician or qualified health care professional who is not a representative of the agency are nonfacility services. |
| **Introduction Time** | The CPT code set contains many codes with a time basis for code selection. The following standards shall apply to time measurement, unless there are code or code-range–specific instructions in guidelines, parenthetical instructions, or code descriptors to the contrary. Time is the face-to-face time with the patient. Phrases such as "interpretation and report" in the code descriptor are not intended to indicate in all cases that report writing is part of the reported time. A unit of time is attained when the mid-point is passed. For example, an hour is attained when 31 minutes have elapsed (more than midway between zero and sixty minutes). A second hour is attained when a total of 91 minutes have elapsed. When codes are ranked in sequential typical times and the actual time is between two typical times, the code with the typical time closest to the actual time is used. See also the Evaluation and Management (E/M) Services Guidelines. |

| CPT Code/Section/Subsection | Revision/Addition/Deletion |
|---|---|
| **Introduction Time** *(continued)* | When another service is performed concurrently with a time-based service, the time associated with the concurrent service should not be included in the time used for reporting the time-based service. Some services measured in units other than days extend across calendar dates. When this occurs, a continuous service does not reset and create a first hour. However, any disruption in the service does create a new initial service. For example, if intravenous hydration (96360, 96361) is given from 11 PM to 2 AM, 96360 would be reported once and 96361 twice. <u>For facility reporting on a single date of service or for continuous services that last beyond midnight (ie, over a range of dates), report the total units of time provided continuously.</u> <br><br> However, if instead of a continuous infusion, a medication was given by intravenous push at 10 PM and 2 AM, as the service was not continuous, both administrations would be reported as initial (96374) <u>and sequential (96376) as: 1) no other infusion services were performed; and 2) the push of the same drug was performed more than 30 minutes beyond the initial administration. For facility reporting per single calendar date, both administrations would be reported as initial (96374). For continuous services that last beyond midnight, use the date in which the service began and report the total units of time provided continuously.</u> ~~For continuous services that last beyond midnight, use the date in which the service began and report the total units of time provided continuously.~~ |
| **Classification of Evaluation and Management (E/M) Services** | The E/M section is divided into broad categories such as office visits, hospital visits, and consultations. Most of the categories are further divided into two or more subcategories of E/M services. For example, there are two subcategories of office visits (new patient and established patient) and there are two subcategories of hospital visits (initial and subsequent). This classification is important because the nature of ~~physician~~ work varies by type of service, place of service, and the patient's status. |
| **Evaluation and Management (E/M) Services Guidelines Definitions of Commonly Used Terms New and Established Patient** | Solely for the purposes of distinguishing between new and established patients, **professional services** are those face-to-face services rendered by ~~a~~ physician<u>s and other qualified health care professionals who may report evaluation and management services</u> reported by a specific CPT code(s). A new patient is one who has not received any professional services from the physician<u>/qualified health care professional</u> or another physician<u>/qualified health care professional</u> of the **exact** same specialty **and subspecialty** who belongs to the same group practice, within the past three years. <br><br> An established patient is one who has received professional services from the physician<u>/qualified health care professional</u> or another physician<u>/qualified health care professional</u> of the **exact** same specialty **and subspecialty** who belongs to the same group practice, within the past three years. See Decision Tree. <br><br> In the instance where a physician<u>/qualified health care professional</u> is on call for or covering for another physician<u>/qualified health care professional</u>, the patient's encounter will be classified as it would have been by the physician<u>/qualified health care professional</u> who is not available. <u>When advanced practice nurses and physician assistants are working with physicians, they are considered as working in the exact same specialty and exact same subspecialties as the physician.</u> <br><br> *No distinction is made between new and established . . .* <br> *The decision tree on page . . . . .* <br> _____Coding Tip _____ <br><br> **Instructions for Use of the CPT Codebook** <br> When advanced practice nurses and physician assistants are working with physicians they are considered as working in the exact same specialty and exact same subspecialties as the physicians. A "physician or other qualified health care professional" is an individual who is qualified by education, training, licensure/regulation (when applicable), and facility privileging (when applicable) who performs a professional service within his or her scope of practice and independently reports that professional services. These professionals are distinct from "clinical staff." A clinical staff member is a person who works under the supervision of a physician or other qualified health care professional, and who is allowed by law, regulation and facility policy to perform or assist in the performance of a specific professional service, but who does not individually report that professional service. Other policies may also affect who may report specific services. <br><br> *CPT Coding Guidelines, Introduction, Instructions for Use of the CPT Codebook* |

| CPT Code/Section/Subsection | Revision/Addition/Deletion |
|---|---|
| **Evaluation and Management (E/M) Services Guidelines Concurrent Care and Transfer of Care** | Concurrent care is the provision of similar services (eg, hospital visits) to the same patient by more than one physician <u>or other qualified health care professional</u> on the same day. When concurrent care is provided, no special reporting is required. Transfer of care is the process whereby a physician <u>or other qualified health care professional</u> who is providing management for some or all of a patient's problems relinquishes this responsibility to another physician <u>or other qualified health care professional</u> who explicitly agrees to accept this responsibility and who, from the initial encounter, is not providing consultative services. The physician <u>or other qualified health care professional</u> transferring care is then no longer providing care for these problems though he or she may continue providing care for other conditions when appropriate. Consultation codes should not be reported by the physician <u>or other qualified health care professional</u> who has agreed to accept transfer of care before an initial evaluation but are appropriate to report if the decision to accept transfer of care cannot be made until after the initial consultation evaluation, regardless of site of service. |
| **Evaluation and Management (E/M) Services Guidelines Levels of E/M Services** | *Within each category or subcategory...*<br><br>The levels of E/M services include examinations, evaluations, treatments, conferences with or concerning patients, preventive pediatric and adult health supervision, and similar medical services, such as the determination of the need and/or location for appropriate care. Medical screening includes the history, examination, and medical decision-making required to determine the need and/or location for appropriate care and treatment of the patient (eg, office and other outpatient setting, emergency department, nursing facility). The levels of E/M services encompass the wide variations in skill, effort, time, responsibility, and medical knowledge required for the prevention or diagnosis and treatment of illness or injury and the promotion of optimal health. Each level of E/M services may be used by all physicians <u>or other qualified health care professionals.</u><br><br>*The descriptors for the levels of E/M...*<br><br>*The first three of these components...*<br><br>*The next three components (counseling...*<br><br>Coordination of care with other ~~providers~~ <u>physicians, other health care professionals,</u> or agencies without a patient encounter on that day is reported using the case management codes.<br><br>*The final component, time, is discussed...*<br><br>*Any specifically identifiable procedure . . . .*<br><br>*The actual performance and/or interpretation . . .*<br><br>*The physician may need to indicate that on the day a procedure . . .* |
| **Evaluation and Management (E/M) Services Guidelines/ Nature of Presenting Problem** | ***Minimal***: A problem that may not require the presence of the physician <u>or other qualified health care professional</u>, but service is provided under the physician's <u>or other qualified health care professional's</u> supervision. |
| **Evaluation and Management (E/M) Services Guidelines Time** | The inclusion of time in the definitions of levels of E/M services has been implicit in prior editions of the CPT codebook. The inclusion of time as an explicit factor beginning in *CPT 1992* is done to assist ~~physicians~~ in selecting the most appropriate level of E/M services. It should be recognized that the specific times expressed in the visit code descriptors are averages and, therefore, represent a range of times that may be higher or lower depending on actual clinical circumstances.<br><br>Time is **not** a descriptive component for the emergency department levels of E/M services because emergency department services are typically provided on a variable intensity basis, often involving multiple encounters with several patients over an extended period of time. Therefore, it is often difficult ~~for physicians~~ to provide accurate estimates of the time spent face-to-face with the patient. |

◎=Modifier 51 Exempt  ◉=Moderate Sedation  ✛=Add-on Code  ✗=FDA approval pending

| CPT Code/Section/Subsection | Revision/Addition/Deletion |
|---|---|
| **Evaluation and Management (E/M) Services Guidelines** **Time** *(continued)* | Studies to establish levels of E/M services employed surveys of practicing physicians to obtain data on the amount of time and work associated with typical E/M services. Since "work" is not easily quantifiable, the codes must rely on other objective, verifiable measures that correlate with physicians' estimates of their "work." It has been demonstrated that ~~physi-cians'~~ estimations of **intraservice** time (as explained on the next page), both within and across specialties, is a variable that is predictive of the "work" of E/M services. This same research has shown there is a strong relationship between intraservice time and total time for E/M services. Intraservice time, rather than total time, was chosen for inclusion with the codes because of its relative ease of measurement and because of its direct correlation with measurements of the total amount of time and work associated with typical E/M services.

*Intraservice times are defined as* **face-to-face** *time...*

**Face-to-face time (office and other outpatient visits and office consultations):** For coding purposes, face-to-face time for these services is defined as only that time spent ~~that the physician spends~~ face-to-face with the patient and/or family. This includes the time spent performing ~~in which the physician performs~~ such tasks as obtaining a history, performing an examination, and counseling the patient.

~~Physicians also spend t~~ Time is also spent doing work before or after the face-to-face time with the patient, performing such tasks as reviewing records and tests, arranging for further services, and communicating further with other professionals and the patient through written reports and telephone contact.

This **non-face-to-face** time for office services-also called pre- and post-encounter time-is not included in the time component described in the E/M codes. However, the pre- and post-non-face-to-face work associated with an encounter was included in calculating the total work of typical services in physician surveys.

*Thus, the face-to-face time associated with the services...*

**Unit/floor time (hospital observation services, inpatient hospital care, initial inpatient hospital consultations, nursing facility):** For reporting purposes, intraservice time for these services is defined as unit/floor time, which includes the time ~~that the physician is~~ present on the patient's hospital unit and at the bedside rendering services for that patient. This includes the time ~~in which the physician~~ to establishes and/or ~~reviews~~ the patient's chart, examines the patient, writes notes, and communicates with other professionals and the patient's family.

*In the hospital, pre- and post-time includes time...*

This pre- and post-visit time is not included in the time component described in these codes. However, the pre- and post-work performed during the time spent off the floor or unit was included in calculating the total work of typical services in physician surveys. |
| **Evaluation and Management (E/M) Services Guidelines** **Clinical Examples** | Clinical examples of the codes for E/M services are provided to assist ~~physicians~~ in under-standing the meaning of the descriptors and selecting the correct code. The clinical examples are listed in Appendix C. Each example was developed by ~~physicians in~~ the specialties shown.

The same problem, when seen by ~~physicians in~~ different specialties, may involve different amounts of work. Therefore, the appropriate level of encounter should be reported using the descriptors rather than the examples.

The examples have been tested for validity and approved by the CPT Editorial Panel. ~~Physicians~~ Specialties were given the examples and asked to assign a code or assess the amount of time and work involved. Only examples that were rated consistently have been included in Appendix C. |
| **Evaluation and Management (E/M) Services Guidelines** **Instructions for Selecting a Level of E/M Service** **Select the Appropriate Level of E/M Services Based on the Following** | *1. For the following categories/subcategories...*

*2. For the following categories/subcategories,* **two...**

3. When counseling and/or coordination of care dominates (more than 50%) the ~~physician/encounter with the~~ patient and/or family ~~encounter~~ (face-to-face time in the office or other outpatient setting or floor/unit time in the hospital or nursing facility), then **time** shall be considered the key or controlling factor to qualify for a particular level of E/M services. This includes time spent with parties who have assumed responsibility for the care of the patient or decision making whether or not they are family members (eg, foster parents, person acting in loco parentis, legal guardian). The extent of counseling and/or coordination of care must be documented in the medical record. |

| CPT Code/Section/Subsection | Revision/Addition/Deletion |
|---|---|
| **Evaluation and Management (E/M) Services Office or Other Outpatient Services** | The following codes are used to report evaluation and management services provided in the ~~physician's~~ office or in an outpatient or other ambulatory facility. A patient is... <br><br> *To report services provided to a patient who is admitted to a hospital or nursing facility.......* <br><br> For services provided ~~by physicians~~ in the emergency department, see 99281-99285. |
| **Evaluation and Management (E/M) Services Office or Other Outpatient Services** <br><br> ***Counseling and Coordination of Care/Typical Time* Revisions** <br> **99201-99205, 99212-99215, 99218-99220, 99224-99226, 99221-99223, 99231-99236, 99241-99245, 99251-99255, 99281-99285, 99304-99306, 99307-99310, 99318, 99324-99328, 99334-99337, 99341-99345, 99347-99350** | The following refinements to the "counseling and coordination of care" and "typical time" language are also applicable to the E/M codes listed in the left column. Due to the number and length of these refinements, only the 99203 revision has been included to illustrate the revised text. (For further information, refer to *CPT 2013*). <br><br> ▲99203 **Office or other outpatient visit....** <br><br> Counseling and/or coordination of care with other <u>physicians, other health care professionals,</u> ~~providers~~ or agencies are provided consistent with the nature of the problem(s) and the patient's and/or family's needs. <br><br> Usually, the presenting problem(s) are of moderate severity. ~~Physicians t~~Typically, ~~spend~~ 30 minutes <u>are spent</u> face-to-face with the patient and/or family. |
| **Evaluation and Management (E/M) Services Office or Other Outpatient Services Established Patient** | ▲99211 **Office or other outpatient visit** for the evaluation and management of an established patient, that may not require the presence of a physician <u>or other qualified health care professional</u>..... |
| **Evaluation and Management (E/M) Services Hospital Observation Services Initial Observation Care New or Established Patient** | The following codes are used to report the encounter(s) by the supervising <u>physician or other qualified health care professional</u> with the patient when designated as "observation status." This refers to the initiation of observation status, supervision of the care plan for observation and performance of periodic reassessments. For ~~other~~ observation encounters by other physicians, see office or other outpatient consultation codes (99241-99245) or subsequent observation care codes (99224-99226) as appropriate. <br><br> *To report services provided to a patient who is admitted...* <br><br> When "observation status" is initiated in the course of an encounter in another site of service (eg, hospital emergency department, ~~physician's~~ office, nursing facility) all evaluation and management services provided by the supervising physician <u>or other qualified health care professional</u> in conjunction with initiating "observation status" are considered part of the initial observation care when performed on the same date. The observation care level of service reported by the supervising physician <u>or other qualified health care professional</u> should include the services related to initiating "observation status" provided in the other sites of service as well as in the observation setting. <br><br> *Evaluation and management services...* <br><br> *These codes may not be utilized for post-operative recovery....* |
| **Evaluation and Management (E/M) Services Hospital Observation Services Observation Care Discharge Services** | ▲99217 **Observation care discharge** day management (This code is to be utilized ~~by the physician~~ to report all services provided to a patient on discharge from "observation status" if the discharge is on other than the initial date of "observation status."....... |
| **Evaluation and Management (E/M) Services Hospital Observation Services Subsequent Observation Care** | All levels of subsequent observation care include reviewing the medical record and reviewing the results of diagnostic studies and changes in the patient's status (ie, changes in history, condition, and response to management) since the last assessment ~~by the physician~~. |
| **Evaluation and Management (E/M) Services Hospital Inpatient Services Subsequent Hospital Care** | All levels of subsequent hospital care include reviewing the medical record and reviewing the results of diagnostic studies and changes in the patient's status (ie, changes in history, physical condition and response to management) since the last assessment ~~by the physician~~. <br><br> 99231 *Subsequent hospital care,* per day, for the evaluation and management of a patient, which requires at least 2 of these 3 key components: |

⊘=Modifier 51 Exempt ⊙=Moderate Sedation ✚=Add-on Code ⋏=FDA approval pending

| CPT Code/Section/Subsection | Revision/Addition/Deletion |
|---|---|
| **Evaluation and Management (E/M) Services**<br>**Observation or Inpatient Care Services (Including Admission and Discharge Services)** | The following codes are used to report observation or inpatient hospital care services provided to patients admitted and discharged on the same date of service. When a patient is admitted to the hospital from observation status on the same date, only the initial hospital care code ~~the physician~~ should be reported ~~only the initial hospital care code~~. The initial hospital care code reported by the admitting physician or other qualified health care professional should include the services related to the observation status services he/she provided on the same date of inpatient admission.<br><br>When "observation status" is initiated in the course of an encounter in another site of service (eg, hospital emergency department, ~~physician's~~ office, nursing facility) all evaluation and management services provided by the supervising physician or other qualified health care professional in conjunction with initiating "observation status" are considered part of the initial observation care when performed on the same date. The observation care level of service should include the services related to initiating "observation status" provided in the other sites of service as well as in the observation setting when provided by the same individual ~~physician~~.<br><br>*For patients admitted to observation...*<br><br>*99234    Observation or inpatient hospital care,.....* |
| **Evaluation and Management (E/M) Services**<br>**Hospital Discharge Services** | The hospital discharge day management codes . . .<br><br>*99238    **Hospital discharge day management;** 30 minutes or less*<br><br>*99239        more than 30 minutes*<br><br>(These codes are to be utilized by the physician to report all services provided to a patient on the date of discharge, if other than the initial date of inpatient status. To report services to a patient who is admitted as an inpatient and discharged on the same date, see codes 99234-99236 for observation or inpatient hospital care including the admission and discharge of the patient on the same date. To report concurrent care services provided by a physician[s] other than the ~~attending~~ ordering physician or another qualified health care professional, use subsequent hospital care codes [99231-99233] on the day of discharge.) |
| **Evaluation and Management (E/M) Services**<br>**Consultations** | A consultation is a type of evaluation and management service provided ~~by a physician~~ at the request of another physician or appropriate source to either recommend care for a specific condition or problem or to determine whether to accept responsibility for ongoing management of the patient's entire care or for the care of a specific condition or problem.<br><br>*A physician consultant...*<br><br>*A "consultation" initiated by a patient and/or family...*<br><br>*The written or verbal request for consult may be made...*<br><br>*If consultation is mandated...*<br><br>*Any specifically identifiable procedure...*<br><br>If subsequent to the completion of a consultation the consultant assumes responsibility for management of a portion or all of the patient's condition(s), the appropriate **Evaluation and Management** services code for the site of service should be reported. In the hospital or nursing facility setting, the ~~consulting physician~~ consultant should use the appropriate inpatient consultation code for the initial encounter and then subsequent hospital or nursing facility care codes. In the office setting, the ~~physician~~ consultant should use the appropriate office or other outpatient consultation codes and then the established patient office or other outpatient services codes.<br><br>*To report services provided...*<br><br>*For definitions of key components...* |

| CPT Code/Section/Subsection | Revision/Addition/Deletion |
|---|---|
| **Evaluation and Management (E/M) Services** **Office or Other Outpatient Consultations** | The following codes are used to report consultations provided in the ~~physician's~~ office or in an outpatient or other ambulatory facility, including hospital observation services, home services, domiciliary, rest home, or emergency department (see the preceding consultation definition above). Follow-up visits in the consultant's office or other outpatient facility that are initiated by the ~~physician~~ consultant or patient are reported using the appropriate codes for established patients, office visits (99211-99215), domiciliary, rest home (99334-99337), or home (99347-99350). If an additional request for an opinion or advice regarding the same or a new problem is received from another physician or other appropriate source and documented in the medical record, the office consultation codes may be used again. Services that constitute transfer of care (ie, are provided for the management of the patient's entire care or for the care of a specific condition or problem) are reported with the appropriate new or established patient codes for office or other outpatient visits, domiciliary, rest home services, or home services. <br><br> 99241    **Office consultation** *for a new or established patient, which requires these 3 key components:...* |
| **Evaluation and Management (E/M) Services** **Inpatient Consultations** | The following codes are used to report physician <u>or other qualified health care professional</u> consultations provided to hospital inpatients, residents of nursing facilities, or patients in a partial hospital setting..... <br> When an inpatient consultation is performed... <br><br> 99251    **Inpatient consultation** *for a new or established patient, which requires these 3 key components:...* |
| **Evaluation and Management (E/M) Services** **Other Emergency Services** | In ~~physician~~ directed emergency care, advanced life support, the physician <u>or other qualified health care professional</u> is located in a hospital emergency or critical care department, and is in two-way voice communication with ambulance or rescue personnel outside the hospital. ~~The physician directs~~ <u>Direction of</u> the performance of necessary medical procedures, <u>includes</u> ~~including~~ but <u>is</u> not limited to:..... <br><br> ▲99288    **Physician <u>or other qualified health care professional</u> direction of** emergency medical systems (EMS) emergency care, advanced life support |
| **Evaluation and Management (E/M) Services** **Critical Care Services** | Critical care is the direct delivery by a physician(s) <u>or other qualified health care professional</u> of medical care for a critically ill or critically injured patient. A critical illness or injury acutely impairs one or more vital organ systems such that there is a high probability of imminent or life threatening deterioration in the patient's condition. Critical care involves high complexity decision making to assess, manipulate, and support vital system function(s) to treat single or multiple vital organ system failure and/or to prevent further life threatening deterioration of the patient's condition. Examples of vital organ system failure include, but are not limited to: central nervous system failure, circulatory failure, shock, renal, hepatic, metabolic, and/or respiratory failure. Although critical care typically requires interpretation of multiple physiologic parameters and/or application of advanced technology(s), critical care may be provided in life threatening situations when these elements are not present. Critical care may be provided on multiple days, even if no changes are made in the treatment rendered to the patient, provided that the patient's condition continues to require the level of <u>~~the individual's~~</u> ~~physician~~ attention described above. <br><br> *Providing medical care to a critically...* <br><br> Inpatient critical care services provided to infants 29 days through 71 months of age are reported with pediatric critical care codes 99471-99476. The pediatric critical care codes are reported as long as the infant/young child qualifies for critical care services during the hospital stay through 71 months of age. Inpatient critical care services provided to neonates (28 days of age or younger) are reported with the neonatal critical care codes 99468 and 99469. The neonatal critical care codes are reported as long as the neonate qualifies for critical care services during the hospital stay through the 28th postnatal day. The reporting of the pediatric and neonatal critical care services is not based on time or the type of unit (eg, pediatric or neonatal critical care unit) and it is not dependent upon the type of <u>physician or other qualified health care professional</u> ~~provider~~ delivering the care. To report critical care services provided in the outpatient setting (eg, emergency department or office), for neonates and pediatric patients up through 71 months of age, see the critical care codes 99291, 99292. If the same <u>individual</u> ~~physician~~ provides critical care services for a neonatal or pediatric patient in both the outpatient and inpatient settings on the same day, report only the appropriate neonatal or pediatric critical care code 99468-99472 for all critical care services provided on that day. |

| CPT Code/Section/Subsection | Revision/Addition/Deletion |
|---|---|
| **Evaluation and Management (E/M) Services**<br>**Critical Care Services**<br>*(continued)* | Also report 99291-99292 for neonatal or pediatric critical care services provided by the individual ~~physician~~ providing critical care at one facility but transferring the patient to another facility. Critical care services provided by a second individual ~~physician~~ of a different specialty not reporting a per day neonatal or pediatric critical care code can be reported with codes 99291, 99292. For additional instructions on reporting these services, see the Neonatal and Pediatric Critical Care section and codes 99468-99476.<br><br>*Services for a patient who is not critically ill...*<br><br>Critical care and other E/M services may be provided to the same patient on the same date by the same individual ~~physician~~.<br><br>*For reporting by professionals, the following services are included...*<br><br>Codes 99291, 99292 should be reported for the ~~physician's~~ attendance during the transport of critically ill or critically injured patients older than 24 months of age to or from a facility or hospital. For ~~physician~~ transport services of critically ill or critically injured pediatric patients 24 months of age or younger, see 99466, 99467.<br><br>*Codes 99291, 99292 should be reported...*<br><br>Codes 99291, 99292 are used to report the total duration of time spent ~~by a physician providing~~ in provision of critical care services to a critically ill or critically injured patient, even if the time spent providing care ~~by the physician~~ on that date is not continuous. For any given period of time spent providing critical care services, the individual ~~physician~~ must devote his or her full attention to the patient and, therefore, cannot provide services to any other patient during the same period of time.<br><br>*Time spent with the individual patient...*<br><br>Time spent in activities that occur outside of the unit or off the floor (eg, telephone calls whether taken at home, in the office, or elsewhere in the hospital) may not be reported as critical care since the individual ~~physician~~ is not immediately available to the patient. Time spent in activities that do not directly contribute to the treatment of the patient may not be reported as critical care, even if they are performed in the critical care unit (eg, participation in administrative meetings or telephone calls to discuss other patients). Time spent performing separately reportable procedures or services should not be included in the time reported as critical care time. No individual ~~physician~~ may report remote real-time interactive video-conferenced critical care services (0188T, 0189T) for the period in which any other physician or qualified health care professional reports codes 99291, 99292 ~~are reported~~.<br><br>Code 99291 is used to report the first 30-74 minutes of critical care on a given date. It should be used only once per date even if the time spent by the individual ~~physician~~ is not continuous on that date. Critical care of less than 30 minutes total duration on a given date should be reported with the appropriate E/M code.<br><br>*Code 99292 is used to report the...* |
| **Evaluation and Management (E/M) Services**<br>**Nursing Facility Services** | *The following codes are used...*<br><br>*These codes should also be used...*<br><br>*Nursing facilities that provide...*<br><br>Physicians and other qualified health care professionals have a central role in assuring that all residents receive thorough assessments and that medical plans of care are instituted or revised to enhance or maintain the residents' physical and psychosocial functioning. This role includes providing input in the development of the MDS and a multi-disciplinary plan of care, as required by regulations pertaining to the care of nursing facility residents.<br><br>*Two major subcategories of nursing facility services...*<br><br>*For definitions of key components...* |

| CPT Code/Section/Subsection | Revision/Addition/Deletion |
|---|---|
| **Evaluation and Management (E/M) Services**<br>**Nursing Facility Services**<br>**Initial Nursing Facility Care**<br>**New or Established Patient** | When the patient is admitted to the nursing facility in the course of an encounter in another site of service (eg, hospital emergency department, ~~physician's~~ office), all evaluation and management services provided by that physician in conjunction with that admission are considered part of the initial nursing facility care when performed on the same date as the admission or readmission. The nursing facility care level of service reported by the admitting physician should include the services related to the admission he/she provided in the other sites of service as well as in the nursing facility setting.<br>*Hospital discharge or observation discharge...*<br><br>99304   *Initial nursing facility care, per day, for the evaluation and management of a patient, which requires these 3 key components:...* |
| **Evaluation and Management (E/M) Services**<br>**Nursing Facility Services**<br>**Evaluation and Management (E/M) Services**<br>**Subsequent Nursing Facility Care** | All levels of subsequent nursing facility care include reviewing the medical record and reviewing the results of diagnostic studies and changes in the patient's status (ie, changes in history, physical condition, and response to management) since the last assessment by the physician <u>or other qualified health care professional</u>.<br><br>99307   *Subsequent nursing facility care, per day, for the evaluation and management of a patient, which requires at least 2 of these 3 key components:...* |
| **Evaluation and Management (E/M) Services**<br>**Nursing Facility Discharge Services** | The nursing facility discharge day management codes are to be used to report the total duration of time spent by a physician <u>or other qualified health care professional</u> for the final nursing facility discharge of a patient. The codes include, as appropriate, final examination of the patient, discussion of the nursing facility stay, even if the time spent ~~by the physician~~ on that date is not continuous. Instructions are given for continuing care to all relevant caregivers, and preparation of discharge records, prescriptions and referral forms.<br><br>99315   *Nursing facility discharge day management; 30 minutes or less* |
| **Evaluation and Management (E/M) Services**<br>**Domiciliary, Rest Home (eg, Boarding Home), or Custodial Care Services** | *The following codes are used to report evaluation and management services ...*<br><br>*The facility's services do not include a medical component.*<br><br>*For definitions of key components and commonly used terms...*<br><br>(For care plan oversight services provided to a patient in a domiciliary facility under the care of a home health agency, see 99374, 99375<u>, and for hospice agency, see 99377, 99378. For care plan oversight provided to a patient under hospice or home health agency care, see 99339-99340</u>)<br><br>~~(For care plan oversight services provided to a patient in a domiciliary facility under the individual supervision of a physician~~ <u>~~or other qualified health care professional~~</u>~~, see 99339, 99340)~~ |
| **Evaluation and Management (E/M) Services**<br>**Home Services/New Patient** | *The following codes are used to report evaluation and management services provided in a private residence.*<br><br>*For definitions of key components and commonly used terms, please see **Evaluation and Management Services Guidelines**.*<br><br>(For care plan oversight services provided to a patient in the home under the care of a home health agency, see 99374, 99375<u>, and for hospice agency, see 99377, 99378. For care plan oversight provided to a patient under hospice or home health agency care, see 99339, 99340</u>)<br><br>~~(For care plan oversight services provided to a patient in the home under the individual supervision of a physician,~~ <u>~~or other qualified health care professional~~</u>~~, see 99339, 99340)~~<br><br>99341   ***Home visit** for the evaluation and management of a new patient, which requires these three key components:...* |

| CPT Code/Section/Subsection | Revision/Addition/Deletion |
|---|---|
| **Evaluation and Management (E/M) Services** <br> **~~Physician~~ Standby Service** | Code 99360 is used to report physician <u>or other qualified health care professional</u> standby services that are requested by another <u>individual</u> ~~physician~~ and that involves prolonged ~~physician~~ attendance without direct (face-to-face) patient contact. ~~The physician may not be providing eCare~~ or services <u>may not be provided </u>to other patients during this period. This code is not used to report time spent proctoring another <u>individual</u> ~~physician~~. It is also not used if the period of standby ends with the performance of a procedure, subject to a surgical package by the <u>individual</u> ~~physician~~ who was on standby. <br><br> Code 99360 is used to report the total duration of time spent ~~by a physician~~ on a given date on standby. Standby service of less than 30 minutes total duration on a given date is not reported separately. <br><br> ▲99360    ~~Physician~~ **Standby service,** requiring prolonged ~~physician~~ attendance, each 30 minutes (eg, operative standby, standby for frozen section, for cesarean/high risk delivery, for monitoring EEG) |
| **Evaluation and Management (E/M) Services** <br> **Case Management Services** <br> **Medical Team Conferences** | *Medical team conferences include face-to-face participation by a minimum of three qualified health care professionals …* <br><br> Physicians <u>or other qualified health care professionals who may report evaluation and management services </u>~~may~~<u> should </u>report their time spent in a team conference with the patient and/or family present using evaluation and management (E/M) codes (and time as the key controlling factor for code selection when counseling and/or coordination of care dominates the service). These introductory guidelines do not apply to services reported using E/M codes (see E/M services guidelines). However, the ~~physician~~<u>individual </u>must be directly involved with the patient, providing face-to-face services outside of the conference visit with other <u>physicians, qualified health care professionals,</u> ~~providers~~ or agencies. <br><br> *Reporting participants shall document their participation…* <br><br> *No more than one individual from the same specialty…* <br><br> Individuals should not report 99366-99368 when their participation in the medical team conference is part of a facility or organizational service contractually provided by the organizationa~~l~~ or facility ~~provider~~. <br><br> The team conference starts at the beginning of the review of an individual patient and ends at the conclusion of the review. Time related to record keeping and report generation is not reported. The reporting participant shall be present for all time reported. The time reported is not limited to the time that the participant is communicating to the other team members or patient and/or family. Time reported for medical team conferences may not be used in the determination of time for other services such as care plan oversight (99374-99380), home, domiciliary, or rest home care plan oversight (99339-99340), prolonged services (99354-99359), psychotherapy, or any E/M service. For team conferences where the patient is present for any part of the duration of the conference, nonphysician qualified health care professionals (~~ie,~~ <u>eg,</u> speech-language pathologists, physical therapists, occupational therapists, social workers, dietitians)</u> report the team conference face-to-face code 99366. |

| CPT Code/Section/Subsection | Revision/Addition/Deletion |
|---|---|
| **Evaluation and Management (E/M) Services**<br>**Care Plan Oversight Services** | ... The complexity and approximate ~~physician~~ time of the care plan oversight services.....<br>Only one individual ~~physician~~ may report services for a given period of time, to reflect <u>the</u> ~~that physician's~~ sole or predominant...<br><br>(For care plan oversight services of patients in the home, domiciliary, or rest home (eg, assisted living facility) ~~under the individual supervision of a physician~~, see 99339, 99340, <u>and for hospice agency, see 99377, 99378</u>)<br><br>▲99374   ~~Physician s~~**S**upervision of a patient .....involving regular ~~physician~~ development and/or revision of care plans<u> by that individual</u>,...<br><br>▲99375   30 minutes or more<br><br>▲99377   ~~Physician s~~**S**upervision of a hospice patient (patient not present) requiring complex and multidisciplinary care modalities involving regular ~~physician~~ development and/or revision of care plans<u> by that individual</u>,...<br><br>▲99378   30 minutes or more<br><br>▲99379   ~~Physician s~~**S**upervision of a nursing facility patient (patient not present) requiring complex and multidisciplinary care modalities involving regular ~~physician~~ development and/or revision of care plans<u> by that individual</u>,...<br><br>▲99380   30 minutes or more |
| **Evaluation and Management (E/M) Services**<br>**Preventive Medicine Services** | *The following codes are used to report...*<br><br>*The extent and focus of the services will largely...*<br><br>If an abnormality is encountered or a preexisting problem is addressed in the process of performing this preventive medicine evaluation and management service, and if the problem or abnormality is significant enough to require additional work to perform the key components of a problem-oriented E/M service, then the appropriate Office/Outpatient code 99201-99215 should also be reported. Modifier 25 should be added to the Office/Outpatient code to indicate that a significant, separately identifiable evaluation and management service was provided ~~by the same physician~~ on the same day as the preventive medicine service. The appropriate preventive medicine service is additionally reported.<br><br>*An insignificant or trivial problem/abnormality that is ...* |
| **Evaluation and Management (E/M) Services**<br>**Non-Face-to-Face ~~Physician~~ Services**<br>**Telephone Services** | Telephone services are non-face-to-face evaluation and management (E/M) services provided to a patient using the telephone by a physician <u>or other qualified health care professional, who may report evaluation and management services</u>. These codes are used to report episodes of <u>patient </u>care ~~by the physician~~ initiated by an established patient or guardian of an established patient. If the telephone service ends with a decision to see the patient within 24 hours or next available urgent visit appointment, the code is not reported; rather the encounter is considered part of the preservice work of the subsequent E/M service, procedure, and visit. Likewise if the telephone call refers to an E/M service performed and reported by <u>that individual</u> ~~the physician~~ within the previous seven days (either ~~physician~~ requested or unsolicited patient follow-up) or within the postoperative period of the previously completed procedure, then the service(s) are considered part of that previous E/M service or procedure. (Do not report 99441-99443 if reporting 99441-99444 performed in the <u>previous</u> seven days.)<br><br>(For telephone services provided by a qualified nonphysician health care professional <u>who may not report evaluation and management services (eg, speech-language pathologists, physical therapists, occupational therapists, social workers, dietitians)</u>, see 98966-98968)<br><br>▲99441   Telephone evaluation and management service ~~provided~~ by a physician <u>or other qualified health care professional who may report evaluation and management services provided</u> to an established patient, parent, or guardian not originating from a related E/M service provided within the previous 7 days nor leading to an E/M service or procedure within the next 24 hours or soonest available appointment; 5-10 minutes of medical discussion<br><br>▲99442   11-20 minutes of medical discussion<br><br>▲99443   21-30 minutes of medical discussion |

| CPT Code/Section/Subsection | Revision/Addition/Deletion |
|---|---|
| **Evaluation and Management (E/M) Services**<br>**Newborn Care Services** | *The following codes are used to report the services provided…*<br><br>*Evaluation and Management (E/M) services for the newborn …*<br><br>*When delivery room attendance services (99464) or…*<br><br>For E/M services provided to newborns who are other than normal, see codes for hospital inpatient services (99221-99233) and neonatal intensive and critical care services (99466-99469, 99477-99480). When normal newborn services are provided by the same <u>individual</u> ~~physician~~ on the same date that the newborn later becomes ill and receives additional intensive or critical care services, report the appropriate E/M code with modifier 25 for these services in addition to the normal newborn code.<br><br>*Procedures (eg, 54150, newborn circumcision) are not…*<br><br>*When newborns are seen in follow-up after the date of discharge…*<br><br>    *99460   Initial hospital or birthing center care, per day, for evaluation and management of normal newborn infant* |
| **Evaluation and Management (E/M) Services**<br>**Newborn Care Services**<br>**Delivery/Birthing Room Attendance and Resuscitation Services** | ▲99464   Attendance at delivery (when requested by the delivering physician <u>or other qualified health care professional</u>) and initial stabilization of newborn |
| **Evaluation and Management (E/M) Services**<br>**Inpatient Neonatal Intensive Care Services and Pediatric and Neonatal Critical Care Services**<br>**Inpatient Neonatal and Pediatric Critical Care** | *The same definitions for critical care services apply for the adult, child, and neonate.*<br><br>Codes 99468, 99469 are used to report <u>the</u> services <u>of</u> ~~provided by a physician~~ directing the inpatient care of a critically ill neonate or infant 28 days of age or younger. They represent care starting with the date of admission (99468) <u>to a critical care unit</u> and subsequent day(s) (99469) that the neonate remains critical. These codes may be reported only by a single <u>individual</u> ~~physician~~ and only once per day, per patient, <u>per hospital stay in a given facility. If readmitted to the neonatal critical care unit during the same day, report the subsequent day(s) code 99469 for the first day of readmission to critical care, and 99469 for each day of critical care following readmission.</u><br><br>The initial day neonatal critical care code (99468) can be used in addition to 99464 or 99465 as appropriate, when the physician <u>or other qualified healthcare professional</u> is present for the delivery (99464) or resuscitation (99465) is required. Other procedures performed as a necessary part of the resuscitation (eg, endotracheal intubation [31500]) are also reported separately when performed as part of the pre-admission delivery room care. In order to report these procedures separately, they must be performed as a necessary component of the resuscitation and not simply as a convenience before admission to the neonatal intensive care unit.<br><br>Codes 99471-99476 are used to report ~~services provided by a physician directing~~ <u>direction of</u> the inpatient care of a critically ill infant or young child from 29 days of postnatal age through ~~five~~ <u>less than 6</u> years of age. They represent care starting with the date of admission (99471, 99475) ~~and~~ to <u>all</u> subsequent day(s) (99472, 99476) the infant or child remains critical. These codes may be reported only by a single <u>individual</u> ~~physician~~ and only once per day, per patient in a given setting. Services<u>_</u>for the critically ill or critically injured child ~~older than five years of age~~ <u>6 years of age or older</u> would be reported with <u>the time based</u> critical care codes (99291, 99292). <u>Report 99471, 99475 only once per hospital stay in a given facility. If readmitted to the pediatric critical care unit during the same stay, report 99472 or 99476 for the first day of readmission to critical care and 99472 for each day of critical care following readmission.</u> |

| CPT Code/Section/Subsection | Revision/Addition/Deletion |
|---|---|
| **Evaluation and Management (E/M) Services**<br>**Inpatient Neonatal Intensive Care Services and Pediatric and Neonatal Critical Care Services**<br>**Inpatient Neonatal and Pediatric Critical Care**<br>(continued) | *The pediatric and neonatal critical care codes include…*<br><br>*Any services performed that are not included in these listings…*<br><br>*Facilities may report….*<br><br>*Invasive or non-invasive electronic monitoring of vital signs*<br><br>*Vascular access procedures….*<br><br>*Airway and ventilation management….*<br><br>*Any services performed which are not listed above may be reported separately.*<br><br>*When a neonate or infant is not critically ill but requires intensive observation…..*<br><br>To report critical care services provided in the outpatient setting (eg, emergency department or office) for neonates and pediatric patients of any age, see the Critical Care codes 99291, 99292. If the same <u>individual</u> ~~physician~~ provides critical care services for a neonatal or pediatric patient <u>less than 6 years of age</u> in both the outpatient and inpatient settings on the same day, report only the appropriate Neonatal or Pediatric Critical Care codes 99468-99476 for all critical care services provided on that day. Critical care services provided by a second <u>individual</u> ~~physician~~ of a different specialty not reporting a per-day neonatal or pediatric critical care code can be reported with 99291, 99292.<br><br>When critical care services are provided to neonates or pediatric patients less than ~~five~~ <u>6</u> years of age at two separate institutions by <u>an</u> <u>individual</u> ~~physician~~ from a different group on the same date of service, the <u>individual</u> ~~physician~~ from the referring institution should report their critical care services with the time-based critical care codes (99291, 99292) and the receiving institution should report the appropriate <u>initial day of care</u> ~~global admission~~ code ~~(99468, 99471, 99475, 99476)~~ for the same date of service.<br><br>*Critical care services to a pediatric patient 6 years of age or older are reported with the time based critical care codes 99291, 99292.*<br><br>When the critically ill neonate or pediatric patient improves and is transferred to a lower level of care~~,~~ <u>to another individual</u> ~~physician~~ <u>in another group within the same facility</u>, the transferring <u>individual</u> ~~physician~~ does not report a per day critical care service. Subsequent hospital care (99231-99233) or <u>time-based</u> critical care services (99291-99292) is reported, as appropriate based upon the condition of the neonate or child. The receiving ~~physician~~ <u>individual</u> reports ~~a~~ subsequent intensive care (99478-99480) or subsequent hospital care (99231-99233) <u>services</u>, as appropriate based upon the condition of the neonate or child. The receiving ~~physician~~ <u>individual</u> reports ~~a~~ subsequent intensive care (99478-99480) or subsequent hospital care (99231-99233) <u>services</u>, as appropriate based upon the condition of the neonate or child.<br><br><u>When the neonate or infant becomes critically ill on a day when initial or subsequent intensive care services (99477-99480), hospital services (99221-99233), or normal newborn services (99460, 99461, 99462) have been performed by one individual</u> ~~physician~~ <u>and is transferred to a critical care level of care provided by a different individual</u> ~~physician~~ <u>in a different group, the transferring individual</u> ~~physician~~ <u>reports either the time-based critical care services performed (99291, 99292) for the time spent providing critical care to the patient, the intensive care service (99477-99480), hospital care services (99221-99233), or normal newborn service (99460, 99461, 99462) performed, but only one service. The receiving individual</u> ~~physician~~ <u>reports initial or subsequent inpatient neonatal or pediatric critical care (99468-99476), as appropriate based upon the patient's age and whether this is the first or subsequent admission to the critical care unit for the hospital stay.</u><br><br><u>When a newborn becomes critically ill on the same day they have already received normal newborn care (99460, 99461, 99462) and the same individual</u> ~~physician~~ <u>or group assumes critical care, report initial critical care service (99468) with modifier 25 in addition to the normal newborn code.</u> |

| CPT Code/Section/Subsection | Revision/Addition/Deletion |
|---|---|
| **Evaluation and Management (E/M) Services** <br> **Inpatient Neonatal Intensive Care Services and Pediatric and Neonatal Critical Care Services** <br> **Inpatient Neonatal and Pediatric Critical Care** <br> *(continued)* | When a neonate, infant, or child requires initial critical care services on the same day the patient already has received hospital care or intensive care services by the same individual or group, only the initial critical care service code (99468, 99471, 99475) is reported. <br><br> Time-based critical care services (99291, 99292) are not reportable by the same individual or different individual within the same group when neonatal or pediatric critical care services (99468-99476) are reported for the same patient on the same day. <br><br> No individual ~~physician~~ may report remote real-time videoconferenced critical care (0188T, 0189T) when neonatal or pediatric intensive or critical care services (99468-99476) are reported. <br><br> 99468    **Initial inpatient neonatal critical care,** *per day, for the evaluation and management of a critically ill neonate, 28 days of age or younger* |
| **Evaluation and Management (E/M) Services** <br> **Inpatient Neonatal Intensive Care Services and Pediatric and Neonatal Critical Care Services** <br> **Initial and Continuing Intensive Care Services** | Code 99477 represents the initial day of inpatient care for the child who is not critically ill but requires intensive observation, frequent interventions, and other intensive care services. Codes 99478-99480 are used to report the subsequent day services ~~provided by a physician~~ of directing the continuing intensive care of the low birth weight (LBW 1500-2500 grams) present body weight infant, very low birth weight (VLBW less than 1500 grams) present body weight infant, or normal (2501-5000 grams) present body weight newborn who does not meet the definition of critically ill but continues to require intensive observation, frequent interventions, and other intensive care services. These services are for infants and neonates who are not critically ill but continue to require intensive cardiac and respiratory monitoring, continuous and/or frequent vital sign monitoring, heat maintenance, enteral and/or parenteral nutritional adjustments, laboratory and oxygen monitoring, and constant observation by the health care team under direct ~~physician~~ supervision of the physician or other qualified health care professional. Codes 99477-99480 may be reported by ~~only one~~ a single ~~physician~~ individual and only once per day, per patient in a given facility. If readmitted to the intensive care unit during the same hospital stay, report 99478-99480 for the first ~~initial~~ day of intensive care and for each successive day that the child requires intensive care services. <br><br> *These codes include the same procedures that are outlined in the* **Neonatal and Pediatric Critical Care Services** *section and these services should not be separately reported.* <br><br> The initial day neonatal intensive care code (99477) can be used in addition to 99464 or 99465 as appropriate, when the physician or other qualified health care professional is present for the delivery (99464) or resuscitation (99465) is required. In this situation, report 99477 with modifier 25. Other procedures performed as a necessary part of the resuscitation (eg, endotracheal intubation [31500]) are also reported separately when performed as part of the pre-admission delivery room care. In order to report these procedures separately, they must be performed as a necessary component of the resuscitation and not simply as a convenience before admission to the neonatal intensive care unit. <br><br> The same procedures... <br><br> When the neonate or infant improves after the initial day and no longer requires intensive care services and is transferred to a lower level of care, the transferring ~~physician~~ individual does not report a per day intensive care service. Subsequent hospital care (99231-99233) or subsequent normal newborn care (99460, 99462) is reported as appropriate based upon the condition of the neonate or infant. If the transfer to a lower level of care occurs on the same day as initial intensive care services were provided by the transferring individual, 99477 may be reported. <br><br> When the neonate or infant is transferred after the initial day within the same facility to the care of another individual in a different group, both individuals report subsequent hospital care (99231-99233) services. The receiving individual reports subsequent hospital care (99231-99233) or subsequent normal newborn care (99462). |

| CPT Code/Section/Subsection | Revision/Addition/Deletion |
|---|---|
| **Evaluation and Management (E/M) Services** <br> **Inpatient Neonatal Intensive Care Services and Pediatric and Neonatal Critical Care Services** <br> **Initial and Continuing Intensive Care Services** *(continued)* | When the neonate or infant becomes critically ill on a day when initial or subsequent intensive care services (99477-99480) have been ~~performed~~ reported by one individual and is transferred to a critical care level of care ~~performed~~ provided by a different ~~physician~~ individual from a different group, the transferring ~~physician~~ individual reports either the time-based critical care services performed (99291, 99292) for the time spent providing critical care to the patient or the initial or subsequent intensive care (99477-99480) ~~S~~service ~~performed~~, but not both. The receiving ~~physician~~ individual reports initial or subsequent inpatient neonatal or pediatric critical care (~~99469, 99472~~ 99468-99476) based upon the patient's age and whether this is the first or subsequent admission to critical care for the same hospital stay. <br><br> When the neonate or infant becomes critically ill on a day when initial or subsequent intensive care services (99477-99480) have been performed by the same individual or group, report only initial or subsequent inpatient neonatal or pediatric critical care (99468-99476) based upon the patient's age and whether this is the first or subsequent admission to critical care for the same hospital stay. <br><br> *For the subsequent care of the sick neonate younger than 28 days of age but more than 5000 grams who does not require intensive or critical care services, use codes 99231-99233.* <br><br> **99477** **Initial hospital care,** *per day, for the evaluation and management of the neonate, 28 days of age or younger, who requires intensive observation, frequent interventions, and other intensive care services* |
| **Anesthesia Guidelines** <br> **Anesthesia** ~~Physician's~~ **Services** | ~~Physician's s~~Services rendered in the office, home, or hospital; consultation; and other medical services are listed in the **Evaluation and Management**.... |
| **Supplied Materials** ~~Supplied by~~ ~~Physician~~ | Supplies and materials provided ~~by the physician~~ (eg, sterile trays, drugs) over and above.... |
| **Anesthesia** <br> **Other Procedures** | ▲ 01991 Anesthesia for diagnostic or therapeutic nerve blocks and injections (when block or injection is performed by a different physician or other qualified health care professional ~~provider~~); other than the prone position |
| **Surgery Guidelines** | Guidelines to direct general ~~Items used by all physicians in~~ reporting of ~~their~~ services are presented... Some of the commonalities are repeated here for the convenience of those ~~physicians~~ referring... |
| **Surgery Guidelines** <br> **Physician's Services** | ~~Physicians' s~~Services rendered in the office, home, or hospital, consultations... |
| **Surgery Guidelines** <br> **CPT Surgical Package Definition** | By their very nature, ~~T~~the services ~~provided by the physician~~ to any patient ~~by their very nature~~ are variable... <br> • Immediate postoperative care, including dictating operative notes, talking with the family and other physicians or other qualified health care professionals |
| **Surgery Guidelines** <br> **Supplied Materials** ~~Supplied by~~ ~~Physician~~ | Supplies and materials ~~provided by the physician~~ (eg, sterile trays/drugs)... |
| **Surgery Guidelines** <br> **Reporting More Than One Procedure/Service** | When ~~a physician performs~~ more than one procedure/service is performed on the same date, |
| **Surgery** <br> **Skin, Subcutaneous and Acccessory Structures** <br> **Excision-Benign Lesions** | *Excision (including simple closure) of benign lesions...* <br><br> Excision is defined as full-thickness (through the dermis) removal of a lesion, including margins, and includes simple (non-layered) closure when performed. Report separately each benign lesion excised. Code selection is determined by measuring the greatest clinical diameter of the apparent lesion plus that margin required for complete excision (lesion diameter plus the most narrow margins required equals the excised diameter). The margins refer to the most narrow margin required to adequately excise the lesion, based on individual ~~the physician's~~ judgment. The measurement of lesion plus margin is made prior to excision. The excised diameter is the same whether the surgical defect is repaired in a linear fashion, or reconstructed (eg, with a skin graft). <br><br> *The closure of defects created by incision, excision,...* <br><br> 11400 *Excision, benign lesion including margins, except skin tag (unless listed elsewhere), trunk, arms or legs; excised diameter 0.5 cm or less* |

| CPT Code/Section/Subsection | Revision/Addition/Deletion |
|---|---|
| **Surgery**<br>**Integumentary System**<br>**Skin Replacement Surgery** | Skin replacement surgery consists of ***surgical preparation*** and topical placement of an ***autograft*** (including tissue cultured autograft) or ***skin substitute graft*** (ie, homograft, allograft, xenograft). The graft is anchored using the <u>individual's</u> ~~provider's~~ choice of fixation. When services are performed in the office, routine dressing supplies are not reported separately. |
| **Surgery**<br>**Integumentary System**<br>**Destruction**<br>**Mohs Micrographic Surgery** | Mohs micrographic surgery is a technique for the removal of complex or ill-defined skin cancer with histologic examination of 100% of the surgical margins. It requires <u>the integration of an individual functioning</u> ~~a single physician to act~~ in two ~~integrated but~~ separate and distinct capacities: surgeon and pathologist. If either of these responsibilities is delegated to another physician<u> or other qualified health care professional</u> who reports the services separately, these codes should not be reported. The Mohs surgeon removes the tumor tissue and maps and divides the tumor specimen into pieces, and each piece is embedded into an individual tissue block for histopathologic examination. Thus a tissue block in Mohs surgery is defined as an individual tissue piece embedded in a mounting medium for sectioning.<br><br>*If repair is performed, use separate repair, flap,...*<br><br>    *17311   Mohs micrographic technique, including removal of all gross tumor, surgical excision of tissue specimens, mapping, color coding of specimens, microscopic examination of specimens by the surgeon,...* |
| **Surgery**<br>**Musculoskeletal System** | *Cast and strapping procedures appear at the end of this section...*<br><br>*The services listed below include the application ...*<br><br>***Definitions***<br><br>*The terms "closed treatment," "open treatment,...*<br><br>***Closed treatment*** *specifically means that the fracture ...*<br><br>***Open treatment*** *is used when the fractured bone is ...*<br><br>***Percutaneous skeletal fixation*** *describes fracture ...*<br>Re-reduction of a fracture and/or dislocation performed by the primary physician <u>or other qualified healthcare professional </u>may be identified by the addition of the modifier 76 to the usual procedure number to indicate "Repeat Procedure or Service by Same Physician <u>or Other Qualified Healthcare Professional</u>." (See Appendix A guidelines.)<br><br>*Codes for external fixation...*<br><br>*All codes for suction irrigation...*<br><br>***Manipulation*** *is used throughout the ...*<br><br>***Excision of subcutaneous soft tissue tumors*** *(including simple or intermediate repair) involves the simple or marginal resection of tumors confined to subcutaneous tissue below the skin but above the deep fascia.......*<br><br>***Excision of fascial or subfascial soft tissue tumors*** *(including simple or intermediate repair) involves the resection of tumors confined to the tissue within or below the deep fascia, but not involving the bone. These tumors are usually benign, are often intramuscular, and are resected without removing a significant amount of surrounding normal tissue. Code selection is based on size and location of the tumor. Code selection is determined by measuring the greatest diameter of the tumor plus that margin required for complete excision of the tumor. The margins refer to the most narrow margin required to adequately excise the tumor, based on* <u>individual</u> ~~the physician's~~ *judgment. The measurement of the tumor plus margin is made at the time of the excision. Appreciable vessel exploration and/or neuroplasty should be reported separately. Extensive undermining or other techniques to close a defect created by skin excision may require a complex repair which should be reported separately. Dissection or elevation of tissue planes to permit resection of the tumor is included in the excision.*<br><br>*Digital (ie, fingers and toes) subfascial tumors are defined...* |

| CPT Code/Section/Subsection | Revision/Addition/Deletion |
|---|---|
| **Surgery**<br>**Musculoskeletal System**<br>*(continued)* | ***Radical resection of soft tissue tumors*** (including simple or intermediate repair) involves the resection of the tumor with wide margins of normal tissue. Appreciable vessel exploration and/or neuroplasty repair or reconstruction (eg, adjacent tissue transfer[s], flap[s]) should be reported separately. Extensive undermining or other techniques to close a defect created by skin excision may require a complex repair which should be reported separately. Dissection or elevation of tissue planes to permit resection of the tumor is included in the excision. Although these tumors may be confined to a specific layer (eg, subcutaneous, subfascial), radical resection may involve removal of tissue from one or more layers. Radical resection of soft tissue tumors is most commonly used for malignant tumors or very aggressive benign tumors. Code selection is based on size and location of the tumor. Code selection is determined by measuring the greatest diameter of the tumor plus that margin required for complete excision of the tumor. The margins refer to the most narrow margin required to adequately excise the tumor, based on <u>individual</u> ~~the physician's~~ judgment. The measurement of the tumor plus margin is made at the time of the excision. For radical resection of tumors of cutaneous origin, (eg, melanoma), see 11600-11646.<br><br>***Radical resection of bone tumors*** *(including simple or intermediate…* |
| **Musculoskeletal System**<br>**General**<br>**Introduction or Removal** | ▲20665    Removal of tongs or halo applied by another <u>individual</u> ~~physician~~ |
| **Surgery**<br>**Head**<br>**Head Prosthesis** | Codes 21076-21089 describe professional services for the rehabilitation of patients with oral, facial, or other anatomical deficiencies by means of prostheses such as an artificial eye, ear, or nose or intraoral obturator to close a cleft. Codes 21076-21089 should only be used when the physician <u>or other qualified health care professional</u> actually designs and prepares the prosthesis (ie, not prepared by an outside laboratory).<br><br>*21076    Impression and custom preparation; surgical obturator prosthesis* |
| **Surgery**<br>**Head**<br>**Introduction or Removal** | *21110    Application of interdental…*<br><br>(For removal of interdental fixation by another <u>individual</u> ~~physician~~, see 20670-20680) |
| **Surgery**<br>**Spine (Vertebral Column)**<br>**Arthrodesis**<br>**Anterior or Anterolateral**<br>**Approach Technique** | *22554    Arthrodesis, anterior interbody technique,….*<br><br>(Do not report 22554 in conjunction with 63075, even if performed by a separate <u>individual</u> ~~providers~~……)<br><br>*22585    each additional interspace…*<br><br>(Use 22585 in conjunction with 22554, 22556, 22558)<br><br>(Do not report 22585 in conjunction with 63075, even if performed by a separate <u>individual</u> ~~providers~~……) |
| **Surgery**<br>**Foot and Toes**<br>**Other Procedures** | ▲28890    Extracorporeal shock wave, high energy, performed by a physician <u>or other qualified health care professional</u>, requiring anesthesia other than local, incuding ultrasound guidance, involving the plantar fasica<br><br>▶<u>(For extracorporeal shock wave therapy involving integumentary system no otherwise specified, see 0299T, 0300T)</u>◀<br><br>▶<u>(Do not report 28890 in conjunction with 0299T, 0300T when treating the same area)</u>◀ |
| **Surgery**<br>**Application of Casts and**<br>**Strapping** | The listed procedures apply when the cast application or strapping is a replacement procedure used during or after the period of follow-up care, or when the cast application or strapping is an initial service performed without a restorative treatment or procedure(s) to stabilize or protect a fracture, injury, or dislocation and/or to afford comfort to a patient. Restorative treatment or procedure(s) rendered by another <u>individual</u> ~~physician~~ following the application of the initial cast/splint/strap may be reported with a treatment of fracture and/or dislocation code.<br><br>An <u>individual</u> ~~physician~~ who applies the initial cast, strap, or splint and also assumes all of the subsequent fracture, dislocation, or injury care cannot use the application of casts and strapping codes as an initial service, since the first cast/splint or strap application is included in the treatment of fracture and/or dislocation codes. (See notes under Musculoskeletal System, page 92.) A temporary cast/splint/strap is not considered to be part of the preoperative care, and the use of the modifier 56 is not applicable. Additional evaluation and management services are reportable only if significant identifiable further services are provided at the time of the cast application or strapping |

⊘=Modifier 51 Exempt  ⊙=Moderate Sedation  ✛=Add-on Code  ⋀=FDA approval pending

| CPT Code/Section/Subsection | Revision/Addition/Deletion |
|---|---|
| **Surgery**<br>**Application of Casts and**<br>**Strapping** *(continued)* | .If cast application or strapping is provided as an initial service (eg, casting of a sprained ankle or knee) in which no other procedure or treatment (eg, surgical repair, reduction of a fracture, or joint dislocation) is performed or is expected to be performed by an individual ~~physician~~ rendering the initial care only, use the casting, strapping, and/or supply code (99070) in addition to an evaluation and management code as appropriate.<br><br>*Listed procedures include removal of cast or strapping.* |
| **Surgery**<br>**Application of Casts and**<br>**Strapping**<br>**Removal or Repair** | Codes for cast removals should be employed only for casts applied by another individual ~~physician~~.<br><br>29700   *Removal or bivalving; gauntlet, boot or body cast* |
| **Surgery**<br>**Cardiovascular System**<br>**Arteries and Veins**<br>**Venous** | *Venipuncture, needle or catheter for diagnostic study or intravenous therapy…*<br><br>▲36400   Venipuncture, younger than age 3 years, necessitating ~~physician's~~ the skill of a physician or other qualified health care professional, not to be used for routine venipuncture; femoral or jugular vein<br><br>▲36410   Venipuncture, age 3 years or older, necessitating ~~physician's~~ the skill of a physician or other qualified health care professional (separate procedure), for diagnostic or therapeutic purposes (not to be used for routine venipuncture)<br><br>36511   *Therapeutic apheresis; for white blood cells*<br><br>36516   *with extracorporeal selective adsorption or selective filtration and plasma reinfusion*<br><br>(For professional ~~physician~~ evaluation, use modifier 26)<br><br>_____ ***Coding Tip***_____<br><br>**Instructions for Use of the CPT Codebook**<br><br>When advanced practice nurses and physician assistants are working with physicians they are considered as working in the exact same specialty and exact same subspecialties as the physician. A "physician or other qualified health care professional" is an individual who is qualified by education, training, licensure/regulation (when applicable), and facility privileging (when applicable) who performs a professional service within his or her scope of practice and independently reports that professional services. These professionals are distinct from "clinical staff." A clinical staff member is a person who works under the supervision of a physician or other qualified health care professional, and who is allowed by law, regulation and facility policy to perform or assist in the performance of a specific professional service, but does not individually report that professional service. Other policies may also affect who may report specific services.<br><br>*CPT Coding Guidelines, Introduction, Instructions for Use of the CPT Codebook* |
| **Surgery**<br>**Urinary System**<br>**Bladder**<br>**Urodynamics** | *The following section (51725-51798) lists procedures that may be used separately or in many and varied combinations.*<br><br>*When multiple procedures are performed in the same investigative session, modifier 51 should be employed.*<br><br>All procedures in this section imply that these services are performed by, or are under the direct supervision of, a physician or other qualified health care professional and that all instruments, equipment, fluids, gases, probes, catheters, technician's fees, medications, gloves, trays, tubing, and other sterile supplies be provided by that individual ~~the physician~~. When the individual ~~physician~~ only interprets the results and/or operates the equipment, a professional component, modifier 26, should be used to identify these ~~physicians'~~ services.<br><br>51725   *Simple cystometrogram (CMG) (eg, spinal manometer)* |
| **Surgery**<br>**Female Genital System**<br>**Corpus Uteri**<br>**Introduction** | 58350   *Chromotubation of oviduct, including materials*<br><br>(~~For~~ To report the supply of any materials ~~supplied by physician~~, use 99070) |

| CPT Code/Section/Subsection | Revision/Addition/Deletion |
|---|---|
| **Surgery**<br>**Maternity Care and Delivery** | *For surgical complications…*<br><br>If ~~a physician provides~~ all or part of the antepartum and/or postpartum patient care <u>is provided except</u> ~~but does not perform~~ delivery due to termination of pregnancy by abortion or referral to another physician <u>or other qualified health care professional </u>for delivery….. |
| **Surgery**<br>**Maternity Care and Delivery**<br>**Repair** | ▲59300   Episiotomy or vaginal repair, by other than attending ~~physician~~ |
| **Surgery**<br>**Nervous System**<br>**Skull, Meninges, and Brain**<br>**Stereotaxis** | ✚ *61781*   *Stereotactic computer-assisted (navigational) procedure; cranial, intradural (List separately in addition to code for primary procedure)*<br><br>*(Do not report 61781 in conjunction with 61720-61791, 61796-61799, 61863-61868, 62201, 77371-77373, 77432)*<br><br>✚ *61782*     *cranial, extradural (List separately in addition to code for primary procedure)*<br><br>(Do not report 61781, 61782 by the same <u>individual</u> ~~provider~~ during the same surgical session) |
| **Surgery**<br>**Nervous System**<br>**Skull, Meninges, and Brain**<br>**Stereotactic Radiosurgery**<br>**(Cranial)** | Cranial stereotactic radiosurgery is a distinct procedure that utilizes externally generated ionizing radiation to inactivate or eradicate defined target(s) in the head without the need to make an incision. The target is defined by and the treatment is delivered using high-resolution stereotactic imaging. Stereotactic radiosurgery codes and headframe application procedures are reported by the neurosurgeon. The radiation oncologist reports the appropriate code(s) for clinical treatment planning, physics and dosimetry, treatment delivery, and management from the **Radiation Oncology** section (77261-77790). Any necessary planning, dosimetry, targeting, positioning, or blocking by the neurosurgeon is included in the stereotactic radiation surgery services. The same<u> individual</u> ~~physician~~ should not report stereotactic radiosurgery services with radiation treatment management codes (77427-77435).<br><br>*Cranial stereotactic radiosurgery is typically performed …*<br><br>*Codes 61796 and 61797 involve stereotactic radiosurgery …*<br><br>*Codes 61798 and 61799 involve stereotactic radiosurgery …*<br><br>*Do not report codes 61796-61800 in conjunction with …*<br><br>*Codes 61796-61799 include computer-assisted planning…* |
| **Surgery**<br>**Nervous System**<br>**Skull, Meninges, and Brain**<br>**Neurostimulators (Intracranial)** | *Codes 61850-61888 apply to both simple …*<br><br>Microelectrode recording, when performed by the operating surgeon in association with implantation of neurostimulator electrode arrays, is an inclusive service and should not be reported separately. If another ~~physician~~<u>individual</u> participates in neurophysiological mapping during a deep brain stimulator implantation procedure, this service may be reported by the ~~other physician~~<u>second individual</u> with codes 95961-95962.<br><br>*61850*   *Twist drill or burr hole(s) for implantation of neurostimulator electrodes, cortical* |
| **Surgery**<br>**Nervous System**<br>**Spine and Spinal Cord**<br>**Reservoir/Pump Implantation** | *62367*   *Electronic analysis of programmable, implanted pump for intrathecal or epidural drug infusion (includes evaluation of reservoir status, alarm status, drug prescription status); without reprogramming or refill*<br><br>*62368*   *with reprogramming*<br><br>*(For refilling and maintenance of an implantable infusion pump for spinal or brain drug therapy, see 95990-95991)*<br><br>*62369*     *with reprogramming and refill*<br><br>▲*62370*     *with reprogramming and refill (requiring* ~~physician's~~ *skill* <u>*of a physician or other qualified health care professional*</u>*)*<br><br>*(Do not report 62367-62370 in conjunction with 95990, 95991. For refilling and maintenance of a reservoir or an implantable infusion pump for spinal or brain drug delivery without reprogramming, see 95990, 95991)* |

| CPT Code/Section/Subsection | Revision/Addition/Deletion |
|---|---|
| **Surgery**<br>**Nervous System**<br>**Spine and Spinal Cord**<br>**Anterior or Anterolateral**<br>**Approach for Extradural**<br>**Exploration/Decompression** | *63075*   *Discectomy, anterior, with decompression of spinal cord and/or nerve root(s), including osteophytectomy; cervical, single interspace*<br><br>(Do not report 63075 in conjunction with 22554, even if performed by separate individuals ~~providers~~. To report anterior cervical discectomy and interbody fusion at the same level during the same session, use 22551)<br><br>*+63076*   *cervical, each additional interspace (List separately in addition to code for primary procedure)*<br><br>(Do not report 63076 in conjunction with 22554, even if performed by separate individuals ~~providers~~. To report anterior cervical discectomy and interbody fusion at the same level during the same session, use 22552) |
| **Surgery**<br>**Nervous System**<br>**Spine and Spinal Cord**<br>**Stereotactic Radiosurgery**<br>**(Spinal)** | Spinal stereotactic radiosurgery is a distinct procedure that utilizes externally generated ionizing radiation to inactivate or eradicate defined target(s) in the spine without the need to make an incision. The target is defined by and the treatment is delivered using high-resolution stereotactic imaging. These codes are reported by the surgeon. The radiation oncologist reports the appropriate code(s) for clinical treatment planning, physics and dosimetry, treatment delivery and management from the **Radiation Oncology** section (77261-77790). Any necessary planning, dosimetry, targeting, positioning, or blocking by the neurosurgeon is included in the stereotactic radiation surgery services. The same individual ~~physician~~ should not report stereotactic radiosurgery services with radiation treatment management codes (77427-77432).<br><br>*Spinal stereotactic radiosurgery is typically performed …*<br><br>*Stereotactic spinal surgery is only used when the tumor …*<br><br>*Codes 63620, 63621 include computer-assisted planning…*<br><br>*63620*   *Stereotactic radiosurgery (particle beam, gamma ray, or linear accelerator); 1 spinal lesion* |
| **Surgery**<br>**Eye and Ocular Adnexa**<br>**Anterior Segment**<br>**Intraocular Lens Procedures** | *66985*   *Insertion of intraocular lens prosthesis (secondary implant), not associated with concurrent cataract removal*<br><br>*(To code implant at time of concurrent cataract surgery, see 66982, 66983, 66984)*<br><br>*(To report supply of ~~For~~ intraocular lens prosthesis ~~supplied by physician~~, use 99070)*<br><br>*(For ultrasonic determination of intraocular lens power, use 76519)*<br><br>*(For removal of implanted material from anterior segment, use 65920)*<br><br>*(For secondary fixation (separate procedure), use 66682)*<br><br>*(For use of ophthalmic endoscope with 66985, use 66990)* |
| **Radiology Guidelines**<br>**(Including Nuclear Medicine**<br>**and Diagnostic Ultrasound)** | Guidelines to direct general ~~Items used by all physicians in~~ reporting of ~~their~~ services are presented in the **Introduction**. Some of the commonalities are repeated here for the convenience of those ~~physicians~~ referring to this section…. |
| **Radiology Guidelines**<br>**(Including Nuclear Medicine**<br>**and Diagnostic Ultrasound)**<br>**Subject Listings** | Subject listings apply when radiological services are performed by or under the responsible supervision of a physician or other qualified health care professional. |

| CPT Code/Section/Subsection | Revision/Addition/Deletion |
|---|---|
| **Radiology Guidelines (Including Nuclear Medicine and Diagnostic Ultrasound) Supervision and Interpretation** | Imaging may be required during the performance of certain procedures or certain imaging procedures may require surgical procedures to access the imaged area. Many services include image guidance, which is not separately reportable and is so stated in the descriptor or guidelines. When imaging is not included in a surgical procedure or procedure from the **Medicine** section, image guidance codes or codes labeled "radiological supervision and interpretation" may be reported for the portion of the service that requires imaging. Both services require image documentation and radiological supervision, interpretation, and report services require a separate interpretation.<br><br>When a procedure is performed by two ~~individuals~~ physicians, the radiologic portion of the procedure is designated as "radiological supervision and interpretation." When a physician ~~the same individual~~ performs both the procedure and provides imaging supervision and interpretation, a combination of procedure codes outside the 70000 series and imaging supervision and interpretation codes are to be used. |
| **Radiology Guidelines (Including Nuclear Medicine and Diagnostic Ultrasound) Written Report(s)** | A written report signed by the interpreting individual ~~physician~~ should be considered an integral part of a radiologic procedure or interpretation. |
| **Radiology Diagnostic Radiology (Diagnostic Imaging) Heart** | *Cardiac magnetic imaging differs from traditional ...*<br><br>*Cardiac MRI for velocity flow mapping can be reported...*<br><br>Listed procedures may be performed independently or in the course of overall medical care. If the individual ~~physician~~ providing these services is also responsible for diagnostic workup and/or follow-up care of the patient, also see appropriate sections. Only one procedure in the series 75557-75563 is appropriately reported per session. Only one add-on code for flow velocity can be reported per session.<br><br>*Cardiac MRI studies may be performed at rest...*<br><br>*Cardiac computed tomography (CT) and coronary...*<br><br>75557  *Cardiac magnetic resonance imaging for morphology and function without contrast material;* |
| **Radiology Diagnostic Radiology (Diagnostic Imaging) Other Procedures** | ▲76000  Fluoroscopy (separate procedure), up to 1 hour physician or other qualified health care professional time,....<br><br>▲76001  Fluoroscopy, physician or other qualified health care professional time more than 1 hour, assisting a nonradiologic physician or other qualified health care professional.....<br><br>76140  *Consultation on X-ray examination made elsewhere, written report*<br><br>~~(76376, 76377 require concurrent physician supervision of image postprocessing 3D manipulation of volumetric data set and image rendering)~~<br><br>▲76376  3D rendering with interpretation and reporting of computed tomography, magnetic resonance imaging, ultrasound, or other tomographic modality with image post processing under concurrent supervision;...<br><br>▲76377  rendering image postprocessing on an independent workstation<br><br>(76376, 76377 require concurrent supervision of image postprocessing 3D manipulation of volumetric data set and image rendering) |
| **Radiology Diagnostic Ultrasound Extremities** | ▲76885  Ultrasound, infant hips, real time with imaging documentation; dynamic (requiring physician or other qualified health care professional manipulation)<br><br>▲76886  limited, static (not requiring physician or other qualified health care professional manipulation) |
| **Radiology Breast, Mammography** | ✚▲77051  Computer-aided detection (computer algorithm analysis of digital image data for lesion detection) with further ~~physician~~ review for interpretation, with or without digitization of film radiographic images; diagnostic mammography (List separately in addition to code for primary procedure) |

| CPT Code/Section/Subsection | Revision/Addition/Deletion |
|---|---|
| **Radiology**<br>**Bone/Joint Studies** | ▲77071    Manual application of stress performed by physician <u>or other qualified health care</u> <u>professional</u> for joint radiography, including contralateral joint if indicated |
| **Radiology**<br>**Nuclear Medicine** | Listed procedures may be performed independently or in the course of overall medical care. If the <u>individual</u> ~~physician~~ providing these services is also responsible for diagnostic workup and/or follow-up care of patient, see appropriate sections also.<br><br>*Radioimmunoassay tests are found in the* **Clinical Pathology** *section…*<br><br>The services listed do not include the radiopharmaceutical or drug. <u>To separately report supply</u> <u>of d</u>~~D~~iagnostic and therapeutic radiopharmaceuticals and drugs, ~~supplied by the physician~~ ~~should be reported separately using~~ <u>use</u> the appropriate supply code(s), in addition to the procedure code.<br><br>•78012    Thyroid uptake, single or multiple quantitative measurement(s) (including stimulation, suppression, or discharge, when performed) |
| **Pathology and Laboratory**<br>**Guidelines** | <u>Guidelines to direct general</u> ~~Items used by~~ <u>all</u> ~~physicians~~ <u>in</u> reporting <u>of</u> ~~their~~ services are presented in the **Introduction.** Some of the commonalities are repeated here for the convenience of those ~~physicians~~ referring to this section… |
| **Pathology and Laboratory**<br>**Evocative/Suppresssion Testing** | The following test panels involve the administration of evocative or suppressive agents and the baseline and subsequent measurement of their effects on chemical constituents. These codes are to be used for the reporting of the laboratory component of the overall testing protocol. For the ~~physician's~~ administration of the evocative or suppressive agents, see <u>Hydration, Therapeutic, Prophylactic, Diagnostic Injections and Infusions, and Chemotherapy</u> <u>and Other Highly Complex Drug or Highly Complex Biologic Agent Administration (eg,</u> ~~96360,~~ ~~96361,~~ <u>96365, 96366, 96367, 96368, 96372, 96374, 96375, 96376)</u>; ~~for the supplies and drugs,~~ ~~see 99070. To report physician attendance and monitoring during the testing~~ <u>by a physician</u> <u>or other qualified health care professional,</u> ~~use the appropriate evaluation and management~~ ~~code~~<u>,</u> <u>including the prolonged physician care codes (99354-99357)</u> if required. Prolonged ~~physician~~ <u>services</u> ~~care codes (99354-99357)~~ are not separately reported when evocative/ suppression testing involves prolonged infusions reported with ~~96360, 96361,~~ <u>96365, 96366,</u> ~~96367~~. In the code descriptors where reference is made to a particular analyte (eg, Cortisol: 82533 x 2) the "x 2" refers to the number of times the test for that particular analyte is performed. |
| **Pathology and Laboratory**<br>**Consultations (Clinical**<br>**Pathology)** | A clinical pathology consultation is a service, including a written report, rendered by the pathologist in response to a request from a <u>physician or qualified health care professional</u> ~~in~~ ~~attending physician~~ in relation to a test result(s)… |
| **Medicine Guidelines**<br><u>**Supplied**</u> **Materials** ~~Supplied by~~<br>~~Physician~~ | Supplies and materials ~~provided by the physician~~ (eg, ~~sterile trays/drugs~~ <u>trays</u>,… reported separately <u>using code</u> ~~. List drugs, trays, supplies, and materials provided. Identify as~~ 99070 or <u>a</u> specific supply code. |
| **Medicine**<br>**Immunization Administration**<br>**for Vaccines/Toxoids** | Report codes 90460 and 90461 only when the physician or qualified health care professional provides face-to-face counseling of the patient/family during the administration of a vaccine. For immunization administration of any vaccine that is not accompanied by face-to-face physician or qualified health care professional counseling to the patient/family or for administration of vaccines to patients over 18 years of age, report codes 90471-90474. <u>(See also</u> **Instructions for Use of the CPT Codebook** <u>for definition of reporting qualifications)</u> If a significant separately identifiable Evaluation and Management…<br><br>90460    *Immunization administration through 18 years of age via any route of administration, with counseling by physician or other qualified health care professional;* *first…* |
| **Other Psychiatric Services or**<br>**Procedures** | ▲90889    Preparation of report of patient's psychiatric status, history, treatment, or progress (other than for legal or consultative purposes) for other <u>individuals</u> ~~physicians~~, agencies, or insurance carriers |

| CPT Code/Section/Subsection | Revision/Addition/Deletion |
|---|---|
| **Medicine**<br>**Dialysis**<br>**Hemodialysis** | Codes 90935, 90937 are reported to describe the hemodialysis procedure…<br><br>*(For home visit hemodialysis services performed by a non-physician health care professional, use 99512)*<br><br>*(For cannula declotting, see 36831, 36833, 36860, 36861)*<br><br>*(For declotting of implanted vascular access device or catheter by thrombolytic agent, use 36593)*<br><br>*(For collection of blood specimen from a partially or completely implantable venous access device, use 36591)*<br><br>(For prolonged ~~physician~~ attendance <u>by a physician or other qualified health care professional</u>, see 99354-99360)<br><br>▲90935   Hemodialysis procedure with single ~~physician~~ evaluation <u>by a physician or other qualified health care professional</u> |
| **Medicine**<br>**Dialysis**<br>**Miscellaneous Dialysis**<br>**Procedures** | (For prolonged ~~physician~~ attendance <u>by a physician or other qualified health care professional</u>, see 99354-99360)<br><br>▲90945   Dialysis procedure other than hemodialysis (eg, peritoneal dialysis, hemofiltration, or other continuous renal replacement therapies), with single ~~physician~~ evaluation<u> by a physician or other qualified health care professional</u><br><br>▲90947   Dialysis procedure other than hemodialysis (eg, peritoneal dialysis, hemofiltration, or other continuous renal replacement therapies) requiring repeated ~~physician~~ evaluation<u> by a physician or other qualified health care professional</u>, with or without substantial revision of dialysis prescription |
| **Medicine**<br>**Dialysis**<br>**End Stage Renal Disease**<br>**Services** | Codes 90951-90962 are reported **once** per month to distinguish age-specific services related to the patient's end-stage renal disease (ESRD) performed in an outpatient setting with three levels of service based on the number of face-to-face visits. ESRD-related ~~physician~~ services <u>by a physician or other qualified health care professional </u>include establishment of a dialyzing cycle, outpatient evaluation and management of the dialysis visits, telephone calls, and patient management during the dialysis provided during a full month. In the circumstances in which the patient has had a complete assessment visit during the month and services are provided over a period of less than a month, 90951-90962 may be used according to the number of visits performed.<br><br>*Codes 90963-90966 are reported once per month for…*<br><br>*For ESRD and non-ESRD dialysis services performed in…*<br><br>*Evaluation and management services unrelated to ESRD services…*<br><br>*Codes 90967-90970 are reported to distinguish age-specific…* |

⊘=Modifier 51 Exempt ⊙=Moderate Sedation ✚=Add-on Code 〆=FDA approval pending

| CPT Code/Section/Subsection | Revision/Addition/Deletion |
|---|---|
| **Medicine**<br>**Dialysis**<br>**End Stage Renal Disease**<br>**Services** *(continued)* | *Examples:*<br><br>*ESRD-related services:*<br><br>ESRD-related services are initiated on July 1 for a 57-year-old male. On July 11, he is admitted to the hospital as an inpatient and is discharged on July 27. He has had a complete assessment and the physician or other qualified health care professional has performed two face-to-face visits prior to admission. Another face-to-face visit occurs after discharge during the month.<br><br>*In this example, 90961 is reported for the three face-to-face...*<br><br>*If the patient did not have a complete assessment...*<br><br>*ESRD-related services for the home dialysis...*<br><br>*Home ESRD-related services are initiated on...*<br><br>*In this example, 90970 should be reported for each day...* |

▲90951    End-stage renal disease (ESRD) related services monthly, for patients younger than 2 years of age to include monitoring for the adequacy of nutrition, assessment of growth and development, and counseling of parents; with 4 or more face-to-face ~~physician~~ visits by a physician or other qualified health care professional per month

▲90952    with 2-3 face-to-face ~~physician~~ visits by a physician or other qualified health care professional per month

▲90953    with 1 face-to-face ~~physician~~ visit by a physician or other qualified health care professional per month

▲90954    End-stage renal disease (ESRD) related services monthly, for patients 2-11 years of age to include monitoring for the adequacy of nutrition, assessment of growth and development, and counseling of parents; with 4 or more face-to-face ~~physician~~ visits by a physician or other qualified health care professional per month

▲90955    with 2-3 face-to-face ~~physician~~ visits by a physician or other qualified health care professional per month

▲90956    with 1 face-to-face ~~physician~~ visit by a physician or other qualified health care professional per month

▲90957    End-stage renal disease (ESRD) related services monthly, for patients 12-19 years of age to include monitoring for the adequacy of nutrition, assessment of growth and development, and counseling of parents; with 4 or more face-to-face ~~physician~~ visits by a physician or other qualified health care professional per month

▲90958    with 2-3 face-to-face ~~physician~~ visits by a physician or other qualified health care professional per month

▲90959    with 1 face-to-face ~~physician~~ visit by a physician or other qualified health care professional per month

▲90960    End-stage renal disease (ESRD) related services monthly, for patients 20 years of age and older; with 4 or more face-to-face ~~physician~~ visits by a physician or other qualified health care professional per month

▲90961    with 2-3 face-to-face ~~physician~~ visits by a physician or other qualified health care professional per month

▲90962    with 1 face-to-face ~~physician~~ visit by a physician or other qualified health care professional per month

| **Medicine**<br>**Gastroenterology** | ▲91110    Gastrointestinal tract imaging, intraluminal (eg, capsule endoscopy), esophagus through ileum, with ~~physician~~ interpretation and report ~~by a physician~~ |
|---|---|
| | ▲91111    Gastrointestinal tract imaging, intraluminal (eg, capsule endoscopy), esophagus with ~~physician~~ interpretation and report ~~by a physician~~ |

| CPT Code/Section/Subsection | Revision/Addition/Deletion |
|---|---|
| **Medicine**<br>**Ophthalmology** | *(For surgical procedures, see* **Surgery***, Eye and Ocular Adnexa, 65091 et seq)*<br><br>**Definitions**<br><br>***Intermediate ophthalmological services*** *describes an evaluation…*<br><br>*For example:*<br>    *a.  Review of history, external examination…*<br>    *b.  Review of interval history, external examination…*<br><br>***Comprehensive ophthalmological services*** *describes a general evaluation…*<br><br>Intermediate and comprehensive ophthalmological services…<br><br>*For example:*<br><br>The comprehensive services required for diagnosis and treatment of a patient…<br>*Initiation of diagnostic and treatment program includes the prescription…*<br><br>***Special ophthalmological services*** *describes services in which…*<br><br>*For example:*<br><br>*Fluorescein angioscopy, quantitative visual field examination, refraction or…*<br>*Prescription of lenses, when required, is included…*<br><br>Interpretation and report by the physician <u>or other qualified health care professional</u> is an integral part of special ophthalmological services where indicated. Technical procedures (which may or may not be performed ~~by the physician~~ personally) are often part of the service… |
| **Medicine**<br>**Ophthalmology**<br>**General Ophthalmological**<br>**Services**<br>**New Patient** | (For distinguishing between new and established patients, see **Evaluation and Management** guidelines)<br><br>~~Solely for the purposes of distinguishing between new and established patients,~~ **professional services** ~~are those face-to-face services rendered by a physician and reported by a specific code(s). A new patient is one who has not received any professional services from the physician or another physician of the same specialty who belongs to the same group practice within the past three years.~~<br><br>    *92002   Ophthalmological services: medical examination and evaluation with initiation of diagnostic and treatment program; intermediate, new patient* |
| **Medicine**<br>**Ophthalmology**<br>**General Ophthalmological**<br>**Services**<br>**Established Patient** | (For distinguishing between new and established patients, see **Evaluation and Management** guidelines)<br><br>~~Solely for the purposes of distinguishing between new and established patients,~~ **professional services** ~~are those face-to-face services rendered by a physician and reported by a specific code(s). An established patient is one who has received professional services from the physician or another physician of the same specialty who belongs to the same group practice within the past three years.~~<br><br>    *92012   Ophthalmological services: medical examination and evaluation, with initiation or continuation of diagnostic and treatment program; intermediate, established patient* |
| **Medicine**<br>**Ophthalmology**<br>**Spectacle Services (Including Prosthesis for Aphakia)** | *Prescription of lenses, when required, is included…*<br><br><u>When provided ~~by the physician~~, fitting</u> ~~Fitting~~ of spectacles is a separate service; ~~when provided by the physician, it~~ <u>and</u> is reported as indicated by 92340-92371.<br><br>Fitting includes measurement of anatomical facial characteristics, the writing of laboratory specifications, and the final adjustment of the spectacles to the visual axes and anatomical topography. Presence of <u>the</u> physician <u>or other qualified health care professional</u> is not required.<br><br>*Supply of materials is a separate service component; it is…*<br><br>    *92340   Fitting of spectacles, except for aphakia; monofocal* |

| CPT Code/Section/Subsection | Revision/Addition/Deletion |
|---|---|
| **Medicine**<br>**Special Otorhinolaryngologic Services**<br>**Evaluative and Therapeutic Services** | *92612  Flexible fiberoptic endoscopic evaluation of swallowing by cine or video recording;*<br><br>▲92613  ~~physician~~ interpretation and report only<br><br>*92614  Flexible fiberoptic endoscopic evaluation, laryngeal sensory testing by cine or video recording;*<br><br>▲92615  ~~physician~~ interpretation and report only<br><br>*92616  Flexible fiberoptic endoscopic evaluation of swallowing and laryngeal sensory testing by cine or video recording;*<br><br>▲92617  ~~physician~~ interpretation and report only |
| **Medicine**<br>**Cardiovascular**<br>**Therapeutic Services and Procedures** | *92953  Temporary transcutaneous pacing*<br><br>(For ~~physician~~ direction of ambulance or rescue personnel outside the hospital <u>by a physician or other qualified health care professional</u>, use 99288) |
| **Medicine**<br>**Cardiovascular**<br>**Cardiography** | ▲93015  Cardiovascular stress test using maximal or submaximal treadmill or bicycle exercise, continuous electrocardiographic monitoring, and/or pharmacological stress; with ~~physician~~ supervision, ~~with~~ interpretation and report<br><br>▲93016  ~~physician~~ supervision only, without interpretation and report |
| **Medicine**<br>**Cardiovascular**<br>**Cardiography**<br>**Cardiovascular Monitoring Services** | *Cardiovascular monitoring services are diagnostic medical procedures…*<br><br>***Attended surveillance:*** *is the immediate availability of a remote technician to respond……*<br><br>***Electrocardiographic rhythm derived elements:*** *elements derived…….*<br><br>***Mobile cardiovascular telemetry (MCT):*** continuously records the electrocardiographic rhythm from external electrodes placed on the patient's body. Segments of the ECG data are automatically (without patient intervention) transmitted to a remote surveillance location by cellular or landline telephone signal. The segments of the rhythm, selected for transmission, are triggered automatically (MCT device algorithm) by rapid and slow heart rates or by the patient during a symptomatic episode. There is continuous real time data analysis by preprogrammed algorithms in the device and attended surveillance of the transmitted rhythm segments by a surveillance center technician to evaluate any arrhythmias and to determine signal quality. The surveillance center technician reviews the data and notifies the physician <u>or other qualified health care professional</u> depending on the prescribed criteria.<br><br>*ECG rhythm derived elements are distinct from physiologic data,…*<br><br>▲93224  External electrocardiographic …~~physician~~ review and interpretation <u>by a physician or other qualified health care professional</u><br><br>*93225      recording (includes connection, recording, and disconnection)*<br><br>*93226      scanning analysis with report* |

| CPT Code/Section/Subsection | Revision/Addition/Deletion |
|---|---|
| **Medicine**<br>**Cardiovascular**<br>**Cardiovascular Monitoring**<br>**Services** *(continued)* | ▲93227 ~~physician~~ review and interpretation <u>by a physician or other qualified health care professional</u><br><br>▲93228 External mobile cardiovascular telemetry …for up to 30 days; ~~physician~~ review and interpretation with report <u>by a physician or other qualified health care professional</u><br><br>▲93229 technical support for connection and patient instructions for use, attended surveillance, analysis and ~~physician prescribed~~ transmission of daily and e emergent data reports <u>as prescribed by a physician or other qualified health care professional</u><br><br>▲93268 External …….24-hour attended monitoring; includes transmission, ~~physician~~ review and interpretation <u>by a physician or other qualified health care professional</u><br><br>93270 *recording (includes connection, recording, and disconnection)*<br><br>93271 *transmission download and analysis*<br><br>▲93272 ~~physician~~ review and interpretation <u>by a physician or other qualified health care professional</u> |
| **Medicine**<br>**Cardiovascular**<br>**Implantable and Wearable**<br>**Cardiac Device Evaluations** | Cardiac device evaluation services are diagnostic medical procedures using in-person and remote technology to assess device therapy and cardiovascular physiologic data. Codes 93279-93299 describe this technology and technical/professional ~~physician~~ and service center practice. Codes 93279-93292 are reported per procedure. Codes 93293-93296 are reported no more than **once** every 90 days. Do not report 93293-93296 if the monitoring period is less than 30 days. Codes 93297, 93298 are reported no more than **once** up to every 30 days. Do not report 93297-93299 if the monitoring period is less than 10 days.<br><br>A service center may report 93296 or 93299 during a period in which a physician <u>or other qualified health care professional</u> performs an in-person interrogation device evaluation. <u>The same individual</u> ~~A physician~~ may not report an in-person and remote interrogation of the same device during the same period. Report only remote services when an in-person interrogation device evaluation is performed during a period of remote interrogation device evaluation. A period is established by the initiation of the remote monitoring or the 91st day of a pacemaker or implantable cardioverter-defibrillator (ICD) monitoring or the 31st day of an implantable loop recorder (ILR) or implantable cardiovascular monitor (ICM) monitoring and extends for the subsequent 90 or 30 days, respectively, for which remote monitoring is occurring. Programming device evaluations and in-person interrogation device evaluations may not be reported on the same date by the same <u>individual</u> ~~physician~~. Programming device evaluations and remote interrogation device evaluations may both be reported during the remote interrogation device evaluation period.<br><br>*For monitoring by wearable devices, see …*<br><br>*ECG rhythm derived elements are distinct …*<br><br>*Do not report 93268-93272 when performing 93279…*<br><br>The pacemaker and ICD interrogation device evaluations, peri-procedural device evaluations and programming, and programming device evaluations may not be reported in conjunction with pacemaker or ICD device and/or lead insertion or revision services by the same <u>individual</u> ~~physician~~. |

| CPT Code/Section/Subsection | Revision/Addition/Deletion |
|---|---|
| **Medicine**<br>**Cardiovascular**<br>**Implantable and Wearable**<br>**Cardiac Device Evaluations**<br>*(continued)* | *The following definitions and instructions apply …*<br><br>***Attended surveillance:*** the immediate availability of a remote technician to respond to rhythm or device alert transmissions from a patient, either from an implanted or wearable monitoring or therapy device, as they are generated and transmitted to the remote surveillance location or center.<br><br>***Device, single lead:*** *a pacemaker or …*<br><br>***Device, dual lead:*** *a pacemaker or …*<br><br>***Device, multiple lead:*** *a pacemaker or …*<br><br>***Electrocardiographic rhythm derived elements:*** *elements derived …*<br><br>***Implantable cardiovascular monitor (ICM):*** an implantable cardiovascular device used to assist the physician in the management of non-rhythm related cardiac conditions such as heart failure. The device collects longitudinal physiologic cardiovascular data elements from one or more internal sensors (such as right ventricular pressure, left atrial pressure or an index of lung water) and/or external sensors (such as blood pressure or body weight) for patient assessment and management. The data are stored and transmitted ~~to the physician~~ by either local telemetry or remotely to an Internet-based file server or surveillance technician. The function of the ICM may be an additional function of an implantable cardiac device (eg, implantable cardioverter-defibrillator) or a function of a stand-alone device. When ICM functionality is included in an ICD device or pacemaker, the ICM data and the ICD or pacemaker heart rhythm data such as sensing, pacing, and tachycardia detection therapy are distinct and therefore, the monitoring processes are distinct.<br><br>***Implantable cardioverter-defibrillator (ICD):*** *an implantable device …*<br><br>***Implantable loop recorder (ILR):*** an implantable device that continuously records the electrocardiographic rhythm triggered automatically by rapid and slow heart rates or by the patient during a symptomatic episode. The ILR function may be the only function of the device or it may be part of a pacemaker or implantable cardioverter-defibrillator device. The data are stored and transmitted ~~to the physician~~ by either local telemetry or remotely to an Internet-based file server or surveillance technician. Extraction of data and compilation or report for ~~individual~~ physician <u>or qualified health care professional</u> interpretation is usually performed in the office setting.<br><br>***Interrogation device evaluation:*** *an evaluation of …*<br><br>*The components that must be evaluated…*<br><br>***Interrogation device evaluation (remote):*** *a procedure…*<br><br>***Pacemaker:*** *an implantable device that provides low…*<br><br>***Peri-procedural device evaluation and programming:*** an evaluation of an implantable device system (either a pacemaker or implantable cardioverter defibrillator) to adjust the device to settings appropriate for the patient prior to a surgery, procedure, or test. The device system data are interrogated to evaluate the lead(s), sensor(s), and battery in addition to review of stored information, including patient and system measurements. The device is programmed to settings appropriate for the surgery, procedure, or test, as required. A second evaluation and programming are performed after the surgery, procedure, or test to provide settings appropriate to the post procedural situation, as required. If one ~~provider~~ performs both the pre- and post-evaluation and programming service, the appropriate code, either 93286 or 93287, would be reported two times. If one ~~provider~~ performs the pre-surgical service and a separate <u>individual</u> ~~provider~~ performs the post-surgical service, each reports either 93286 or 93287 only one time. |

| CPT Code/Section/Subsection | Revision/Addition/Deletion |
|---|---|
| **Medicine**<br>**Cardiovascular**<br>**Implantable and Wearable**<br>**Cardiac Device Evaluations**<br>*(continued)* | ▲93279 Programming device evaluation (in person)....... with ~~physician~~ analysis, review and report by a physician or other qualified health care professional; single lead pacemaker system |
| | ▲93280      dual lead pacemaker system |
| | ▲93281      multiple lead pacemaker system |
| | ▲93282      single lead implantable cardioverter-defibrillator |
| | ▲93283      dual lead implantable cardioverter-defibrillator system |
| | ▲93284      multiple lead implantable cardioverter-defibrillator system |
| | ▲93285      implantable loop recorder system |
| | ▲93286 Peri-procedural device evaluation (in person).... review and report by a physician or other qualified health care professional; single, dual, or multiple lead pacemaker system |
| | ▲93287      single, dual, or multiple lead implantable cardioverter-defibrillator system |
| | ▲93288 Interrogation device evaluation (in person) with ~~physician~~ analysis, review and report by a physician or other qualified health care professional, includes connection, recording and disconnection per patient encounter; single, dual, or multiple lead pacemaker system |
| | ▲93289      single, dual, or multiple lead implantable cardioverter defibrillator system, including analysis of heart rhythm derived data elements |
| | ▲93293 Transtelephonic rhythm strip pacemaker evaluation(s) ......by a physician or other qualified health care professional, up to 90 days |
| | ▲93294 Interrogation device evaluation(s) (remote..... by a physician or other qualified health care professional |
| | ▲93295      single, dual, or multiple lead....interim ~~physician~~ analysis, review(s) and report(s) by a physician or other qualified health care professional |
| | 93296      *single, dual, or multiple lead pacemaker system...* |
| | ▲93297 Interrogation device evaluation(s), (remote) up to 30 days; ......~~physician~~ analysis, review(s) and report(s) by a physician or other qualified health care professional |
| | ▲93298      implantable loop recorder system, .....by a physician or other qualified health care professional |
| | 93299      *implantable cardiovascular monitor system or implantable loop recorder system, remote data acquisition(s), receipt of transmissions and technician review, technical support and distribution of results* |
| **Medicine**<br>**Cardiovascular**<br>**Echocardiography** | *Echocardiography includes obtaining ultrasonic signals from the heart...*<br><br>*A complete transthoracic echocardiogram without ...*<br><br>*A complete transthoracic echocardiogram with ...*<br><br>*A follow-up or limited echocardiographic study (93308) is...*<br><br>*In stress echocardiography, echocardiographic images are recorded from multiple...*<br><br>When a stress echocardiogram is performed with a complete cardiovascular stress test (continuous electrocardiographic monitoring, ~~physician~~ supervision, interpretation and report by a physician or other qualified health care professional), use 93351... |

⊘=Modifier 51 Exempt ⊙=Moderate Sedation ✚=Add-on Code ⋔=FDA approval pending

| CPT Code/Section/Subsection | Revision/Addition/Deletion |
|---|---|
| **Medicine**<br>**Cardiovascular**<br>**Echocardiography**<br>*(continued)* | *93350    Echocardiography, transthoracic, real-time with image documentation (2D), includes M-mode recording, when performed, during rest and cardiovascular stress test using treadmill, bicycle exercise and/or pharmacologically induced stress, with interpretation and report;*<br><br>▲93351         including performance of continuous electrocardiographic monitoring, with ~~physician~~ supervision <u>by a physician</u> or other qualified health care professional |
| **Medicine**<br>**Cardiovascular**<br>**Peripheral Arterial Disease**<br>**Rehabilitation** | Peripheral arterial disease (PAD) rehabilitative physical exercise consists of a series of sessions, lasting 45-60 minutes per session, involving use of either a motorized treadmill or a track to permit each patient to achieve symptom-limited claudication. Each session is supervised by an exercise physiologist or nurse. The supervising provider monitors the individual patient's claudication threshold and other cardiovascular limitations for adjustment of workload.<br><br>During this supervised rehabilitation program, the development of new arrhythmias, symptoms that might suggest angina or the continued inability of the patient to progress to an adequate level of exercise may require ~~physician~~ review and examination of the patient <u>by a physician or other qualified health care professional</u>. These ~~physician~~ services would be separately reported with an appropriate level E/M service code <u>including office or other outpatient services (99201-99215), initial hospital care (99221-99223), subsequent hospital care (99231-99233), critical care services (99291-99292).</u><br><br>*93668    Peripheral arterial disease (PAD) rehabilitation, per session* |
| **Medicine**<br>**Cardiovascular**<br>**Noninvasive Physiologic**<br>**Studies and Procedures** | ▲93745   Initial set-up and programming by a physician <u>or other qualified health care professional</u> of wearable cardioverter-defibrillator…<br><br>▲93750   Interrogation of ventricular assist device (VAD), in person, with <u>physician or other qualified health care professional</u> ~~physician~~ analysis of device parameters ~~by a physician or other qualified health care professional~~ (eg, drivelines, alarms, power surges), review of device function…<br><br>▲93790   ~~physician~~ review with interpretation and report |
| **Medicine**<br>**Cardiovascular**<br>**Other Procedures** | ▲93797   Physician <u>or other qualified health care professional</u> services for outpatient cardiac rehabilitation; without continuous ECG monitoring (per session) |
| **Medicine**<br>**Pulmonary**<br>**Ventilator Management** | *94005         Home ventilator management care plan oversight….*<br><br>(Ventilator management care plan oversight is reported separately from home or domiciliary, rest home [eg, assisted living] services. A physician <u>or other qualified health care professional</u> may report 94005, when performed, including when a different <u>individual</u> ~~physician~~ reports 99339, 99340, 99374-99378 for the same 30 days) |
| **Medicine**<br>**Pulmonary**<br>**Other Procedures** | ▲94014   Patient-initiated spirometric recording per 30-day period of time; includes reinforced education, transmission of spirometric tracing, data capture, analysis of transmitted data, periodic recalibration and ~~physician~~ review and interpretation <u>by a physician or other qualified health care professional</u><br><br>▲94016   ~~physician~~ review and interpretation only <u>by a physician or other qualified health care professional</u><br><br>▲94452   High altitude simulation test (HAST), with ~~physician~~ interpretation and report <u>by a physician or other qualified health care professional</u>;<br><br>▲94610   Intrapulmonary surfactant administration by a physician <u>or other qualified health care professional</u> through endotracheal tube<br><br>▲94774   Pediatric home apnea monitoring event recording……….download of data, ~~physician~~ review, interpretation, and preparation of a report <u>by a physician or other qualified health care professional</u><br><br>▲94777   ~~physician~~ review, interpretation and preparation of report only <u>by a physician or other qualified health care professional</u> |

| CPT Code/Section/Subsection | Revision/Addition/Deletion |
|---|---|
| **Medicine**<br>**Allergy and Clinical**<br>**Immunology**<br>**Allergy Testing** | ▲95004 Percutaneous tests (scratch, puncture, prick) with allergenic extracts, immediate type reaction, including test interpretation and report ~~by a physician~~, specify number of tests |
| | •95017 Allergy testing, any combination of percutaneous (scratch, puncture, prick) and intracutaneous (intradermal), sequential and incremental, with venoms, immediate type reaction, including test interpretation and report, specify number of tests |
| | •95018 Allergy testing, any combination of percutaneous (scratch, puncture, prick) and intracutaneous (intradermal), sequential and incremental, with drugs or biologicals, immediate type reaction, including test interpretation and report, specify number of tests |
| | ▲95024 Intracutaneous (intradermal) tests with allergenic extracts, immediate type reaction, including test interpretation and report ~~by a physician~~, specify number of tests |
| | ▲95027 Intracutaneous (intradermal) tests, sequential and incremental, with allergenic extracts for airborne allergens, immediate type reaction, including test interpretation and report ~~by a physician~~, specify number of tests |
| **Medicine Allergy and**<br>**Clinical Immunology Allergen**<br>**Immunotherapy** | ▲95120 Professional services for allergen immunotherapy in <u>the office or institution of the</u> prescribing physician<u>s or other qualified health care professional</u> ~~office or institution~~, including provision of allergenic extract; single injection |
| | ▲95125 2 or more injections |
| | ▲95130 single stinging insect venom |
| | ▲95131 2 stinging insect venoms |
| | ▲95132 3 stinging insect venoms |
| | ▲95133 4 stinging insect venoms |
| | ▲95134 5 stinging insect venoms . |
| **Medicine Neurology and**<br>**Neuromuscular Procedures** | *Neurologic services are typically consultative, and any …*<br><br>*In addition, services and skills outlined under …*<br><br>The EEG, autonomic function, evoked potential, reflex tests, EMG, NCV, and MEG services (95812-95829 and 95860-95967) include recording, interpretation<u>, and report</u> by a physician<u>,</u> ~~and report~~ <u>or other qualified health care professional</u>. For interpretation only, use modifier 26. For EMG guidance, see 95873, 95874.<br><br>Codes 95812-95822~~, 95920~~, 95950-95953 and 95956 use recording time as a basis for code use. Recording time is when the recording is underway and data is being collected. Recording time excludes set up and take down time. Codes 95961-95962 use physician <u>or other qualified health care professional attendance</u> time as a basis for code use. |
| **Medicine Neurology**<br>**and Neuromuscular**<br>**Procedures Routine**<br>**Electroencephalography** | ▲95830 Insertion by physician <u>or other qualified health care professional</u> of sphenoidal electrodes for electroencephalographic (EEG) recording |
| **Medicine**<br>**Neurology and Neuromuscular**<br>**Procedures**<br>**Special EEG Tests** | Codes 95961 and 95962 use physician <u>or other qualified health care professional</u> time as a basis for unit of service. ~~Report for each hour of individual physician attendance.~~ Report 95961 for the first hour of ~~physician~~ attendance. Use modifier 52 with 95961 for 30 minutes or less. Report 95962 for each additional hour of ~~physician~~ attendance.<br><br>▲95954 Pharmacological or physical activation requiring physician <u>or other qualified health care professional</u> attendance…<br><br>▲95961 Functional cortical and subcortical mapping …brain structures; initial hour of ~~physician~~ attendance <u>by a physician or other qualified health care professional</u><br><br>▲95962 each additional hour of ~~physician~~ attendance <u>by a physician or other qualified health care professional</u> (List separately in addition to code for primary procedure) |

| CPT Code/Section/Subsection | Revision/Addition/Deletion |
|---|---|
| **Medicine**<br>**Neurology and Neuromuscular**<br>**Procedures**<br>**Other Procedures** | *95990*     *Refilling and maintenance of implantable pump or reservoir for drug delivery, spinal (intrathecal, epidural) or brain (intraventricular), includes electronic analysis of pump, when performed;*<br><br>▲95991        ~~requiring physician's skill~~ <u>requiring skill</u> of <u>a physician or other qualified health care professional</u><br><br>(Do not report 95990-95991 in conjunction with 62367-62370. For analysis and/or reprogramming of implantable infusion pump, see 62367-62370)<br><br>(For refill and maintenance of implanted infusion pump or reservoir for systemic drug therapy [eg, chemotherapy], use 96522)<br><br>_____Coding Tip_____<br><br>**Instructions for Use of the CPT Codebook**<br><u>When advanced practice nurses and physician assistants are working with physicians, they are considered as working in the exact same specialty and exact same subspecialties as the physician. A "physician or other qualified health care professional" is an individual who is qualified by education, training, licensure/regulation (when applicable), and facility privileging (when applicable) who performs a professional service within his or her scope of practice and independently reports that professional service. These professionals are distinct from "clinical staff." A clinical staff member is a person who works under the supervision of a physician or other qualified health care professional, and who is allowed by law, regulation and facility policy to perform or assist in the performance of a specific professional service, but does not individually report that professional service. Other policies may also affect who may report specific services.</u><br><br>*CPT Coding Guidelines, Introduction, Instructions for Use of the CPT Codebook* |
| **Medicine**<br>**Motion Analysis** | ▲96004     ~~Physician r~~<u>R</u>eview and interpretation by physician <u>or other qualified health care professional</u> of comprehensive computer-based motion analysis,....... |
| **Medicine**<br>**Functional Brain Mapping** | ▲96020     Neurofunctional testing selection ....by a physician or <u>other qualified health care professional (ie, psychologist)</u>, with review of test results and report |
| **Medicine**<br>**Medical Genetics and Genetic**<br>**Counseling Services** | *These services are provided by trained genetic counselors and may include obtaining a structured family genetic history, pedigree construction, analysis for genetic risk assessment, and counseling of the patient and family. These activities may be provided during one or more sessions and may include review of medical data and family information, face-to-face interviews, and counseling services.*<br><br>*96040*     *Medical genetics and genetic counseling services, each 30 minutes face-to-face with patient/family*<br><br>(For genetic counseling and education provided ~~by a physician~~ to an individual~~,~~ <u>by a physician or other qualified health care professional who may report evaluation and management services,</u> see the appropriate Evaluation and Management codes)<br><br>(For genetic counseling and education ~~provided by a physician~~ to a group~~,~~ <u>by a physician or other qualified health care professional,</u> use 99078)<br><br>(For education regarding genetic risks by a nonphysician to a group, see 98961, 98962)<br><br>(For genetic counseling and/or risk factor reduction intervention provided ~~by a physician~~ to patient(s) without symptoms or established disease, <u>by a physician or other qualified health care professional who may report evaluation and management services,</u> see 99401-99412. |
| **Medicine**<br>**Health and Behavior**<br>**Assessment/Intervention** | (For health and behavior assessment and/or intervention performed by a physician <u>or other qualified health care professional who may report evaluation and management services,</u> see evaluation and management or preventive medicine services codes)<br><br>*96150*     *Health and behavior assessment (eg, health-focused clinical interview, behavioral observations, psychophysiological monitoring, health-oriented questionnaires), each 15 minutes face-to-face with the patient; initial assessment* |

| CPT Code/Section/Subsection | Revision/Addition/Deletion |
|---|---|
| **Medicine**<br>**Hydration, Therapeutic, Prophylactic, Diagnostic Injections and Infusions, and Chemotherapy and Other Highly Complex Drug or Highly Complex Biologic Agent Administration** | Physician <u>or other qualified health care professional</u> work related to hydration, injection, and infusion services predominantly involves affirmation of treatment plan and direct supervision of staff.<br><br>*Codes 96360-96379, 96401, 96402, 96409-96425...*<br><br>*If performed to facilitate the infusion or injection, the following...*<br><br>*When multiple drugs are administered, report the service(s)...*<br><br>*When administering multiple infusions, injections or combinations...*<br><br>**Initial infusion:** For physician <u>or other qualified health care professional</u> reporting, an initial infusion is the *key or primary reason for the encounter* reported irrespective of the temporal order in which the infusion(s) or injection(s) are administered. For facility reporting, an initial infusion is based using the hierarchy. For both physician <u>or other qualified health care professional</u> and facility reporting, only one *initial* service code (eg, 96365) should be reported unless the protocol or patient condition requires that two separate IV sites must be utilized. The difference in time and effort in providing this second IV site access is also reported using the *initial* service code with modifier 59 appended (eg, 96365, 96365-59).<br><br>**Sequential infusion:** *A sequential infusion is an infusion ...*<br><br>**Concurrent infusion:** *A concurrent infusion is an ...*<br><br>In order to determine which service should be reported as the initial service when there is more than one type of service, hierarchies have been created. These vary by whether the physician or o<u>ther qualified health care professional</u> or a facility is reporting. The order of selection for <u>reporting</u> ~~physicians~~ is based upon the physician<u>'s or other qualified health care professional's</u> knowledge of the clinical condition(s) and treatment(s). The hierarchy that facilities are to use is based upon a structural algorithm. When these codes are reported by the physician <u>or other qualified health care professional</u>, the "initial" code that best describes the key or primary reason for the encounter should always be reported irrespective of the order in which the infusions or injections occur.<br><br>*When these codes are reported by the facility, the following...*<br><br>*When reporting multiple infusions of the same drug/ substance ...* |
| **Medicine**<br>**Hydration, Therapeutic, Prophylactic, Diagnostic Injections and Infusions, and Chemotherapy and Other Highly Complex Drug or Highly Complex Biologic Agent Administration**<br>**Hydration** | Codes 96360-96361 are intended to report a hydration IV infusion to consist of a pre-packaged fluid and electrolytes (eg, normal saline, D5-1/2 normal saline+30mEq KCl/liter), but are not used to report infusion of drugs or other substances. Hydration IV infusions typically require direct ~~physician~~ supervision for purposes of consent, safety oversight, or intraservice supervision of staff. Typically such infusions require little special handling to prepare or dispose of, and staff that administer these do not typically require advanced practice training. After initial set-up, infusion typically entails little patient risk and thus little monitoring. These codes are not intended to be reported by the physician <u>or other qualified health care professional</u> in the facility setting.<br><br>*Some chemotherapeutic agents and other therapeutic agents require pre- and/or post-hydration....*<br><br>*96360    Intravenous infusion, hydration; initial, 31 minutes to 1 hour* |

| CPT Code/Section/Subsection | Revision/Addition/Deletion |
|---|---|
| **Medicine**<br>**Hydration, Therapeutic,**<br>**Prophylactic, Diagnostic**<br>**Injections and Infusions, and**<br>**Chemotherapy and Other**<br>**Highly Complex Drug or Highly**<br>**Complex Biologic Agent**<br>**Administration**<br><br>**Therapeutic, Prophylactic,**<br>**and Diagnostic Injections**<br>**and Infusions (Excludes**<br>**Chemotherapy and Other**<br>**Highly Complex Drug or Highly**<br>**Complex Biologic Agent**<br>**Administration)** | A therapeutic, prophylactic, or diagnostic IV infusion or injection (other than hydration) is for the administration of substances/drugs. When fluids are used to administer the drug(s), the administration of the fluid is considered incidental hydration and is not separately report-able. These services typically require direct ~~physician~~ supervision for any or all purposes of patient assessment, provision of consent, safety oversight, and intra-service supervision of staff. Typically, such infusions require special consideration to prepare, dose or dispose of, require practice training and competency for staff who administer the infusions, and require periodic patient assessment with vital sign monitoring during the infusion. These codes are not intended to be reported by the physician <u>or other qualified health care professional</u> in the facility setting.<br><br>See codes 96401-96549 for the administration of chemotherapy or other highly complex drug or highly complex biologic agent services. These highly complex services require advanced practice training and competency for staff who provide these services; special considerations for preparation, dosage or disposal; and commonly, these services entail significant patient risk and frequent monitoring. Examples are frequent changes in the infusion rate, prolonged presence of nurse administering the solution for patient monitoring and infusion adjustments, and frequent conferring with the physician <u>or other qualified health care professional</u> about `these issues.<br><br>96365   *Intravenous infusion, for therapy, prophylaxis, or diagnosis (specify substance or drug); initial, up to 1 hour*<br><br>✚96366   *each additional hour (List separately in addition to code for primary procedure)*<br><br>96372   *Therapeutic, prophylactic, or diagnostic injection (specify substance or drug); subcutaneous or intramuscular*<br><br>*(For administration of vaccines/toxoids, see 96365, 96366, 90471, 90472)*<br><br>*(Report 96372 for non-antineoplastic hormonal therapy injections)*<br><br>*(Report 96401 for anti-neoplastic nonhormonal injection therapy)*<br><br>*(Report 96402 for anti-neoplastic hormonal injection therapy)*<br><br>(~~Physicians d~~<u>D</u>o not report 96372 for injections given without direct physician <u>or other quali-fied health care professional</u> supervision. To report, use 99211. Hospitals may report 96372 when the physician <u>or other qualified health care professional</u> is not present) |

| CPT Code/Section/Subsection | Revision/Addition/Deletion |
|---|---|
| **Medicine**<br>**Hydration, Therapeutic, Prophylactic, Diagnostic Injections and Infusions, and Chemotherapy and Other Highly Complex Drug or Highly Complex Biologic Agent Administration**<br><br>**Chemotherapy and Other Highly Complex Drug or Highly Complex Biologic Agent Administration** | Chemotherapy administration codes 96401-96549 apply to parenteral administration of non-radionuclide anti-neoplastic drugs; and also to anti-neoplastic agents provided for treatment of noncancer diagnoses (eg, cyclophosphamide for auto-immune conditions) or to substances such as certain monoclonal antibody agents, and other biologic response modifiers. The highly complex infusion of chemotherapy or other drug or biologic agents requires physician <u>or other qualified health care professional</u> work and/or clinical staff monitoring well beyond that of therapeutic drug agents (96360-96379) because the incidence of severe adverse patient reactions are typically greater. These services can be provided by any physician <u>or other qualified health care professional</u>. Chemotherapy services are typically highly complex and require direct ~~physician~~ supervision for any or all purposes of patient assessment, provision of consent, safety oversight, and intraservice supervision of staff. Typically, such chemotherapy services require advanced practice training and competency for staff who provide these services; special considerations for preparation, dosage, or disposal; and commonly, these services entail significant patient risk and frequent monitoring. Examples are frequent changes in the infusion rate, prolonged presence of the nurse administering the solution for patient monitoring and infusion adjustments, and frequent conferring with the physician <u>or other qualified health care professional</u> about these issues. When performed to facilitate the infusion of injection, preparation of chemotherapy agent(s), highly complex agent(s), or other highly complex drugs is included and is not reported separately. To report infusions that do not require this level of complexity, see 96360-96379. Codes 96401-96402, 96409-96425, 96521-96523 are not intended to be reported by the <u>individual</u> physician <u>or other qualified health care professional</u> in the facility setting.<br><br>*The term "chemotherapy" in 96401-96549 includes other highly...*<br><br>*Report separate codes for each parenteral method...*<br><br>*Report both the specific service as well as code(s)...*<br><br>*Regional (isolation) chemotherapy perfusion should...*<br><br>**Other Injection and Infusion Services**<br><br>Code 96523 does not require direct ~~physician~~ supervision. Codes 96521-96523 may be reported when these devices are used for therapeutic drugs other than chemotherapy.<br><br>96440   *Chemotherapy administration into pleural cavity, requiring and including thoracentesis* |
| **Medicine**<br>**Physical Medicine and Rehabilitation** | The work of the <u>physician or other</u> qualified health care professional consists of face-to-face time with the patient (and caregiver, if applicable)... |
| **Medicine**<br>**Physical Medicine and Rehabilitation**<br>**Supervised** | The application of a modality that does not require direct (one-on-one) patient contact ~~by the provider~~.<br><br>97010   *Application of a modality to 1 or more areas; hot or cold packs* |
| **Medicine**<br>**Physical Medicine and Rehabilitation**<br>**Constant Attendance** | The application of a modality that requires direct (one-on-one) patient contact ~~by the provider~~.<br><br>97032   *Application of a modality to 1 or more areas; electrical stimulation (manual), each 15 minutes* |

| CPT Code/Section/Subsection | Revision/Addition/Deletion |
|---|---|
| **Medicine**<br>**Physical Medicine and Rehabilitation**<br>**Therapeutic Procedures** | *A manner of effecting change through the application of …*<br>Physician or other qualified health care professional (ie, therapist) required to have direct (one-on-one) patient contact.<br><br>97150   *Therapeutic procedure(s), group (2 or more individuals)*<br><br>(Report 97150 for each member of group)<br><br>(Group therapy procedures involve constant attendance of the physician or other qualified health care professional (ie, therapist), but by definition do not require one-on-one patient contact by the same physician or other qualified health care professional therapist)<br><br>▲97530   Therapeutic activities, direct (one-on-one) patient contact by the provider ……<br><br>▲97532   Development of cognitive skills …… contact by the provider, each 15 minutes<br><br>▲97533   Sensory integrative techniques …..direct (one-on-one) patient contact by the provider, each 15 minutes<br><br>▲97535   Self-care/home management training ….direct one-on-one contact by provider, each 15 minutes<br><br>▲97537   Community/work reintegration training (eg, shopping, transportation, money management, ….., direct one-on-one contact by provider, each 15 minutes |
| **Medicine**<br>**Physical Medicine and Rehabilitation**<br>**Active Wound Care Management** | Active wound care procedures are performed to remove devitalized and/or necrotic tissue and promote healing. Services Provider is required to have direct (one-on-one) patient contact with the patient. |
| **Medicine**<br>**Physical Medicine and Rehabilitation**<br>**Tests and Measurements** | ▲97755   Assistive technology assessment… one-on-one contact by provider, with written report, each 15 minutes |
| **Medicine**<br>**Medical Nutrition Therapy** | 97802   *Medical nutrition therapy; initial assessment and intervention, individual, face-to-face with the patient, each 15 minutes*<br><br>97803   *re-assessment and intervention, individual, face-to-face with the patient, each 15 minutes*<br><br>97804   *group (2 or more individual(s)), each 30 minutes*<br><br>(For medical nutrition therapy assessment and/or intervention performed by a physician, see<br><br>**Evaluation and Management** or **Preventive Medicine** service codes)<br><br>(Physicians and other qualified health care professionals who may report evaluation and management services should use the appropriate Evaluation and Management codes) |

| CPT Code/Section/Subsection | Revision/Addition/Deletion |
|---|---|
| **Medicine**<br>**Acupuncture** | *Acupuncture is reported based on 15-minute …*<br><br>*If no electrical stimulation is used during …*<br><br>*Only one code may be reported for …*<br><br>Evaluation and Management services may be reported in addition to acupuncture procedures when performed by physicians or other health care professionals who may report evaluation and management services Evaluation and Management Service codes including new or established patient office or other outpatient services (99201-99215), hospital observation care (99217-99220, 99224-99226), hospital care (99221-99223, 99231-99233), office or other outpatient consultations (99241-99245), inpatient consultations (99251-99255), critical care services (99291, 99292), inpatient neonatal intensive care services and pediatric and neonatal critical care services (99466-99480), emergency department services (99281-99285), nursing facility services (99304-99318), domiciliary, rest home, or custodial care services (99324-99337), and home services (99341-99350), may be reported separately, using modifier 25, if the patient's condition requires a significant, separately identifiable E/M service, above and beyond the usual preservice and postservice work associated with the acupuncture services. The time of the E/M service is not included in the time of the acupuncture service. |
| **Medicine**<br>**Osteopathic Manipulative Treatment** | Osteopathic manipulative treatment (OMT) is a form of manual treatment applied by a physician or other qualified health care professional to eliminate or alleviate somatic dysfunction and related disorders. This treatment may be accomplished by a variety of techniques |
| **Medicine**<br>**Education and Training for Patient Self-Management** | The following codes are used to report educational and training services prescribed by a physician or other qualified health care professional and provided by a qualified, nonphysician health care professional using a standardized curriculum to an individual or a group of patients…<br><br>…(For counseling and education provided by a physician to an individual, see the appropriate evaluation and management codes… (See also **Instructions for Use of the CPT Codebook** for definition of reporting qualifications). |
| **Medicine**<br>**Special Services, Procedures and Reports** | Code 99091 should be reported no more than once in a 30-day period to include the physician or other qualified health care professional care provider time involved with data accession, review and interpretation, modification of care plan as necessary (including communication to patient and/or caregiver), and associated documentation. |
| **Medicine**<br>**Miscellaneous Services** | ▲99000 Handling and/or conveyance of specimen for transfer from the physician's office to a laboratory<br><br>▲99001 Handling and/or conveyance of specimen for transfer from the patient in other than an physician's office to a laboratory (distance may be indicated)<br><br>▲99002 Handling, conveyance, …by the attending physician or other qualified health care professional<br><br>(For physician standby services requiring prolonged physician attendance, use 99360, as appropriate. Time spent performing separately reportable procedure(s) or service(s) should not be included in the time reported as mandated on-call service)<br><br>▲99070 Supplies and materials (except spectacles), provided by the physician or other qualified health care professional over and above ……<br><br>▲99071 Educational supplies, such as books, tapes, and pamphlets, provided by the physician for the patient's education at cost to physician or other qualified health care professional<br><br>▲99078 Physician or other qualified health care professional qualified by education, training, licensure/regulation (when applicable) educational services rendered to patients in a group setting (eg, prenatal, obesity, or diabetic instructions)<br>(For physician/or other qualified health care care professional qualified by education, training, licensure/regulation [when applicable] collection and interpretation of physiologic data stored/transmitted by patient/caregiver, see 99091)<br><br>▲99091 Collection and interpretation of physiologic data ……to the physician or other qualified health care care professional, qualified by education, training, licensure/regulation (when applicable) requiring a minimum of 30 minutes of time |

| CPT Code/Section/Subsection | Revision/Addition/Deletion |
|---|---|
| **Medicine**<br>**Moderate (Conscious) Sedation** | When a second physician <u>or other qualified health care professional</u> other than the health care professional performing the diagnostic or therapeutic services provides moderate sedation...... the second physician <u>or other qualified health care professional</u> reports 99148-99150. However, for the circumstance in which these services are performed by the second physician <u>or other qualified health care professional</u> in the nonfacility setting (eg, ~~physician~~ office, freestanding imaging center), codes 99148-99150 are not reported. <u>See also</u> **Instructions for Use of the CPT Codebook** <u>for definition of reporting qualifications.</u> |
|  | ▲99143    Moderate sedation services (other than those services described by codes 00100-01999) provided by the same physician <u>or other qualified health care professional</u> performing the diagnostic or therapeutic service... |
|  | ▲99148    Moderate sedation services (other than those services described by codes 00100-01999), provided by a physician <u>or other qualified health care professional</u> other than the health care professional... |
| **Medicine**<br>**Other Services and Procedures** | ▲99183    Physician <u>or other qualified health care professional</u> attendance and supervision of hyperbaric oxygen therapy, per session |
| **Category II Codes**<br>**Follow-up or Other Outcomes** | 1005F    Asthma symptoms evaluated (includes ~~physician~~ documentation of numeric... |
|  | 2060F    Patient interviewed directly ~~by evaluating clinician~~ on or before date of diagnosis... |
|  | 4240F    Instruction in therapeutic exercise with follow-up ~~by the physician~~ provided to patients... |
|  | 5010F    Findings of dilated macular or fundus exam communicated to the physician <u>or other qualified health care professional</u> managing the diabetes care (EC)[5] |
|  | 5020F    Treatment summary report communicated to physician(s) <u>or other qualified health care professional(s)</u> managing continuing .... |
|  | 5100F    Potential risk for fracture communicated to the referring physician <u>or other qualified health care professional</u> within 24 hours of completion of the imaging study (NUC_MED)[1] |
| **Category III** | *The following section contains a set of temporary codes for emerging technology...* |
|  | *The inclusion of a service or procedure in this...* |
|  | New <u>or revised codes</u> ~~in this section~~ are released semi-annually via the AMA/CPT internet site, to expedite dissemination for reporting....... |

| CPT Code/Section/Subsection | Revision/Addition/Deletion |
|---|---|
| **Category III**<br>**Remote Real-Time Interactive**<br>**Videoconferenced Critical Care**<br>**Services** | Remote real-time interactive video-conferenced critical care is the direct delivery by a physician(s) or other qualified health care professional(s) of medical care…<br><br>In order to report remote real-time interactive video-conferenced critical care, the physician(s) or other qualified health care professional(s) in the remote location…The remote physician or other qualified health care professional must have real-time capability…<br><br>The review and interpretation…<br><br>The remote real-time interactive video-conferenced critical care codes 0188T and 0189T…. time spent by the individual a physician providing remote real-time interactive video-conferenced critical care services to a critically ill or critically injured patient, even if the time spent by the individual physician on that date is not continuous. For any given period of time spent providing remote real-time interactive video-conferenced critical care services, the physician or other qualified health care professional must devote his or her full attention to the patient…..<br><br>*Time spent with the individual…*<br><br>Time spent in activities that occur away from the bedside when the individual physician does not have the real-time capabilities described above may not be reported as remote real-time interactive video-conferenced critical care because the individual physician is not immediately available to the patient…… Only one physician or other qualified health care professional may report either critical care services (99291, 99292)….. Do not report remote real-time interactive video-conferenced critical care if another individual physician reports pediatric or neonatal critical care or intensive care services (99468-99476)……<br><br>Code 0188T is used to report the first 30 to 74 minutes of remote real-time interactive video-conferenced, critical care on a given date. It should be used only once per date even if the time spent by the physician or other qualified health care professional is not continuous on that date…<br><br>*Code 0189T is used to report the first…* |

| CPT Code/Section/Subsection | Revision/Addition/Deletion |
|---|---|

<table>
<tr><td>Appendix A</td><td>24</td><td>Unrelated Evaluation and Management Service by the Same Physician or Other Qualified Health care Professional During a Postoperative Period: The physician or other qualified health care professional may need to indicate…</td></tr>
<tr><td></td><td>25</td><td>Significant, Separately Identifiable Evaluation and Management Service by the Same Physician or Other Qualified Health care Professional on the Same Day of the Procedure or Other Service: It may be necessary…</td></tr>
<tr><td></td><td>26</td><td>Professional Component: Certain procedures are a combination of a physician or other qualified health care professional component and a technical component. When the physician or other qualified health care professional component is reported separately, the service may be identified by adding modifier 26 to the usual procedure number.</td></tr>
<tr><td></td><td>51</td><td>Multiple Procedures: When multiple procedures, other than E/M services, Physical Medicine and Rehabilitation services or provision of supplies (eg, vaccines), are performed at the same session by the same individual provider, the primary procedure or service may be reported as listed…</td></tr>
<tr><td></td><td>52</td><td>Reduced Services: Under certain circumstances a service or procedure is partially reduced or eliminated at the physician's discretion of the physician or other qualified health care professional…</td></tr>
<tr><td></td><td>53</td><td>Discontinued Procedure: Under certain circumstances, the physician or other qualified health care professional may elect to terminate a surgical or diagnostic procedure…</td></tr>
<tr><td></td><td>54</td><td>Surgical Care Only: When 1 physician or other qualified health care professional performs a surgical procedure and another provides preoperative and/or postoperative management, surgical services may be identified by adding modifier 54 to the usual procedure number.</td></tr>
<tr><td></td><td>55</td><td>Postoperative Management Only: When 1 physician or other qualified health care professional performed the postoperative management and another physician performed the surgical procedure…</td></tr>
<tr><td></td><td>56</td><td>Preoperative Management Only: When 1 physician or other qualified health care professional performed the preoperative care and evaluation and another physician performed the surgical procedure…</td></tr>
<tr><td></td><td>58</td><td>Staged or Related Procedure or Service by the Same Physician or Other Qualified Health Care Professional During the Postoperative Period:…</td></tr>
<tr><td></td><td>63</td><td>Procedure Performed on Infants less than 4 kg: Procedures performed on neonates and infants up to a present body weight of 4 kg may involve significantly increased complexity and individual physician or other qualified health care professional work commonly associated with these patients…</td></tr>
<tr><td></td><td>66</td><td>Surgical Team: Under some circumstances, highly complex procedures (requiring the concomitant services of several physicians or other qualified health care professionals, often of different specialties,… identified by each participating individual physician with the addition of modifier 66 to the basic procedure number used for reporting services.</td></tr>
<tr><td></td><td>79</td><td>Unrelated Procedure or Service by the Same Physician or other Qualified Health care Professional During the Postoperative Period: The individual physician may need to indicate that the performance of a procedure or service…</td></tr>
<tr><td></td><td>90</td><td>Reference (Outside) Laboratory: When laboratory procedures are performed by a party other than the treating or reporting physician or other qualified health care professional, the procedure may be identified by adding modifier 90 to the usual procedure number.</td></tr>
<tr><td>Appendix B<br>Summary of Additions,<br>Deletions, and Revisions</td><td colspan="2">Appendix B shows the actual changes that were made to the code descriptors. New codes appear with a bullet (•) and are indicated as "Code Added."…Codes with which conscious moderate sedation would not be separately reported when performed at the same session by the same individual provider are denoted with the bullseye (⊙)……</td></tr>
</table>

| CPT Code/Section/Subsection | Revision/Addition/Deletion |
|---|---|
| **Appendix C** | As described in *CPT 2013*, clinical examples of the CPT codes for Evaluation and Management (E/M) services… provide a comprehensive and powerful tool for individuals ~~physicians~~ to report the services provided to their patients…<br><br>*The American Medical Association is pleased to provide…*<br><br>*These clinical examples do not encompass…*<br><br>Of utmost importance is that these clinical examples are just that: examples. A particular patient encounter, depending on the specific circumstances, must be judged by the services provided by the physician or other qualified health care professional for that particular patient… |
| **Appendix G**<br>**Summary of CPT Codes That Include Moderate (Conscious) Sedation** | Since these services include moderate sedation, it is not appropriate for the same physician or other qualified health care professional to report both the service and the sedation codes 99143-99145. It is expected that if conscious sedation is provided to the patient as part of one of these services, it is provided by the same physician or other qualified health care professional who is providing the service.<br><br>In the unusual event when a second physician or other qualified health care professional other than the health care professional…… the second individual ~~physician~~ can report 99148-99150. However, for the circumstance in which these services are performed by the second individual ~~physician~~ in the nonfacility setting (eg, ~~physician~~ office, freestanding imaging center), codes 99148-99150 would not be reported……<br><br>The inclusion of a procedure on this list does not prevent separate reporting of an associated anesthesia procedure/service (CPT codes 00100-01999) when performed by a physician or other qualified health care professional other than the health care ~~care~~ professional performing the diagnostic or therapeutic procedure……. the operating physician or other qualified health care professional is not required to report the procedure as a reduced service using modifier 52. |

# Explicit Code Ranges

The recent style for CPT guidelines has moved to greater specificity and transparency. The addition of specific code ranges provides uniform instruction related to each code in the range/series. The format of listing explicit code ranges currently exists in the CPT code set and has been expanded for 2013. The addition of explicit code range listings to many CPT guidelines provides reporting transparency for physician, or other qualified health care professional, administrative staff, and payer claims submission and processing. Commonly, when including code ranges in guidelines, a brief description of the code range is provided to eliminate the need for constant cross-referencing. The format lists the title of a family or series of codes and the corresponding code number(s) or range(s).

# Explicit Code Ranges

## Explicit Code Ranges

There is a growing demand from the health information technology (HIT) community for clear and explicit content within electronic health care tools and initiatives, eg, electronic health records, performance measure reporting, and health information exchange. As a Health Insurance Portability and Accountability Act (HIPAA) designated code set, it is essential that CPT reflect health information technology requirements within the development and maintenance process. To illustrate, the listing of typical Evaluation and Management (E/M) service code(s) enhances development of adaptable electronic formats and computerization. Overall, including explicit code ranges in guidelines provides the following:

- Guidance toward the specific codes that are appropriate to report with the listed procedure.

- A level of transparency for users and payers alike.

- The submission of clean claims.

- A decrease in the number of appeals resulting from incorrect claims submissions.

- Support for existing AMA policy, which vigorously opposes the practice of unilateral, arbitrary recoding and/or bundling by all payers. By providing lists of the applicable codes, the CPT code set provides clear guidance on reporting multiple CPT codes.

- Utilization of existing RUC data to support the validity of the site of service.

- Consistency with the most recent guideline style (eg, Cardiac Cath/Infusions, Cardiac Device/Echo) of a service description.

The CPT code set now reflects the addition of further explicit code ranges in those places in the CPT guidelines where previously users were directed only to the title of specific services (eg, "Evaluation and Management," "Office visit codes," etc), without a specific code range. For those locations where explicit listings were lacking, the addition of explicit code ranges has been made to ensure:

- that the explicit code listings provide transparency

- the accurate representation of the services in the appropriate sites of service

- the integral participation by the national medical specialties in this process

- that the medical specialties understand the significance of this effort

- that the affect on payment policy will be the reduction of costs for claims processing for users and payers alike through the transparency and definitions provided

- that inappropriate codes are excluded from reporting, with opportunities provided through engagement of the CPT process to continue addressing those areas in which the code set lacks transparency or clarity.

Because of the number of refinements, reference is made to the code number, section, or subsection language revised. Therefore, the following revisions include abbreviated guidelines and parenthetical instructions. Underlined text indicates new language, while the stricken text indicates deleted language.
(For complete long descriptors, guidelines, and parenthetical information, refer to the *CPT 2013* codebook).

| CPT Code/Section/Subsection | Revision/Addition/Deletion |
|---|---|
| **Evaluation and Management Hospital Observation Services Initial Observation Care New or Established Patient** | *To report services provided to a patient......*Do not report observation discharge (99217) in conjunction with a hospital admission (99221-99223). *When "observation status".......* Evaluation and management services including new or established patient office or other outpatient services including (99201-99215), emergency department services (99281-99285), nursing facility services (99304-99318), domiciliary, rest home, or custodial care services (99324-99337), home services (99341-99350), and preventive medicine services (99381-99429) on the same date provided in sites that are related to the admission to "observation status" should not be reported separately. |
| **Hospital Inpatient Services Initial Hospital Care New or Established Patient** | *When the patient is admitted to the hospital as an inpatient....* Evaluation and management services including new or established patient office or other outpatient services (99201-99215), emergency department services (99281-99285), nursing facility services (99304-99318), domiciliary, rest home, or custodial care services (99324-99337), home services (99341-99350), and preventive medicine services (99381-99397) on the same date provided in sites that are related to the admission to "observation status" should **not** be reported separately. For a patient admitted and discharged from observation or inpatient status on the same date, the services should be reported with codes 99234-99236 as appropriate. |
| **Inpatient Consultations New or Established Patient** | *When an inpatient consultation is performed on a date that a patient is admitted....* Do not report both an outpatient consultation (99241-99245) and inpatient consultation (99251-99255) for services related to the same inpatient stay. |
| **Prolonged Services Prolonged Service Without Direct Patient Contact** | *Codes 99358 and 99359 are used when a prolonged service is provided that is neither face-to face time in the office or outpatient setting....* *This service is to be reported in relation to other physician or other qualified health care professional services, including evaluation and management services at any level...* *Codes 99358 and 99359 are used to report the total duration of non-face-to-face time spent by a physician or other qualified health care professional on a given date....* *Prolonged service of less than 30 minutes total duration on a given date is not separately reported.* *Code 99359 is used to report each additional 30 minutes beyond the first hour regardless of the place of service....* *Prolonged service of less than 15 minutes beyond the first hour or less than 15 minutes beyond the final 30 minutes is not reported separately.* |

⊘=Modifier 51 Exempt  ⊙=Moderate Sedation  ✚=Add-on Code  ⁄=FDA approval pending

| CPT Code/Section/Subsection | Revision/Addition/Deletion |
|---|---|
| **Prolonged Services**<br>**Prolonged Service Without**<br>**Direct Patient Contact**<br>*(Continued)* | Do not report 99358, 99359 for time spent in care plan oversight services (99339, 99340, 99374-99380), anticoagulant management (99363, 99364), medical team conferences (99366-99368), on-line medical evaluations (99444), or other non-face-to-face services that have more specific codes and no upper time limit in the CPT code set. Codes 99358, 99359 may be reported when related to other non-face-to-face services codes that have a published maximum time (eg, telephone services). |
| **Preventive Medicine Services**<br>**Counseling Risk Factor**<br>**Reduction and Behavior Change**<br>**Intervention** | *Behavior change interventions are for persons who have a behavior that is often considered an illness itself,....*<br><br>Health and Behavior Assessment/Intervention services (96150-96155) should not be reported on the same day as codes 99401-99412. |
| **Surgery**<br>**Maternity Care and Delivery** | *The services normally provided in uncomplicated maternity cases include…*<br><br>*Antepartum care includes the initial and subsequent history, physical examinations, recording of weight, blood pressures, fetal heart tones…,*<br><br>*Postpartum care only services (59430) include office or other outpatient visits following vaginal or cesarean section delivery.*<br><br>Delivery services include admission to the hospital, the admission history and physical examination, management of uncomplicated labor, vaginal delivery (with or without episiotomy, with or without forceps), or cesarean delivery. When reporting delivery only services (59409, 59514, 59612, 59620), report inpatient postdelivery management and discharge services using Evaluation and Management Services codes (99217-99239). Delivery and postpartum services (59410, 59515, 59614, 59622) include delivery services and all inpatient and outpatient postpartum services. Medical complications of pregnancy (eg, cardiac problems, neurological problems, diabetes, hypertension, toxemia, hyperemesis, preterm labor, premature rupture of membranes, trauma) and Mmedical problems complicating labor and delivery management may require additional resources and may be reported separately. and should be identified by utilizing the codes in the **Medicine** and **Evaluation and Management Services** in addition to codes for maternity care.<br><br>For medical complications of pregnancy (eg, cardiac problems, neurological problems, diabetes, hypertension, toxemia, hyperemesis, pre-term labor, premature rupture of membranes), see services in the **Medicine** and **Evaluation and Management Services** section.<br><br>*For surgical complications of pregnancy (eg, appendectomy, hernia, ovarian cyst, Bartholin cyst), see services in the* **Surgery** *section.* |
| **Medicine**<br>**Immunization Administration**<br>**for Vaccines/Toxoids** | *Report vaccine immunization administration codes 90460, 90461, 90471-90474 in addition to the vaccine and toxoid code(s) 90476-90749.*<br><br>*Report codes 90460 and 90461 only when the physician or qualified health care professional provides……*<br><br>If a significant separately identifiable Evaluation and Management service (eg, new or established patient office or other outpatient services [99201-99215], office or other outpatient consultations [99241-99245], emergency department services [99281-99285], preventive medicine services [99381-99429]) is performed, the appropriate E/M service code should be reported in addition to the vaccine and toxoid administration codes. |
| **Medicine**<br>**Dialysis**<br>**Hemodialysis** | Codes 90935, 90937 are reported to describe the hemodialysis procedure with all evaluation and management services related to the patient's renal disease on the day of the hemodialysis procedure. These codes are used for inpatient ESRD and non-ESRD procedures or for outpatient non-ESRD dialysis services. Code 90935 is reported if only one evaluation of the patient is required related to that hemodialysis procedure. Code 90937 is reported when patient re-evaluation(s) is required during a hemodialysis procedure. Use modifier 25 with evaluation and management codes, including new or established patient office or other outpatient services (99201-99215), office or other outpatient consultations (99241-99245), observation care (99217-99220, 99224-99226), observation or inpatient care including admission and discharge (99234-99236), initial hospital care (99221-99226, 99231-99239), new or established patient emergency department services (99281-99285), critical care services (99291, 99292), inpatient neonatal intensive care services and pediatric and neonatal critical care services (99466-99480), nursing facility services (99304-99318), domiciliary, rest home services, or custodial care (99324-99337), and home services (99341-99350), for separately identifiable services unrelated to the dialysis procedure or renal failure which cannot be rendered during the dialysis session. |

| CPT Code/Section/Subsection | Revision/Addition/Deletion |
|---|---|
| **Medicine Dialysis** <br> **Miscellaneous Dialysis** <br> **Procedures** | Codes 90945, 90947 describe dialysis procedures other than hemodialysis (eg, peritoneal dialysis, hemofiltration or continuous renal replacement therapies), and all evaluation and management services related to the patient's renal disease on the day of the procedure. Code 90945 is reported if only one evaluation of the patient is required related to that procedure. Code 90947 is reported when patient re-evaluation(s) is required during a procedure. Use modifier 25 with evaluation and management codes, including <u>office or other outpatient services (99201-99215), office or other outpatient consultations (99241-99245), observation care (99217-99220, 99224-99226), observation or inpatient care including admission and discharge (99234-99239), hospital care (99221-99226, 99231- 99239), new or established patient emergency department services (99281-99285), critical care services (99291, 99292), inpatient neonatal intensive care services and pediatric and neonatal critical care services (99466-99480), nursing facility services (99304-99318), domiciliary, rest home, or custodial care services (99324-99337), and home services (99341-99350)</u> for separately identifiable services unrelated to the procedure or the renal failure which cannot be rendered during the dialysis session. |
| **Medicine Special** <br> **Otorhinolaryngologic Services** | *Diagnostic or treatment procedures that are reported....* <br><br> Special otorhinolaryngologic services are those diagnostic and treatment services not included in an <u>evaluation and management</u> service <u>including office or other outpatient services (99201-99215), or office or other outpatient consultations (99241-99245)</u> . ~~These services are reported separately, using codes 92502-92526, 92533-92700.~~ 92502-92700. <br><br> *Code 92506 is used to report evaluation of speech production, receptive language, and expressive language abilities.....* |
| **Medicine Special** <br> **Otorhinolaryngologic Services** <br> **Vestibular Function Tests,** <br> **Without Electrical Recording** | *92532 Positional nystagmus test* <br><br> (Do not report <u>92531</u>, <u>92532</u> with evaluation and management services <u>including office or other outpatient services [99201-99215], observation care [99218-99220, 99224-99226], observation or inpatient care including admission and discharge [99234-99236], hospital care [99221-99223, 99231-99233], office or other outpatient consultations [99241-99245], nursing facility services [99304-99318], and domiciliary, rest home, or custodial care services [99324-99337]</u>). |
| **Medicine** <br> **Cardiovascular** <br> **Peripheral Arterial Disease** <br> **Rehabilitation** | *Peripheral arterial disease (PAD) rehabilitative physical exercise consists of a series of sessions, lasting 45-60 minutes per session, involving use of either a motorized treadmill or a track to permit each patient to achieve symptom-limited claudication. Each session is supervised by an exercise physiologist or nurse. The supervising provider monitors the individual patient's claudication threshold and other cardiovascular limitations for adjustment of workload.* <br><br> During this supervised rehabilitation program, the development of new arrhythmias, symptoms that might suggest angina or the continued inability of the patient to progress to an adequate level of exercise may require ~~physician~~ review and examination of the patient <u>by a physician or other qualified health care professional</u>. These ~~physician~~ services would be separately reported with an appropriate level E/M service code <u>including office or other outpatient services (99201-99215), initial hospital care (99221-99223), subsequent hospital care (99231-99233), critical care services (99291-99292)</u>. |

⊘=Modifier 51 Exempt   ⊙=Moderate Sedation   ✛=Add-on Code   ⩜=FDA approval pending

| CPT Code/Section/Subsection | Revision/Addition/Deletion |
|---|---|
| **Medicine**<br>**Pulmonary**<br>**Pulmonary Diagnostic**<br>**Testing and Therapies** | Codes 94010-94799 include laboratory procedure(s)and interpretation of test results. If a separate identifiable evaluation and management service is performed, the appropriate E/M service code including <u>new or established patient office or other outpatient services (99201-99215), office or other outpatient consultations (99241-99245), emergency department services (99281-99285), nursing facility services (99304-99318), domiciliary, rest home, or custodial care services (99324-99337), and home services (99341-99350), may</u> be reported in addition to 94010-94799. |
| **Medicine**<br>**Allergy and Clinical**<br>**Immunology** | **Definitions**<br><br>***Immunotherapy (desensitization, hyposensitization)*** *is the parenteral administration of allergenic....*<br><br>**Other therapy:** for medical conferences on the use of mechanical and electronic devices (precipitators, air conditioners, air filters, humidifiers, dehumidifiers), climatotherapy, physical therapy, occupational and recreational therapy, see **Evaluation and Management** <u>services</u> ~~section~~<br><br>Do not report Evaluation and Management (E/M) services for test interpretation and report. If a significant separately identifiable E/M service is performed, the appropriate E/M service code, <u>which may include new or established patient office or other outpatient services (99201-99215), hospital observation services (99217-99220, 99224-99226), hospital care (99221-99223, 99231-99233), consultations (99241-99255),  emergency department services (99281-99285), nursing facility services (99304-99318), domiciliary, rest home, or custodial care services (99324-99337), home services (99341-99350), preventive medicine services (99381-99429)</u> should be reported using modifier 25. |
| **Medicine**<br>**Special Dermatological**<br>**Procedures** | ~~*Dermatologic services are typically consultative, and any of the five levels of consultation (99241-99255) may be appropriate.*~~<br><br><u>See the</u> **Evaluation and Management coding guidelines**<u>, for further instructions on reporting that is appropriate for management of dermatologic illnesses.</u><br><br>~~In addition, services and skills outlined under~~ **Evaluation and Management** ~~levels of service appropriate to dermatologic illnesses should be coded similarly.~~ |
| **Medicine**<br>**Acupuncture** | *Acupuncture is reported based on 15-minute increments of personal....*<br><br>*If no electrical stimulation is used during a 15-minute increment....*<br><br>*Only one code may be reported for each 15-minute increment....*<br><br><u>Evaluation and Management services may be reported in addition to acupuncture procedures when performed by physicians or other health care professionals, who may report evalua-tion and management services,</u> ~~Evaluation and Management Service codes~~ <u>including new or established patient office or other outpatient services (99201-99215), hospital observation care (99217-99220, 99224-99226), hospital care (99221-99223, 99231-99233), office or other outpatient consultations (99241-99245), inpatient consultations (99251-99255), critical care services (99291, 99292), inpatient neonatal intensive care services and pediatric and neonatal critical care services (99466-99480), emergency department services (99281-99285), nursing facility services (99304-99318), domiciliary, rest home, or custodial care services (99324-99337), and home services (99341-99350), may</u> be reported separately, using modifier 25, if the patient's condition requires a significant, separately identifiable E/M service above and beyond the usual preservice and postservice work associated with the acupuncture services. The time of the E/M service is not included in the time of the acupuncture service. |

| CPT Code/Section/Subsection | Revision/Addition/Deletion |
|---|---|
| **Medicine**<br>**Osteopathic**<br>**Manipulative Treatment** | *Osteopathic manipulative treat (OMT) is a form of manual treatment....*<br><br>Evaluation and Management services <u>including new or established patient office or other outpatient services (99201-99215),  hospital observation care (99217-99220, 99224-99226), hospital care (99221-99223, 99231-99233), critical care services (99291, 99292), observation or inpatient care services (99234-99236), office or other outpatient consultations (99241-99245), emergency department services (99281-99285), nursing facility services (99304-99318), domiciliary, rest home, or custodial care services (99324-99337), and home services (99341-99350)</u> may be reported separately using modifier 25 if the patient's condition requires a significant, separately identifiable E/M service above and beyond the usual preservice and postservice work associated with the procedure.  The E/M service may be caused or prompted by the same symptoms or condition for which the OMT service was provided.  As such, different diagnoses are not required for the reporting of the OMT and E/M service on the same date.<br><br>*Body regions referred to are:.......* |
| **Medicine**<br>**Chiropractic**<br>**Manipulative Treatment** | *Chiropractic manipulative treatment (CMT) is a form of manual treatment....*<br><br>The chiropractic manipulative treatment codes include a pre-manipulation patient assessment. Additional evaluation and management services including office or other outpatient services <u>(99201-99215), subsequent observation care (99224-99226), subsequent hospital care (99231-99233), office or other outpatient consultations (99241-99245), subsequent nursing facility services (99307-99310), domiciliary, rest home, or custodial care services (99324-99337), and home services (99341-99350)</u> may be reported separately using modifier 25 if the patient's condition requires a significant, separately identifiable E/M service above and beyond the usual preservice and postservice work associated with the procedure. The E/M service may be caused or prompted by the same symptoms or condition for which the CMT service was provided. As such, different diagnoses are not required for the reporting of the CMT and E/M service on the same date.<br><br>*For purposes of CMT,........* |
| **Medicine**<br>**Education and**<br>**Training for**<br>**Patient Self-Management** | *The following codes are used to report educational and training services....*<br><br>*The purpose of the educational and training services is to teach the patient....*<br><br>*The qualifications of the nonphysician health care..*<br><br>(For counseling and education provided by a physician to an individual, see the appropriate evaluation and management codes including <u>office or other outpatient services [99201-99215], hospital observation care [99217-99220, 99224-99226], hospital care [99221-99223, 99231-99233], new or established patient office or other outpatient consultations [99241-99245], inpatient consultations [99251-99255],emergency department services [99281-99285], nursing facility services [99304-99318], domiciliary, rest home, or custodial care services [99324-99337], home services [99341-99350], and counseling risk factor reduction and behavior change intervention [99401-99429]</u>. See also **Instructions for Use of the CPT Codebook** for definition of reporting qualifications). |

⊘=Modifier 51 Exempt   ⊙=Moderate Sedation   ✚=Add-on Code   𝄢=FDA approval pending

# Evaluation and Management

Numerous changes have been made in the Evaluation and Management Services (E/M) section, some of which include: (1) typical service times added to the observation or inpatient hospital care codes 99234, 99235 and 99236; (2) revised parenthetical notes included in prolonged services that reference psychotherapy codes 90809 and 90815, for consistency with the deletion of these codes; and (3) revisions made to the Inpatient Neonatal and Pediatric Critical Care Services and the Initial and Continuing Intensive Care Service guidelines.

A new coding structure was added in the E/M services section that describes Complex Chronic Care Coordination Services and Transitional Care Management Services. The new structure includes three new codes in the Chronic Care Coordination Services section and two new codes in the Transitional Care Management Services section. Numerous guidelines have been added to these sections to clarify the reporting of these services to define the types of services, professionals, and patients receiving these services. Instructional parenthetical notes were also added throughout the E/M and Medicine subsections to instruct the appropriate reporting of these services in conjunction with other E/M services.

# Evaluation and Management (E/M) Services Guidelines

## Definitions of Commonly Used Terms

### Counseling

Counseling is a discussion with a patient and/or family concerning one or more of the following areas:

- Diagnostic results, impressions, and/or recommended diagnostic studies

- Prognosis

- Risks and benefits of management (treatment) options

- Instructions for management (treatment) and/or follow-up

- Importance of compliance with chosen management (treatment) options

- Risk factor reduction

- Patient and family education

▶(For psychotherapy, see 90832-90834, 90836-90840)◀

### ✐ Rationale

The parenthetical instructional note in the "Counseling" instructions in the Evaluation and Management subsection was revised to remove references to the psychotherapy codes 90809, 90815 for consistency with the deletion of these codes in the CPT 2013 code set.

# Evaluation and Management

## Hospital Inpatient Services

### Subsequent Hospital Care

OBSERVATION OR INPATIENT CARE SERVICES (INCLUDING ADMISSION AND
DISCHARGE SERVICES)

▶The following codes are used to report observation or inpatient hospital care services provided
to patients admitted and discharged on the same date of service. When a patient is admitted to
the hospital from observation status on the same date, only the initial hospital care code should be
reported. The initial hospital care code reported by the admitting physician or other qualified health
care professional should include the services related to the observation status services he/she
provided on the same date of inpatient admission.

When "observation status" is initiated in the course of an encounter in another site of service (eg,
hospital emergency department, office, nursing facility) all evaluation and management services
provided by the supervising physician or other qualified health care professional in conjunction with
initiating "observation status" are considered part of the initial observation care when performed on
the same date. The observation care level of service should include the services related to initiating
"observation status" provided in the other sites of service as well as in the observation setting when
provided by the same individual.◀

▲99234    **Observation or inpatient hospital care,** for the evaluation and management of a patient including
admission and discharge on the same date, which requires these 3 key components:

- **A detailed or comprehensive history;**

- **A detailed or comprehensive examination; and**

- **Medical decision making that is straightforward or of low complexity.**

Counseling and/or coordination of care with other physicians, other qualified health care
professionals, or agencies are provided consistent with the nature of the problem(s) and the patient's
and/or family's needs.

Usually the presenting problem(s) requiring admission are of low severity. Typically, 40 minutes are
spent at the bedside and on the patient's hospital floor or unit.

▲99235    **Observation or inpatient hospital care,** for the evaluation and management of a patient including
admission and discharge on the same date, which requires these 3 key components:

- **A comprehensive history;**

- **A comprehensive examination; and**

- **Medical decision making of moderate complexity.**

Counseling and/or coordination of care with other physicians, other qualified health care
professionals, or agencies are provided consistent with the nature of the problem(s) and the patient's
and/or family's needs.

Usually the presenting problem(s) requiring admission are of moderate severity. Typically, 50 minutes are spent at the bedside and on the patient's hospital floor or unit.

▲99236   **Observation or inpatient hospital care,** for the evaluation and management of a patient including admission and discharge on the same date, which requires these 3 key components:

■ **A comprehensive history;**

■ **A comprehensive examination; and**

■ **Medical decision making of high complexity.**

Counseling and/or coordination of care with other physicians, other qualified health care professionals, or agencies are provided consistent with the nature of the problem(s) and the patient's and/or family's needs.

Usually the presenting problem(s) requiring admission are of high severity. Typically, 55 minutes are spent at the bedside and on the patient's hospital floor or unit.

### ✍ Rationale

Typical service times have been added to the codes for observation or inpatient hospital care services provided to patients admitted and discharged on the same date (99234, 99235, 99236). Data was obtained by the RUC survey for revision of codes 99234-99236 to reflect time according to actual practice patterns. See also discussion on CPT nomenclature reporting neutrality.

## Domiciliary, Rest Home (eg, Assisted Living Facility), or Home Care Plan Oversight Services

99339   Individual physician supervision of a patient (patient not present) in home, domiciliary or rest home (eg, assisted living facility) requiring complex and multidisciplinary care modalities involving regular physician development and/or revision of care plans, review of subsequent reports of patient status, review of related laboratory and other studies, communication (including telephone calls) for purposes of assessment or care decisions with health care professional(s), family member(s), surrogate decision maker(s) (eg, legal guardian) and/or key caregiver(s) involved in patient's care, integration of new information into the medical treatment plan and/or adjustment of medical therapy, within a calendar month; 15-29 minutes

99340          30 minutes or more

(Do not report 99339, 99340 for patients under the care of a home health agency, enrolled in a hospice program, or for nursing facility residents)

▶(Do not report 99339, 99340 during the same month with 99487-99489)◀

▶(Do not report 99339, 99340 when performed during the service time of codes 99495 or 99496)◀

**Rationale**

To support the establishment of new Complex Chronic Care Coordination Services codes 99487-99489 and Transitional Care Management Services codes 99495 and 99496, two exclusionary parenthetical notes were added following Domiciliary, Rest Home (eg, Assisted Living Facility), or Home Care Plan Oversight Services codes 99339 and 99340 to instruct that these services should not be reported in conjunction with the Complex Chronic Care Coordination Services codes 99487-99489 or the Transitional Care Management Services codes 99495 and 99496.

# Prolonged Services

## Prolonged Service With Direct Patient Contact

**+99354** Prolonged service in the office or other outpatient setting requiring direct patient contact beyond the usual service; first hour (List separately in addition to code for office or other outpatient **Evaluation and Management** service)

▶(Use 99354 in conjunction with 99201-99215, 99241-99245, 99324-99337, 99341-99350)◀

### Rationale

The parenthetical instructional note following 99354 has been revised to remove references to the psychotherapy codes 90809, 90815 for consistency with the deletion of these codes in the CPT 2013 code set.

**+99356** Prolonged service in the inpatient or observation setting, requiring unit/floor time beyond the usual service; first hour (List separately in addition to code for inpatient **Evaluation and Management** service)

▶(Use 99356 in conjunction with 99218-99220, 99221-99223, 99224-99226, 99231-99233, 99234-99236, 99251-99255, 99304-99310)◀

### Rationale

The parenthetical listing of applicable codes following code 99356 has been expanded to reflect use of code 99356 in conjunction with the Observation or Inpatient Care Services codes 99224-99226, 99231-99236.

## Prolonged Service Without Direct Patient Contact

Codes 99358 and 99359 are used when a prolonged service is provided that is neither face-to face time in the office or outpatient setting, nor additional unit/floor time in the hospital or nursing facility setting during the same session of an evaluation and management service and is beyond the usual physician or other qualified health care professional service time.

This service is to be reported in relation to other physician or other qualified health care professional services, including evaluation and management services at any level. This prolonged service may be reported on a different date than the primary service to which it is related. For example, extensive

⃠=Modifier 51 Exempt ⊙=Moderate Sedation ✚=Add-on Code 𝑵=FDA approval pending record review may relate to a previous evaluation and management service performed earlier and commences upon receipt of past records. However, it must relate to a service or patient where (face-to-face) patient care has occurred or will occur and relate to ongoing patient management. A typical time for the primary service need not be established within the CPT code set.

Codes 99358 and 99359 are used to report the total duration of non-face-to-face time spent by a physician or other qualified health care professional on a given date providing prolonged service, even if the time spent by the physician or other qualified health care professional on that date is not continuous. Code 99358 is used to report the first hour of prolonged service on a given date regardless of the place of service. It should be used only once per date.

Prolonged service of less than 30 minutes total duration on a given date is not separately reported.

Code 99359 is used to report each additional 30 minutes beyond the first hour regardless of the place of service. It may also be used to report the final 15 to 30 minutes of prolonged service on a given date.

Prolonged service of less than 15 minutes beyond the first hour or less than 15 minutes beyond the final 30 minutes is not reported separately.

▶Do not report 99358, 99359 for time spent in care plan oversight services (99339, 99340, 99374-99380), anticoagulant management (99363, 99364), medical team conferences (99366-99368), on-line medical evaluations (99444), or other non-face-to-face services that have more specific codes and no upper time limit in the CPT code set. Codes 99358, 99359 may be reported when related to other non-face-to-face services codes that have a published maximum time (eg, telephone services).◀

**99358**    **Prolonged evaluation and management service** before and/or after direct patient care; first hour

**+ 99359**      each additional 30 minutes (List separately in addition to code for prolonged service)

(Use 99359 in conjunction with 99358)

▶(Do not report 99358, 99359 during the same month with 99487-99489)◀

▶(Do not report 99358, 99359 when performed during the service time of codes 99495 or 99496)◀

## 🖎 Rationale

To support the establishment of the new Complex Chronic Care Coordination Services codes 99487-99489 and the Transitional Care Management Services codes 99495 and 99496, two exclusionary parenthetical notes were added following Prolonged Services Without Direct Patient Contact codes 99358 and 99359 to instruct that these services should not be reported in conjunction with the Complex Chronic Care Coordination Services codes 99487-99489 or the Transitional Care Management Services codes 99495 and 99496. See also discussion on explicit code ranges.

# Case Management Services

## Anticoagulant Management

**99363** Anticoagulant management for an outpatient taking warfarin, physician review and interpretation of International Normalized Ratio (INR) testing, patient instructions, dosage adjustment (as needed), and ordering of additional tests; initial 90 days of therapy (must include a minimum of 8 INR measurements)

**99364** each subsequent 90 days of therapy (must include a minimum of 3 INR measurements)

▶(Do not report 99363, 99364 during the same month with 99487-99489)◀

▶(Do not report 99363, 99364 when performed during the service time of codes 99495 or 99496)◀

 **Rationale**

To support the establishment of the new Complex Chronic Care Coordination Services codes 99487-99489 and the Transitional Care Management Services codes 99495 and 99496, two exclusionary parenthetical notes were added following the Anticoagulant Management codes 99363 and 99364 to instruct that these services should not be reported in conjunction with the Complex Chronic Care Coordination Services codes 99487-99489 or the Transitional Care Management Services codes 99495 and 99496.

## Medical Team Conferences

### MEDICAL TEAM CONFERENCE, DIRECT (FACE-TO-FACE) CONTACT WITH PATIENT AND/OR FAMILY

**99366** **Medical team conference** with interdisciplinary team of health care professionals, face-to-face with patient and/or family, 30 minutes or more, participation by nonphysician qualified health care professional

(Team conference services of less than 30 minutes duration are not reported separately)

(For team conference services by a physician with patient and/or family present, see Evaluation and Management services)

▶(Do not report 99366 during the same month with 99487-99489)◀

▶(Do not report 99366 when performed during the service time of codes 99495 or 99496)◀

### MEDICAL TEAM CONFERENCE, WITHOUT DIRECT (FACE-TO-FACE) CONTACT WITH PATIENT AND/OR FAMILY

**99367** **Medical team conference** with interdisciplinary team of health care professionals, patient and/or family not present, 30 minutes or more; participation by physician

**99368** participation by nonphysician qualified health care professional

(Team conference services of less than 30 minutes duration are not reported separately)

⊘=Modifier 51 Exempt  ⊙=Moderate Sedation  ✚=Add-on Code  ✔=FDA approval pending

▶(Do not report 99367, 99368 during the same month with 99487-99489)◀

▶(Do not report 99367, 99368 when performed during the service time of codes 99495 or 99496)◀

## 🖎 Rationale

To support the establishment of new Complex Chronic Care Coordination Services codes 99487-99489 and Transitional Care Management Services codes 99495 and 99496, two exclusionary parenthetical notes were added following Medical Team Conferences codes 99366-99368 to instruct that these services should not be reported in conjunction with Complex Chronic Care Coordination Services codes 99487-99489 or Transitional Care Management Services codes 99495 and 99496.

## Care Plan Oversight Services

▶Care plan oversight services are reported separately from codes for office/outpatient, hospital, home, nursing facility or domiciliary, or non-face-to-face services. The complexity and approximate time of the care plan oversight services provided within a 30-day period determine code selection. Only one individual may report services for a given period of time, to reflect the sole or predominant supervisory role with a particular patient. These codes should not be reported for supervision of patients in nursing facilities or under the care of home health agencies unless they require recurrent supervision of therapy.◀

The work involved in providing very low intensity or infrequent supervision services is included in the pre- and post-encounter work for home, office/outpatient and nursing facility or domiciliary visit codes.

▶(For care plan oversight services of patients in the home, domiciliary, or rest home [eg, assisted living facility], see 99339, 99340, and for hospice agency, see 99377, 99378)◀

(Do not report 99374-99380 for time reported with 98966-98969, 99441-99444)

▶(Do not report 99374-99378 during the same month with 99487-99489)◀

▶(Do not report 99374-99380 when performed during the service time of codes 99495 or 99496)◀

## 🖎 Rationale

To support the establishment of new complex chronic care coordination services codes 99487-99489 and transitional care management services codes 99495, 99496, two exclusionary parenthetical notes were added following care plan oversight services guidelines to instruct that these services should not be reported in conjunction with complex chronic care coordination services codes 99487-99489 or transitional care management services codes 99495, 99496. See also discussion on CPT nomenclature reporting neutrality.

## Telephone Services

▲**99441**  Telephone evaluation and management service by a physician or other qualified health care professional who may report evaluation and management services provided to an established patient, parent, or guardian not originating from a related E/M service provided within the previous 7 days nor leading to an E/M service or procedure within the next 24 hours or soonest available appointment; 5-10 minutes of medical discussion

▲**99442**  11-20 minutes of medical discussion

▲**99443**  21-30 minutes of medical discussion

(Do not report 99441-99443 when using 99339-99340, 99374-99380 for the same call[s])

(Do not report 99441-99443 for anticoagulation management when reporting 99363, 99364)

▶(Do not report 99441-99443 during the same month with 99487-99489)◀

▶(Do not report 99441-99443 when performed during the service time of codes 99495 or 99496)◀

### Rationale

To support the establishment of new Complex Chronic Care Coordination Services codes 99487-99489 and Transitional Care Management Services codes 99495 and 99496, two exclusionary parenthetical notes were added following telephone services codes 99441-99443 to instruct that these services should not be reported in conjunction with Complex Chronic Care Coordination Services codes 99487-99489 or Transitional Care Management Services codes 99495 and 99496. See also discussion on CPT nomenclature reporting neutrality.

## On-Line Medical Evaluation

▲**99444**  Online evaluation and management service provided by a physician or other qualified health care professional who may report an evaluation and management services provided to an established patient or guardian, not originating from a related E/M service provided within the previous 7 days, using the Internet or similar electronic communications network

(Do not report 99444 when using 99339, 99340, 99374-99380 for the same communication[s])

(Do not report 99444 for anticoagulation management when reporting 99363, 99364)

▶(Do not report 99444 during the same month with 99487-99489)◀

▶(Do not report 99444 when performed during the service time of codes 99495 or 99496)◀

### Rationale

To support the establishment of new Complex Chronic Care Coordination Services codes 99487-99489 and Transitional Care Management Services codes 99495 and 99496, two exclusionary parenthetical notes were added following online medical evaluation service code 99444 to instruct that this service should not be reported in conjunction with Complex Chronic Care Coordination Services codes 99487-99489 or Transitional Care Management Services codes 99495 and 99496. See also discussion on CPT nomenclature reporting neutrality.

## Inpatient Neonatal Intensive Care Services and Pediatric and Neonatal Critical Care Services

### Pediatric Critical Care Patient Transport

▶Codes 99466, 99467 are used to report the physical attendance and direct face-to-face care by a physician during the interfacility transport of a critically ill or critically injured pediatric patient 24 months of age or younger. Codes 99485, 99486 are used to report the control physician's non-face-to-face supervision of interfacility transport of a critically ill or critically injured pediatric patient 24 months of age or younger. These codes are not reported together for the same patient by the same physician. For the purpose of reporting 99466 and 99467, face-to-face care begins when the physician assumes primary responsibility of the pediatric patient at the referring facility, and ends when the receiving facility accepts responsibility for the pediatric patient's care. Only the time the physician spends in direct face-to-face contact with the patient during the transport should be reported. Pediatric patient transport services involving less than 30 minutes of face-to-face physician care should not be reported using 99466, 99467. Procedure(s) or service(s) performed by other members of the transporting team may not be reported by the supervising physician.

Codes 99485, 99486 are used to report control physician's non-face-to-face supervision of interfacility pediatric critical care transport, which includes all two-way communication between the control physician and the specialized transport team prior to transport, at the referring facility and during transport of the patient back to the receiving facility. The "control" physician is the physician directing transport services. These codes do not include pretransport communication between the control physician and the referring facility before or following patient transport. These codes are only reported for patients 24 months of age or younger who are critically ill or critically injured. The control physician provides treatment advice to a specialized transport team who are present and delivering the hands-on patient care. The control physician does not report any services provided by the specialized transport team. The control physician's non-face-to-face time begins with the first contact by the control physician with the specialized transport team and ends when the patient's care is handed over to the receiving facility team. Refer to 99466 and 99467 for face-to-face transport care of the critically ill/injured patient. Time spent with the individual patient's transport team and reviewing data submissions should be recorded. Code 99485 is used to report the first 16-45 minutes of direction on a given date and should only be used once even if time spent by the physician is discontinuous. Do not report services of 15 minutes or less or any time when another physician is reporting 99466, 99467. Do not report 99485 or 99486 in conjunction with 99466, 99467 when performed by the same physician.◀

For the definition of the critically injured pediatric patient, see the **Neonatal and Pediatric Critical Care Services** section.

▶The non-face-to-face direction of emergency care to a patient's transporting staff by a physician located in a hospital or other facility by two-way communication is not considered direct face-to-face care and should not be reported with 99466, 99467. Physician-directed non-face-to-face emergency care through outside voice communication to transporting staff personnel is reported with 99288 or 99485, 99486 based upon the age and clinical condition of the patient.◄

Emergency department services (99281-99285), initial hospital care (99221-99223), critical care (99291, 99292), initial date neonatal intensive (99477) or critical care (99468) are only reported after the patient has been admitted to the emergency department, the inpatient floor, or the critical care unit of the receiving facility. If inpatient critical care services are reported in the referring facility prior to transfer to the receiving hospital, use the critical care codes (99291, 99292).

►Services provided by the specialized transport team during non-face-to-face transport supervision are not reported by the control physician.◄

Code 99466 is used to report the first 30 to 74 minutes of direct face-to-face time with the transport pediatric patient and should be reported only once on a given date. Code 99467 is used to report each additional 30 minutes provided on a given date. Face-to-face services of less than 30 minutes should not be reported with these codes.

►Code 99485 is used to report the first 30 minutes of non-face-to-face supervision of an interfacility transport of a critically ill or critically injured pediatric patient and should be reported only once per date of service. Code 99486 is used to report each additional 30 minutes beyond the initial 30 minutes. Non-face-to-face interfacility transport of 15 minutes or less is not reported.◄

(For total body cooling of neonates, see 0260T, 0261T)

▲99466 **Critical care** face-to-face services, during an interfacility transport of critically ill or critically injured pediatric patient, 24 months of age or younger; first 30-74 minutes of hands-on care during transport

✚▲99467 each additional 30 minutes (List separately in addition to code for primary service)

(Use 99467 in conjunction with 99466)

(Critical care of less than 30 minutes total duration should be reported with the appropriate E/M code)

#●99485 Supervision by a control physician of interfacility transport care of the critically ill or critically injured pediatric patient, 24 months of age or younger, includes two-way communication with transport team before transport, at the referring facility and during the transport, including data interpretation and report; first 30 minutes

#✚●99486 each additional 30 minutes (List separately in addition to code for primary procedure)

►(Use 99486 in conjunction with 99485)◄

►(For physician direction of emergency medical systems supervision for a pediatric patient older than 24 months of age, or at any age if not critically ill or injured, use 99288)◄

►(Do not report 99485, 99486 with any other services reported by the control physician for the same period)◄

►(Do not report 99485, 99486 in conjunction with 99466, 99467 when performed by the same physician)◄

⊘=Modifier 51 Exempt  ⊙=Moderate Sedation  ✚=Add-on Code  𝒩=FDA approval pending

## ✏️ Rationale

Two codes 99485 and 99486 were established to report non-face-to-face physician supervision of interfacility pediatric critical care transport, 24 months of age or younger. Code 99485 is intended to describe supervision by a control physician of interfacility transport care of the critically ill or critically injured pediatric patient, 24 months of age or younger, includes two-way communication with transport team before transport, at the referring facility and during the transport, including data interpretation and report; first 30 minutes, and add-on code 99486 is intended to describe each additional 30 minutes (List separately in addition to code for primary procedure). Codes 99485 and 99486 appear with a hash symbol (#) to indicate that they are out of numerical sequence.

In order to exemplify the reporting of these services, and to identify age specification the Pediatric Critical Care Patient Transport guidelines were revised to clarify the reporting of these services. It was noted in the guidelines that codes 99485 and 99486 are used to report the control physician's non-face-to-face supervision of interfacility transport of a critically ill or critically injured pediatric patient 24 months of age or younger.

The guidelines further clarify that codes 99485 and 99486 are used to report control physician's non-face-to-face supervision of interfacility pediatric critical care transport, which includes all two-way communication between the control physician and the specialized transport team prior to transport, at the referring facility and during transport of the patient back to the receiving facility. Furthermore, the control physician is the physician directing transport services. In addition, codes 99485 and 99486 do not include pretransport communication between the control physician and the referring facility before or following patient transport. These codes are only intended to be reported for patients 24 months of age or younger who are critically ill or critically injured. The guidelines further instruct that the control physician provides treatment advice to a specialized transport team who are present and delivering the hands-on patient care. In addition, the control physician does not report any services provided by the specialized transport team. Consequently, the control physician's non-face-to-face time begins with the first contact by the control physician with the specialized transport team and ends when the patient's care is handed over to the receiving facility team. For face-to-face transport care of the critically ill/injured patient, report codes 99466 and 99467. Also, time spent with the individual patient's transport team and reviewing data submissions should be recorded. Moreover, code 99485 is used to report the first 16-45 minutes of direction on a given date and should only be used once, even if time spent by the physician is discontinuous. The guidelines further instruct not to report services of 15 minutes or less or any time when another physician is reporting the pediatric critical care patient transport service codes 99466, 99467. In addition, it would not be appropriate to report code 99485 or 99486 in addition to pediatric critical care patient transport codes 99466 and 99467, when performed by the same physician.

In support of the establishment of codes 99485 and 99486, two instructional notes were added following code 99486. The first instructional note instructs users to report code 99486, in addition to code 99485. The second instructional note instructs users to report code 99288 for physician direction of emergency medical systems supervision for a pediatric patient older than 24 months of age or at any age, if not critically ill or injured.

For further clarification, two exclusionary parenthetical notes were also added following code 99486. The first exclusionary parenthetical note precludes the reporting of codes 99485 and 99486 with any other services reported by the control physician for the same period, and the second note precludes the reporting of codes 99485 and 99486 in addition to the pediatric critical care patient transport codes 99466 and 99467, when performed by the same physician. See also discussion on CPT nomenclature reporting neutrality.

###  Clinical Example (99485)

A 34-week critically ill or critically injured neonate is delivered at a level I hospital and the community provider requests a transfer to the physician's hospital. The ground transport team consisting of a nurse and respiratory therapist is dispatched to the level I hospital. After the team evaluates the patient, they contact the control physician to discuss the case. The physician and team remain in two-way communication and decide together on the appropriate management and interventions for the child before and during transport back to the control physician's hospital.

### Description of Procedure (99485)

The transport control physician discusses the planned patient treatment with the specialized transport team before and after leaving the initial facility where care is provided and continues to be in contact with the specialized transport team during the transport to the receiving facility. The control physician maintains two-way communication availability to the transport team throughout the transport.

### Clinical Example (99486)

A 34-week critically ill or critically injured neonate is delivered at a level I hospital, and the community provider requests a transfer to the physician's hospital. The ground transport team consisting of a nurse and respiratory therapist is dispatched to the level I hospital. After the team evaluates the patient, they contact the control physician to discuss the case. The physician and team remain in two-way communication and decide together on the appropriate management and interventions for the child before and during transport back to the control physician's hospital. Code 99485 was reported and code 99486 is reported for each additional 30 minutes. Code 99486 is an add-on code.

Ⓢ=Modifier 51 Exempt   ⊙=Moderate Sedation   ✚=Add-on Code   𝑁=FDA approval pending

## Description of Procedure (99486)

The transport control physician discusses the planned patient treatment with the specialized transport team before and after leaving the initial facility where care is provided and continues to be in contact with the specialized transport team during the transport to the receiving facility. The control physician maintains two-way communication availability to the transport team throughout the transport.

# Inpatient Neonatal and Pediatric Critical Care

The same definitions for critical care services apply for the adult, child, and neonate.

▶Codes 99468, 99469 are used to report the services of directing the inpatient care of a critically ill neonate or infant 28 days of age or younger. They represent care starting with the date of admission (99468) to a critical care unit and subsequent day(s) (99469) that the neonate remains critical. These codes may be reported only by a single individual and only once per day, per patient, per hospital stay in a given facility. If readmitted to the neonatal critical care unit during the same day, report the subsequent day(s) code 99469 for the first day of readmission to critical care, and 99469 for each day of critical care following readmission.

The initial day neonatal critical care code (99468) can be used in addition to 99464 or 99465 as appropriate, when the physician or other qualified health care professional is present for the delivery (99464) or resuscitation (99465) is required. Other procedures performed as a necessary part of the resuscitation (eg, endotracheal intubation [31500]) are also reported separately when performed as part of the pre-admission delivery room care. In order to report these procedures separately, they must be performed as a necessary component of the resuscitation and not simply as a convenience before admission to the neonatal intensive care unit.

Codes 99471-99476 are used to report direction of the inpatient care of a critically ill infant or young child from 29 days of postnatal age through less than 6 years of age. They represent care starting with the date of admission (99471, 99475) to all subsequent day(s) (99472, 99476) the infant or child remains critical. These codes may be reported only by a single individual and only once per day, per patient in a given setting. Services for the critically ill or critically injured child 6 years of age or older would be reported with the time based critical care codes (99291, 99292). Report 99471, 99475 only once per hospital stay in a given facility. If readmitted to the pediatric critical care unit during the same stay, report 99472 or 99476 for the first day of readmission to critical care and 99472 for each day of critical care following readmission.◀

The pediatric and neonatal critical care codes include those procedures listed for the critical care codes (99291, 99292). In addition, the following procedures are also included (and are not separately reported by professionals, but may be reported by facilities) in the pediatric and neonatal critical care service codes (99468-99472, 99475, 99476) and the intensive care services codes (99477-99480):

Any services performed that are not included in these listings may be reported separately. Facilities may report the included services separately.

When a neonate or infant is not critically ill but requires intensive observation, frequent interventions, and other intensive care services, the Continuing Intensive Care Services codes (99477-99480) should be used to report these services.

▶To report critical care services provided in the outpatient setting (eg, emergency department or office) for neonates and pediatric patients of any age, see the Critical Care codes 99291, 99292. If the same individual provides critical care services for a neonatal or pediatric patient less than 6 years of age in both the outpatient and inpatient settings on the same day, report only the appropriate Neonatal or Pediatric Critical Care codes 99468-99476 for all critical care services provided on that day. Critical care services provided by a second individual of a different specialty not reporting a per-day neonatal or pediatric critical care code can be reported with 99291, 99292.

When critical care services are provided to neonates or pediatric patients less than 6 years of age at two separate institutions by an individual from a different group on the same date of service, the individual from the referring institution should report their critical care services with the time-based critical care codes (99291, 99292) and the receiving institution should report the appropriate initial day of care code 99468, 99471, 99475 for the same date of service.◀

Critical care services to a pediatric patient 6 years of age or older are reported with the time based critical care codes 99291, 99292.

▶When the critically ill neonate or pediatric patient improves and is transferred to a lower level of care to another individual in another group within the same facility, the transferring individual does not report a per day critical care service. Subsequent hospital care (99231-99233) or time-based critical care services (99291-99292) is reported, as appropriate based upon the condition of the neonate or child. The receiving individual reports subsequent intensive care (99478-99480) or subsequent hospital care (99231-99233) services, as appropriate based upon the condition of the neonate or child.

When the neonate or infant becomes critically ill on a day when initial or subsequent intensive care services (99477-99480), hospital services (99221-99233), or normal newborn services (99460, 99461, 99462) have been performed by one individual and is transferred to a critical care level of care provided by a different individual in a different group, the transferring individual reports either the time-based critical care services performed (99291, 99292) for the time spent providing critical care to the patient, the intensive care service (99477-99480), hospital care services (99221-99233), or normal newborn service (99460, 99461, 99462) performed, but only one service. The receiving individual reports initial or subsequent inpatient neonatal or pediatric critical care (99468-99476), as appropriate based upon the patient's age and whether this is the first or subsequent admission to the critical care unit for the hospital stay.

When a newborn becomes critically ill on the same day they have already received normal newborn care (99460, 99461, 99462), and the same individual or group assumes critical care, report initial critical care service (99468) with modifier 25 in addition to the normal newborn code.

When a neonate, infant, or child requires initial critical care services on the same day the patient already has received hospital care or intensive care services by the same individual or group, only the initial critical care service code (99468, 99471, 99475) is reported.

Time-based critical care services (99291, 99292) are not reportable by the same individual or different individual within the same group when neonatal or pediatric critical care services (99468-99476) are reported for the same patient on the same day.

No individual may report remote real-time videoconferenced critical care (0188T, 0189T) when neonatal or pediatric intensive or critical care services (99468-99476) are reported.◀

⃠=Modifier 51 Exempt   ⊙=Moderate Sedation   ✚=Add-on Code   ⅄=FDA approval pending

**99468**   **Initial inpatient neonatal critical care,** per day, for the evaluation and management of a critically ill neonate, 28 days of age or younger

### ✎ Rationale

The Neonatal and Pediatric Critical Care guidelines have been revised to provide clarification regarding reporting codes 99468, 99469, and 99471-99476 in relation to other facility codes (newborn care services, time-based critical care services), based on whether the physician or other qualified health care professional is the receiving individual or transferring individual providing care to the patient, and whether the individual(s) is part of the same or different groups within the same facility.

The revised guidelines will aid in the elimination of duplicative reporting of services and inappropriate reporting. For example, the guidelines now make it clear that when an individual provides normal newborn services (99460, 99461, 99462) and the neonate or infant becomes critically ill and treated by a different individual in a different group, the first individual may report either the normal newborn services, or if he or she has provided critical care services, may report code 99291, 99292, but not both the normal newborn care services and the critical care services. The receiving individual reports initial or subsequent inpatient neonatal or pediatric critical care (99468-99476), as appropriate based on the patient's age. However, if the patient becomes critically ill on the same day they received normal newborn care (99460, 99461, 99462) and critical care services are asssumed by the same individual or group, the group or individual may report initial critical care service code 99468 with modifier 25, in addition to the normal newborn code. Also, the guidelines now include instructions that prevent reporting of both time-based critical care services (99291, 99292) and Inpatient Neonatal and Pediatric Critical Care services (99468-99476), when reported by the same individual or different individual within the same group for the same patient on the same day. Clarification has also been provided that the initial Inpatient Pediatric Critical Care codes 99471 and 99475 can only be used once per hospital stay in a given facility, and if a patient is readmitted to pediatric critical care unit during the same stay, the readmission to the unit is coded using the subsequent inpatient pediatric critical care codes 99472 or 99476, depending on the patient's age. The guidelines have also been revised to clarify the intended age range for codes 99291 and 99292, stating that codes are intended for children "6 years of age or older," and not the former definition, "older than five years of age."

# Initial and Continuing Intensive Care Services

▶Code 99477 represents the initial day of inpatient care for the child who is not critically ill but requires intensive observation, frequent interventions, and other intensive care services. Codes 99478-99480 are used to report the subsequent day services of directing the continuing intensive care of the low birth weight (LBW 1500-2500 grams) present body weight infant, very low birth weight (VLBW less than 1500 grams) present body weight infant, or normal (2501-5000 grams) present body weight newborn who does not meet the definition of critically ill but continues to require intensive observation, frequent interventions, and other intensive care services. These services are for infants and neonates who are not critically ill but continue to require intensive cardiac and respiratory monitoring, continuous and/or frequent vital sign monitoring, heat maintenance, enteral and/or parenteral nutritional adjustments, laboratory and oxygen monitoring, and constant observation by the health care team under direct supervision of the physician or other qualified health care professional. Codes 99477-99480 may be reported by a single individual and only once per day, per patient in a given facility. If readmitted to the intensive care unit during the same hospital stay, report 99478-99480 for the first day of intensive care and for each successive day that the child requires intensive care services.

These codes include the same procedures that are outlined in the **Neonatal and Pediatric Critical Care Services** section and these services should not be separately reported.

The initial day neonatal intensive care code (99477) can be used in addition to 99464 or 99465 as appropriate, when the physician or other qualified health care professional is present for the delivery (99464) or resuscitation (99465) is required. In this situation, report 99477 with modifier 25. Other procedures performed as a necessary part of the resuscitation (eg, endotracheal intubation [31500]) are also reported separately when performed as part of the pre-admission delivery room care. In order to report these procedures separately, they must be performed as a necessary component of the resuscitation and not simply as a convenience before admission to the neonatal intensive care unit.

The same procedures are included as bundled services with the neonatal intensive care codes as those listed for the neonatal (99468, 99469) and pediatric (99471-99476) critical care codes.

When the neonate or infant improves after the initial day and no longer requires intensive care services and is transferred to a lower level of care, the transferring individual does not report a per day intensive care service. Subsequent hospital care (99231-99233) or subsequent normal newborn care (99460, 99462) is reported as appropriate based upon the condition of the neonate or infant. If the transfer to a lower level of care occurs on the same day as initial intensive care services were provided by the transferring individual, 99477 may be reported.

When the neonate or infant is transferred after the initial day within the same facility to the care of another individual in a different group, both individuals report subsequent hospital care (99231-99233) services. The receiving individual reports subsequent hospital care (99231-99233) or subsequent normal newborn care (99462).

When the neonate or infant becomes critically ill on a day when initial or subsequent intensive care services (99477-99480) have been reported by one individual and is transferred to a critical care level of care provided by a different individual from a different group, the transferring individual reports either the time-based critical care services performed (99291, 99292) for the time spent providing critical care to the patient or the initial or subsequent intensive care (99477-99480) service, but not both. The receiving individual reports initial or subsequent inpatient neonatal or pediatric critical care

⃠=Modifier 51 Exempt    ⊙=Moderate Sedation    ✚=Add-on Code    𝗡=FDA approval pending

(99468-99476) based upon the patient's age and whether this is the first or subsequent admission to critical care for the same hospital stay.

When the neonate or infant becomes critically ill on a day when initial or subsequent intensive care services (99477-99480) have been performed by the same individual or group, report only initial or subsequent inpatient neonatal or pediatric critical care (99468-99476) based upon the patient's age and whether this is the first or subsequent admission to critical care for the same hospital stay.◄

For the subsequent care of the sick neonate younger than 28 days of age but more than 5000 grams who does not require intensive or critical care services, use codes 99231-99233.

**99477**  **Initial hospital care,** per day, for the evaluation and management of the neonate, 28 days of age or younger, who requires intensive observation, frequent interventions, and other intensive care services

▶Code is out of numerical sequence. See 99466-99486◄

▶Code is out of numerical sequence. See 99466-99486◄

## Rationale

In concert with the revisions to the Inpatient Neonatal and Pediatric Critical Care guidelines, the Initial and Continuing Intensive Care Services guidelines have been revised to clarify the use of codes 99477-99480 in circumstances involving the transfer of care from one individual to another individual within the same group and from different groups, as well as in relation to other services that may be provided on the same day (eg, newborn resuscitation [99465]).

## ▶Complex Chronic Care Coordination Services◄

▶Complex chronic care coordination services are patient centered management and support services provided by physicians, other qualified health care professionals and clinical staff to an individual who resides at home or in a domiciliary, rest home, or assisted living facility. These services typically involve clinical staff implementing a care plan directed by the physician or other qualified health care professional. These services address the coordination of care by multiple disciplines and community service agencies. The reporting individual provides or oversees the management and/or coordination of services, as needed, for all medical conditions, psychosocial needs and activities of daily living.

Patients who require complex chronic care coordination services may be identified by algorithms that utilize reported conditions and services (eg, predictive modeling risk score or repeat admissions or emergency department use) or by clinician judgment. Typical patients have 1 or more chronic continuous or episodic health conditions expected to last at least 12 months, or until the death of the patient, that place the patient at significant risk of death, acute exacerbation/decompensation or functional decline. Because of the complex nature of their diseases and morbidities, these patients commonly require the coordination of a number of specialties and services. Patients may have medical and psychiatric behavioral co-morbidities (eg, dementia and chronic obstructive pulmonary disease or substance abuse and diabetes) that complicate their care. Social support weaknesses or access to care difficulties may cause a need for these services. Medical, functional, and/or psychosocial problems that require medical decision making of moderate or high complexity and extensive clinical staff support are expected. Medical decision making as defined in the Evaluation and Management (E/M) guidelines is not only applied to the face-to-face services, but is determined by the nature of the problems addressed by the reporting individual during the month. A plan of care should be documented and shared with the patient and/or caregiver.

Codes 99487-99489 are reported only **once** per calendar month and include all non-face-to-face complex chronic care coordination services and none or 1 face-to-face office or other outpatient, home, or domiciliary visit. Codes 99487-99489 may only be reported by the single physician or other qualified health care professional who assumes the care coordination role with a particular patient for the calendar month.

Code selection is as follows:

Code 99487 is reported when, during the calendar month, there is no face-to-face visit with the physician or other qualified health care professional and at least 31 minutes of clinical staff time is spent in care coordination activities. 99488 is reported when, during the calendar month, there is a face-to-face visit with the physician or other qualified health care professional and at least 31 minutes of clinical staff time is spent in care coordination activities.

The face-to-face and non-face-to-face time spent by the clinical staff in communicating with the patient and/or family, caregivers, other professionals and agencies; revising, documenting and implementing the care plan; or teaching self management is used in determining the complex chronic care coordination clinical staff time for the month. Note: Do not count any clinical staff time on the date of the first visit or on a day when the physician or qualified health care professional reports an E/M service (office or other outpatient services 99211-99215, domiciliary, rest home services 99334-99337, home services 99347-99350).

Care coordination activities performed by clinical staff may include:

- communication (with patient, family members, guardian or caretaker, surrogate decision makers, and/or other professionals) regarding aspects of care,

- communication with home health agencies and other community services utilized by the patient,

- collection of health outcomes data and registry documentation,

- patient and/or family/caretaker education to support self-management, independent living, and activities of daily living,

- assessment and support for treatment regimen adherence and medication management,

- identification of available community and health resources,

- facilitating access to care and services needed by the patient and/or family,

- development and maintenance of a comprehensive care plan.

If a face-to-face visit was provided during the month by the physician or other qualified health care professional, report 99488. Additional E/M services beyond the first visit may be reported separately by the same physician or other qualified health care professional during the same calendar month. Complex care coordination services include care plan oversight services (99339, 99340, 99374-99378), prolonged services without direct patient contact (99358, 99359), anticoagulant management (99363, 99364), medical team conferences (99366-99368), education and training (98960-98962, 99071, 99078), telephone services (98966-98968, 99441-99443), on-line medical evaluation (98969, 99444), preparation of special reports (99080), analysis of data (99090, 99091), transitional care management services (99495, 99496), medication therapy management services (99605-99607) and, if performed,

⊘=Modifier 51 Exempt   ⊙=Moderate Sedation   ✚=Add-on Code   ⩩=FDA approval pending

these services may not be reported separately during the month for which 99487-99489 are reported. All other services may be reported. Do not report 99487-99489 if reporting ESRD services (90951-90970) during the same month. If the complex chronic care coordination services are performed within the postoperative period of a reported surgery, the same individual may not report 99487-99489.

Complex chronic care coordination can be reported in any calendar month during which the clinical staff time requirements are met. If care coordination resumes after a discharge during a new month, start a new period or report transitional care management services (99495, 99496) as appropriate. If discharge occurs in the same month, continue the reporting period or report Transitional Care Management Services. Do not report 99487-99489 for any post-discharge complex chronic care coordination services for any days within 30 days of discharge, if reporting 99495, 99496.◄

| Total Duration of Staff Care Coordination Services | Code(s) |
|---|---|
| Less than 30 minutes | Not reported separately |
| 31 to 74 minutes (31 minutes - 1 hr. 14 min.) | 99487 or 99488 X 1 |
| 75 - 104 minutes (1 hr. 15 min. - 1 hr. 44 min.) | 99487 or 99488 X 1 and 99489 X 1 |
| 105 minutes or more (1 hr. 45 min. or more) | 99487 or 99488 X 1 and 99489 X 2 or more for each additional 30 minutes |

●99487    Complex chronic care coordination services; first hour of clinical staff time directed by a physician or other qualified health care professional with no face-to-face visit, per calendar month

●99488    first hour of clinical staff time directed by a physician or other qualified health care professional with one face-to-face visit, per calendar month

+●99489    each additional 30 minutes of clinical staff time directed by a physician or other qualified health care professional, per calendar month (List separately in addition to code for primary procedure)

►(Report 99489 in conjunction with 99487, 99488)◄

►(Do not report 99487-99489 during the same month with 90951-90970, 98960-98962, 98966-98969, 99071, 99078, 99080, 99090, 99091, 99339, 99340, 99358, 99359, 99363, 99364, 99366-99368, 99374-99378, 99441-99444, 99495, 99496, 99605-99607)◄

# ►Transitional Care Management Services◄

►Codes 99495 and 99496 are used to report transitional care management services (TCM). These services are for an established patient whose medical and/or psychosocial problems require moderate or high complexity medical decision making during transitions in care from an inpatient hospital setting (including acute hospital, rehabilitation hospital, long-term acute care hospital), partial hospital, observation status in a hospital, or skilled nursing facility/nursing facility, to the patient's community setting (home, domiciliary, rest home, or assisted living). TCM commences upon the date of discharge and continues for the next 29 days.

TCM is comprised of one face-to-face visit within the specified timeframes, in combination with non-face-to-face services that may be performed by the physician or other qualified health care professional and/or licensed clinical staff under his/her direction.

Non-face-to-face services provided by clinical staff, under the direction of the physician or other qualified health care professional, may include:

- communication (with patient, family members, guardian or caretaker, surrogate decision makers, and/or other professionals) regarding aspects of care,

- communication with home health agencies and other community services utilized by the patient,

- patient and/or family/caretaker education to support self-management, independent living, and activities of daily living,

- assessment and support for treatment regimen adherence and medication management,

- identification of available community and health resources,

- facilitating access to care and services needed by the patient and/or family

Non-face-to-face services provided by the physician or other qualified health care provider may include:

- obtaining and reviewing the discharge information (eg, discharge summary, as available, or continuity of care documents);

- reviewing need for or follow-up on pending diagnostic tests and treatments;

- interaction with other qualified health care professionals who will assume or reassume care of the patient's system-specific problems;

- education of patient, family, guardian, and/or caregiver;

- establishment or reestablishment of referrals and arranging for needed community resources;

- assistance in scheduling any required follow-up with community providers and services.

TCM requires a face-to-face visit, initial patient contact, and medication reconciliation within specified timeframes. The first face-to-face visit is part of the TCM service and not reported separately. Additional E/M services after the first face-to-face visit may be reported separately. TCM requires an interactive contact with the patient or caregiver, as appropriate, within two business days of discharge. The contact may be direct (face-to-face), telephonic or by electronic means. Medication reconciliation and management must occur no later than the date of the face-to-face visit.

These services address any needed coordination of care performed by multiple disciplines and community service agencies. The reporting individual provides or oversees the management and/or coordination of services, as needed, for all medical conditions, psychosocial needs and activity of daily living support by providing first contact and continuous access.

Medical decision making and the date of the first face-to-face visit are used to select and report the appropriate TCM code. For 99496, the face-to-face visit must occur within 7 calendar days of the date of discharge and medical decision making must be of high complexity. For 99495, the face-to-face visit must occur within 14 calendar days of the date of discharge and medical decision making must be of at least moderate complexity.

⊘=Modifier 51 Exempt   ⊙=Moderate Sedation   ✚=Add-on Code   𝑵=FDA approval pending

| Type of Medical Decision Making | Face-to-face visit within 7 days | Face to face visit within 8 to 14 days |
| --- | --- | --- |
| Moderate Complexity | 99495 | 99495 |
| High Complexity | 99496 | 99495 |

Medical decision making is defined by the E/M Services Guidelines. The medical decision making over the service period reported is used to define the medical decision making of TCM. Documentation includes the timing of the initial post discharge communication with the patient or caregivers, date of the face-to-face visit, and the complexity of medical decision making.

Only one individual may report these services and only once per patient within 30 days of discharge. Another TCM may not be reported by the same individual or group for any subsequent discharge(s) within the 30 days. The same individual may report hospital or observation discharge services and TCM. The same individual should not report TCM services provided in the postoperative period.

A physician or other qualified health care professional who reports codes 99495, 99496 may not report care plan oversight services (99339, 99340, 99374-99380), prolonged services without direct patient contact (99358, 99359), anticoagulant management (99363, 99364), medical team conferences (99366-99368), education and training (98960-98962, 99071, 99078), telephone services (98966-98968, 99441-99443), end stage renal disease services (90951-90970), online medical evaluation services (98969, 99444), preparation of special reports (99080), analysis of data (99090, 99091), complex chronic care coordination services (99487-99489), medication therapy management services (99605-99607), during the time period covered by the transitional care management services codes.◄

●99495 **Transitional Care Management Services** with the following required elements:

- ■ Communication (direct contact, telephone, electronic) with the patient and/or caregiver within 2 business days of discharge

- ■ Medical decision making of at least moderate complexity during the service period

- ■ Face-to-face visit, within 14 calendar days of discharge

●99496 **Transitional Care Management Services** with the following required elements:

- ■ Communication (direct contact, telephone, electronic) with the patient and/or caregiver within 2 business days of discharge

- ■ Medical decision making of high complexity during the service period

- ■ Face-to-face visit, within 7 calendar days of discharge

▶(Do not report 90951-90970, 98960-98962, 98966-98969, 99071, 99078, 99080, 99090, 99091, 99339, 99340, 99358, 99359, 99363, 99364, 99366-99368, 99374-99380, 99441-99444, 99487-99489, 99605-99607 when performed during the service time of codes 99495 or 99496)◄

## ✍ Rationale

A request was received from the Centers for Medicaid and Medicare Services (CMS) to the AMA/Specialty Society RVS Update Committee (RUC) to review all evaluation and management (E/M) services. In response, a joint CPT/RUC Chronic Care Coordination workgroup was formed and decided to convene the Care Coordination CPT workgroup with the charge to look at new CPT codes for services that are important to chronic care management, especially complex chronic care management of multiple diseases and transitional care management.

The group was asked to define those components of chronic care management and transitional care management that are unrecognized or under recognized in the current Medicare fee for service (FFS) and to create solutions.

In response to these concerns, the workgroup agreed that a new coding structure for the E/M section be created to include guideline language, new codes and descriptors, and instructional parenthetical notes to describe Complex Chronic Care Coordination Services and Transitional Care Management Services.

Specifically, this new coding structure includes a new heading for Complex Chronic Care and new guidelines that define the types of services, professionals, and patients receiving these services. The guidelines also instruct users on how to accurately report these new services. Also, three new codes (99487-99489) were added to describe the work performed by the clinical staff under the direction of a physician or other qualified health care professional. Numerous parenthetical notes were added throughout the E/M and Medicine subsections to instruct appropriate reporting of these services in conjunction with other E/M services.

Similarly, the new coding structure for Transitional Care Management Services includes a new heading and new guidelines that define the types of services, professionals, and patients receiving these services. The guidelines also instruct users on how to accurately report these new services. Code 99495 was added to describe transitional care management with at least moderate complexity medical decision making, and a face-to-face visit within 14 calendar days of discharge. Code 99496 describes transitional care management with high complexity medical decision making, and a face-to-face visit within 7 calendar days of discharge. Numerous parenthetical notes were added throughout the E/M and Medicine subsections to instruct appropriate reporting of these services in conjunction with other E/M services.

Also, several "Coding Tips" were added to offer specific guidance, in addition to the guidelines on how to accurately report or assign these codes.

### Clinical Example 1 (99487)

A 6-year-old child with spastic quadriplegia, gastrostomy, gastroesophageal reflux with recurrent bouts of aspiration pneumonia and reactive airway disease, chronic seizure disorder, failure to thrive and severe neuro development delay. He receives home-occupational, physical- and speech-therapy services.

### Description of Procedure 1 (99487)

The care coordinator/case manager communicates regularly with the family for updates on the child's medical status, any planned or completed specialist visits, significant changes in the goals or frequencies of home-therapy services and any additional unmet needs the family/child are experiencing. Any new medical problems or exacerbation of existing chronic problems, including any medication adjustments or telephone contact with one or more of the child's specialists, are discussed and decided on with the primary care physician (PCP). The case manager reviews any reports received from visits to the child's specialists, any new

⊘=Modifier 51 Exempt   ⊙=Moderate Sedation   ✚=Add-on Code   ✗=FDA approval pending

laboratory, diagnostic or imaging studies and updated goals and interventions instituted by the speech, physical and occupational therapist. This information is shared as needed throughout the month with the PCP and adjustments to the plan of care are developed and discussed with the family and then implemented. He or she reviews any additional visit summaries from the child's medical/surgical specialists and communicates by telephone to clarify any concerns or suggested changes in therapy. He or she communicates regularly with the child's Medicaid case worker and benefits office to assure that needed services are received.

 ## Clinical Example 2 (99487)

An 83-year-old female with congestive heart failure and early cognitive dysfunction, who has been hospitalized twice in the prior 12 months, is becoming increasingly confused and refuses an office visit. She has a certified nursing assistant supervised by a home-care agency, participates in a remote weight- and vital-signs monitoring program, and sees a cardiologist and neurologist.

### Description of Procedure 2 (99487)

The clinical staff nurse obtains the recent weights and vital signs from the monitoring program and obtains a list of medications from the patient's daughter. The physician phones the cardiologist and neurologist and discusses her recent visits with them. He provides additional orders to the home-health agency and changes her medication regimen. The nurse contacts the patient's daughter to confirm the changes in the medication regimen and follow up one week later. The office nurse coordinates with the home-care agency to be sure the medications are taken as directed, and tracks pharmacy utilization data to confirm adherence.

 ## Clinical Example 1 (99488)

A 12-year-old child has severe atopic disease and recurrent asthma, which has led to multiple emergency department visits, hospital admissions, lost school days and behavioral adjustment reactions.

### Description of Procedure 1 (99488)

The care coordinator communicates daily initially, and then every other day with the child by cell phone and text messaging to assure that medications were taken and that atopic and airway symptoms are controlled. She reviews the child's weekly self-obtained spirometry readings and communicates with the child and family, if these values require medication adjustment. She assures that follow-up visits with the allergist and pulmonologist have been made, and that the appointments are kept. She communicates monthly with the child's teacher, school nurse, and psychologist to assure that the care plan is followed, and determines whether adjustments to that plan are needed. She reviews any additional visit-summaries from specialists who are taking care of the child, and communicates by telephone to clarify any concerns or suggested changes in therapy. The physician or other health care professional evaluates the child monthly to determine asthma control and adjusts the care-plan as needed. The clinical staff telephones the family and reviews the changes to the care-plan. She meets with the child to provide encouragement and education and assure that the child understands her disease, and emphasizes her need to continue to develop her self-management skills to maximize her emotional and physical health.

## Clinical Example 2 (99488)

A 92-year-old male living in an assisted-living facility with Parkinsons disease, mild dementia, depression and diabetes mellitus continues to lose weight and remains withdrawn. The patient's family resides out of state, and an attendant sees the patient for 3 hours daily.

### Description of Procedure 2 (99488)

The clinical staff nurse speaks with the son and home-attendant (certified nursing assistant) and determines the medications are not taken correctly. The patient is seen in the office and the family is contacted. Exam reveals an increase in rigidity and tremor. The blood sugar is elevated. The medications are reviewed and changed. Orders are written for the assisted-living facility. The nurse writes a detailed schedule for administration and makes sure the attendant understands the schedule. The nurse explains the schedule for follow-up blood glucose monitoring and asks for glucose and weight reports weekly. The physician makes a referral to an adult day program to reduce social isolation and to increase the hours of observation. The nurse follow up thereafter to make sure the medications are taken properly, the glucose is reasonably controlled, and progress is made toward attending adult day programs.

## Clinical Example (99489)

A 92-year-old male living in an assisted-living facility with Parkinsons disease, mild dementia, depression and diabetes mellitus continues to lose weight and remains withdrawn. The patient's family resides out of state, and an attendant sees the patient for 3 hours daily. The clinical staff has already spent 22 minutes in the month performing care coordination services, and now spends additional time.

### Description of Procedure (99489)

The clinical staff nurse speaks with the son and home attendant (certified nursing assistant) and determines the medications are not being taken correctly. The patient is seen in the office and the family is contacted. Exam reveals an increase in rigidity and tremor. The blood sugar is elevated. The medications are reviewed and changed. Orders are written for the assisted living facility. The nurse writes a detailed schedule for administration and makes sure the attendant understands the schedule. The nurse explains the schedule for follow-up blood glucose monitoring and asks for glucose and weight reports weekly. The physician makes a referral to an adult day-program to reduce social isolation and to increase the hours of observation. The nurse follow up thereafter to make sure the medications are taken properly, the glucose is reasonably controlled, and that progress is made toward attending adult day-programs. The physician speaks to the son about longer term planning, safety vs aging in place and care goals. The physician also addresses concerns raised by the adult day-care staff.

⊘=Modifier 51 Exempt   ⊙=Moderate Sedation   ✚=Add-on Code   𝒩=FDA approval pending

### Clinical Example 1 (99495)

A 6-year-old who is neurologically impaired and developmentally delayed and has a chronic seizure disorder is discharged from the hospital, after an admission for breakthrough seizures.

#### Description of Procedure 1 (99495)

Discuss patient hospital course, medication list, last laboratory values, discharge plan including timing of office visit, need for home services, follow-up laboratory studies. Discuss plan of care with office clinical staff and assure medications are ordered and delivered from local pharmacy, laboratory testing is scheduled, community support services are contacted and requested to re-institute previously delivered or newly requested services, and visits with other specialists in the community are scheduled. The patient is contacted by phone by the physician or office staff to determine his or her medical and psychosocial status within two business days of discharge. The patient's condition is ascertained, and his or her knowledge of his or her condition and treatment is assessed. Patient education is conducted and important self-treatment information is reinforced. A face-to-face office or home visit is scheduled within the next 14 business days.

### Clinical Example 2 (99495)

An 84-year-old female with hypertension and osteoarthritis is discharged from the hospital after a 1-week stay for congestive heart failure.

#### Description of Procedure 2 (99495)

The nurse care manager speaks with the patient's daughter by phone on the day after discharge, reviews her medications and makes an appointment for follow-up. Basics of congestive heart failure self-management are reviewed. The physician reviews the hospital discharge summary and speaks with the two consultants who cared for her in the hospital. At the office visit the next week, the patient's medications are reviewed. The patient is counseled about avoiding nonsteroidal anti-inflamatory drugs (NSAIDs). New prescriptions are written. Based on the discussion with the consultants, recommended follow-up outpatient diagnostic tests are arranged. The physician refers the patient for home-health services. The clinical staff nurse updates the medication list and confirms the medications are correctly administered. The physician and clinical staff monitor the weights by outbound calls/home-care technology data-feeds during the 30-day period.

### Clinical Example 1 (99496)

A 6-month-old child born at 25 weeks gestation with a diagnosis of chronic lung disease on home oxygen, diuretics, bronchodilators and high caloric formula is discharged from the hospital, after admission for respiratory failure.

#### Description of Procedure 1 (99496)

Discuss patient hospital course, medication list, last laboratory values, discharge plan, including timing of office visit, need for home services, and follow-up laboratory studies. Discuss plan of care with office clinical staff and assure medications are ordered and delivered from local pharmacy, laboratory testing is scheduled, community support services are contacted and requested to re-institute previously delivered or newly requested services, and visits with other specialists in the community are scheduled. The patient is contacted by phone by the physician or office staff to determine his or her medical and psychosocial status within two business days of discharge. The patient's condition is ascertained, and his or her knowledge of his or her condition and treatment is assessed. Patient education is conducted and important self-treatment information is reinforced. A face-to-face office or home visit is scheduled within the next 7 business days.

### Clinical Example 2 (99496)

A 93-year-old male is discharged after hospitalization for a myocardial infarction, complicated by hyperglycemia and delirium.

### Description of Procedure 2 (99496)

On the day after discharge, the physician speaks with the wife, who is concerned that the patient remains confused. The physician reviews the medication regimen and instructs the wife to discontinue one of the psychoactive medications. The wife is counseled about avoidance of anticholinergic over-the-counter (OTC) medications. The clinical staff nurse contacts the hospital to obtain the discharge summary to find out who attended the patient during the hospitalization, and which home-health agency received the referral. The physician calls the hospitalist and the consultants to clarify the indications for the medications. The patient comes to the office 3 days later, at which time the physician has received and reviewed additional records, makes further adjustments to the medication regimen, including tapering anti-diabetic medications that are no longer necessary with resolution of the stressors. Care goals are reviewed (resuscitation status, glycemic control and lipid goals in a patient with limited life expectancy). Additional diagnostic/monitoring tests are ordered. The nurse care-manager calls the wife several days later to follow up, and the patient is managed for 30 days with additional nurse-calls to monitor progress in resolution of the delirium and blood glucose testing.

⊘=Modifier 51 Exempt    ⊙=Moderate Sedation    ✚=Add-on Code    ✔=FDA approval pending

# Surgery

Numerous changes have been made to the Surgery section, which include the addition of 47 codes and deletion of 11 codes. Several codes have also been revised, including revisions related to nomenclature neutrality, which is discussed in the CPT Nomenclature Reporting Neutrality section beginning on page 1 of this book.

The Musculoskeletal section includes new codes for revision of total shoulder arthroplasty and revision of total elbow arthroplasty. The Respiratory section includes the addition of four codes to report bronchoscopy services for bronchial valves and two codes for bronchial thermoplasty. Further expansion of the Respiratory section includes new thoracentesis codes, as well as a new heading, code, and guidelines for Thoracic Stereotactic Body Radiation Therapy (SRS/SBRT).

A large number of changes have been made to the Cardiovascular System section, including the addition of codes and guidelines for Transcatheter Aortic Valve Replacement. Other changes include eight new codes that are created to address the duplication of work among the carotid angiography codes. Specific guidelines on the intended use of these eight codes and the appropriate use of modifiers 50 and 59 are also included. Further changes to the Cardiovascular System section include the addition of a new subsection entitled, Transcatheter Thrombolytic Infusion, with guidelines and four new codes that replace deleted thrombolytic infusion codes 37201 and 37209. Other sections with changes include the Digestive System and the Nervous System sections.

# Surgery Guidelines

▶Guidelines to direct general reporting of services are presented in the **Introduction.** Some of the commonalities are repeated here for the convenience of those referring to this section on **Surgery.** Other definitions and items unique to Surgery are also listed.◀

## ▶Services◀

▶Services rendered in the office, home, or hospital, consultations, and other medical services are listed in the **Evaluation and Management Services** section (99201-99499) beginning on page 11. "Special Services and Reports" (99000-99091) are listed in the **Medicine** section.◀

## ▶CPT Surgical Package Definition◀

▶By their very nature, the services to any patient are variable. The CPT codes that represent a readily identifiable surgical procedure thereby include, on a procedure-by-procedure basis, a variety of services. In defining the specific services "included" in a given CPT surgical code, the following services are always included in addition to the operation per se:

- Local infiltration, metacarpal/metatarsal/digital block or topical anesthesia

- Subsequent to the decision for surgery, one related Evaluation and Management (E/M) encounter on the date immediately prior to or on the date of procedure (including history and physical)

- Immediate postoperative care, including dictating operative notes, talking with the family and other physicians or other qualified health care professionals

- Writing orders

- Evaluating the patient in the postanesthesia recovery area

- Typical postoperative follow-up care◀

## ▶Supplied Materials◀

▶Supplies and materials (eg, sterile trays/drugs), over and above those usually included with the procedure(s) rendered are reported separately. List drugs, trays, supplies, and materials provided. Identify as 99070 or specific supply code.◀

## Reporting More Than One Procedure/Service

▶When more than one procedure/service is performed on the same date, same session or during a post-operative period (subject to the "surgical package" concept), several CPT modifiers may apply (see Appendix A [*CPT 2013* codebook] for definition).◀

# Surgery

## Skin, Subcutaneous, and Accessory Structures

### OTHER FLAPS AND GRAFTS

►Code 15740 describes a cutaneous flap, transposed into a nearby but not immediately adjacent defect, with a pedicle that incorporates an anatomically named axial vessel into its design. The flap is typically transferred through a tunnel underneath the skin and sutured into its new position. The donor site is closed directly.◄

Neurovascular pedicle procedures are reported with 15750. This code includes not only skin but also a functional motor or sensory nerve(s). The flap serves to reinnervate a damaged portion of the body dependent on touch or movement (eg, thumb).

Repair of donor site requiring skin graft or local flaps should be reported as an additional procedure.

►For random island flaps, V-Y subcutaneous flaps, advancement flaps, and other flaps from adjacent areas without clearly defined anatomically named axial vessels, see 14000-14302.◄

▲**15740**    Flap; island pedicle requiring identification and dissection of an anatomically named axial vessel

**15750**       neurovascular pedicle

 **Rationale**

As a result of the AMA/Specialty Society RVS Update Committee (RUC) analysis, code 15740 has been identified through the site of service screen and fastest growing screen as potentially misvalued. Therefore, code 15740 has been revised to clearly describe an island pedicle flap by adding the phrase "requiring identification and dissection of an anatomically named axial vessel" to the code descriptor.

To clarify the reporting of this service, the cross-reference note following 15750 has been moved to the introductory guidelines for the Other Flaps and Grafts subsection and revised to include more specific flaps. The introductory guidelines were further modified to include the phrase "anatomically named" within the first sentence by using more specific terminology to describe the flap.

## Breast

### EXCISION

**19271**    Excision of chest wall tumor involving ribs, with plastic reconstruction; without mediastinal lymphadenectomy

**19272**       with mediastinal lymphadenectomy

►(Do not report 19260, 19271, 19272 in conjunction with 32100, 32503, 32504, 32551, 32554, 32555)◄

**Rationale**

In support of the deletion of thoracentesis with insertion of chest tube code 32422 and the establishment of new codes 32554 and 32555, the exclusionary parenthetical note following code 19272 has been revised to include codes 32554 and 32555 as codes that should not be reported in conjunction with codes 19260, 19271, and 19272.

# Musculoskeletal System

## General

### GRAFTS (OR IMPLANTS)

**+ 20930**   Allograft, morselized, or placement of osteopromotive material, for spine surgery only (List separately in addition to code for primary procedure)

▶(Use 20930 in conjunction with 22319, 22532, 22533, 22548-22558, 22590-22612, 22630, 22633, 22634, 22800-22812, 0195T, 0196T)◀

**+ 20931**   Allograft, structural, for spine surgery only (List separately in addition to code for primary procedure)

▶(Use 20931 in conjunction with 22319, 22532-22533, 22548-22558, 22590-22612, 22630, 22633, 22634, 22800-22812)◀

**+ 20936**   Autograft for spine surgery only (includes harvesting the graft); local (eg, ribs, spinous process, or laminar fragments) obtained from same incision (List separately in addition to code for primary procedure)

▶(Use 20936 in conjunction with 22319, 22532, 22533, 22548-22558, 22590-22612, 22630, 22633, 22634, 22800-22812, 0195T, 0196T)◀

**+ 20937**      morselized (through separate skin or fascial incision) (List separately in addition to code for primary procedure)

▶(Use 20937 in conjunction with 22319, 22532, 22533, 22548-22558, 22590-22612, 22630, 22633, 22634, 22800-22812, 0195T, 0196T)◀

**+ 20938**      structural, bicortical or tricortical (through separate skin or fascial incision) (List separately in addition to code for primary procedure)

▶(Use 20938 in conjunction with 22319, 22532, 22533, 22548-22558, 22590-22612, 22630, 22633, 22634, 22800-22812)◀

▶(For needle aspiration of bone marrow for the purpose of bone grafting, use 38220. Do not report 38220-38230 for bone marrow aspiration for platelet rich stem cell injection. For bone marrow aspiration for platelet rich stem cell injection, use 0232T)◀

**Rationale**

Combined arthrodesis codes 22633 and 22634 have been added to the inclusionary parenthetical notes following codes 20930-20938, indicating that 22633 and 22634 may be reported in conjunction with these codes.

In support of changes made to parenthetical notes following code 38220 and Category III code 0232T, the instructional note following Category I code 20938 has been revised to clarify the reporting of code 0232T for the harvest, preparation, and injection of platelet-rich stem cells derived by bone marrow aspiration, as opposed to code 38220.

To differentiate, code 38220 may be used for needle aspiration of bone marrow for the purpose of bone grafting or aspiration of bone marrow for diagnostic purposes. Although the parenthetical instruction following code 20938 directs users to code 38220, in this instance code 38220 involves aspiration of bone marrow for grafting in an arthrodesis procedure. When the bone marrow is obtained prior to the arthrodesis, the placement of the bone marrow aspirate is included as part of the arthrodesis procedure and not reported separately.

## Spine (Vertebral Column)

### VERTEBRAL BODY, EMBOLIZATION OR INJECTION

⊙**22520** Percutaneous vertebroplasty (bone biopsy included when performed), 1 vertebral body, unilateral or bilateral injection; thoracic

⊙**22521**     lumbar

⊙✚▲**22522**     each additional thoracic or lumbar vertebral body (List separately in addition to code for primary procedure)

 **Rationale**

The moderate sedation symbol has been added to percutaneous vertebroplasty add-on code 22522. Moderate sedation is an inclusive component of code 22522 and should not be separately reported.

### ARTHRODESIS

#### Anterior or Anterolateral Approach Technique

**22554** Arthrodesis, anterior interbody technique, including minimal discectomy to prepare interspace (other than for decompression); cervical below C2

▶(Do not report 22554 in conjunction with 63075, even if performed by a separate individual. To report anterior cervical discectomy and interbody fusion at the same level during the same session, use 22551)◄

**22558**     lumbar

▶(For arthrodesis using pre-sacral interbody technique, see 22586, 0195T)◄

**+ 22585**     each additional interspace (List separately in addition to code for primary procedure)

(Use 22585 in conjunction with 22554, 22556, 22558)

▶(Do not report 22585 in conjunction with 63075, even if performed by a separate individual. To report anterior cevical discectomy and interbody fusion at the same level during the same session, use 22552)◀

**●22586**     Arthrodesis, pre-sacral interbody technique, including disc space preparation, discectomy, with posterior instrumentation, with image guidance, includes bone graft when performed, L5-S1 interspace

▶(Do not report 22586 in conjunction with 20930-20938, 22840, 22848, 72275, 77002, 77003, 77011, 77012)◀

## 📝 Rationale

To redirect users regarding the appropriate codes to report to identify arthrodesis using the pre-sacral interbody technique, a parenthetical note has been added following arthrodesis code 22558.

Code 22586 is used to report arthrodesis using a presacral interbody technique. The procedure inherently includes all effort necessary to perform the fusion procedure. This includes preparation of the disc space (at L5-S1), discectomy at this level, posterior instrumentation, imaging necessary for provision of the procedure, and bone grafting performed at the level of arthrodesis for this procedure. As a result, a parenthetical note has been added following code 22586 that restricts use of this code in conjunction with all procedures previously noted (20930-20938, to identify bone grafting at this level; 22840 and 22848, to identify posterior instrumentation at the presacral interbody fusion level; and 72275, 77002, 77003, 77011, and 77012, to identify imaging needed to perform the procedure). An additional parenthetical note has been placed following code 22558, which directs users to appropriate codes to indentify open (22586) and percutaneous (0195T) pre-sacral interbody fusion techniques. In addition, also see the discussion regarding CPT nomenclature reporting neutrality for more information on the change to the parenthetical following code 22554. To further clarify the intention, exclusionary parenthetical notes have been added following the aforementioned imaging code to direct users to the correct codes to identify this procedure.

## SPINAL INSTRUMENTATION

**+ 22840**     Posterior non-segmental instrumentation (eg, Harrington rod technique, pedicle fixation across 1 interspace, atlantoaxial transarticular screw fixation, sublaminar wiring at C1, facet screw fixation) (List separately in addition to code for primary procedure)

▶(Use 22840 in conjunction with 22100-22102, 22110-22114, 22206, 22207, 22210-22214, 22220-22224, 22305-22327, 22532, 22533, 22548-22558, 22590-22612, 22630, 22633, 22634, 22800-22812, 63001-63030, 63040-63042, 63045-63047, 63050-63056, 63064, 63075, 63077, 63081, 63085, 63087, 63090, 63101, 63102, 63170-63290, 63300-63307)◀

**+ 22841**  Internal spinal fixation by wiring of spinous processes (List separately in addition to code for primary procedure)

▶(Use 22841 in conjunction with 22100-22102, 22110-22114, 22206, 22207, 22210-22214, 22220-22224, 22305-22327, 22532, 22533, 22548-22558, 22590-22612, 22630, 22633, 22634, 22800-22812, 63001-63030, 63040-63042, 63045-63047, 63050-63056, 63064, 63075, 63077, 63081, 63085, 63087, 63090, 63101, 63102, 63170-63290, 63300-63307)◀

**+ 22842**  Posterior segmental instrumentation (eg, pedicle fixation, dual rods with multiple hooks and sublaminar wires); 3 to 6 vertebral segments (List separately in addition to code for primary procedure)

▶(Use 22842 in conjunction with 22100-22102, 22110-22114, 22206, 22207, 22210-22214, 22220-22224, 22305-22327, 22532, 22533, 22548-22558, 22590-22612, 22630, 22633, 22634, 22800-22812, 63001-63030, 63040-63042, 63045-63047, 63050-63056, 63064, 63075, 63077, 63081, 63085, 63087, 63090, 63101, 63102, 63170-63290, 63300-63307)◀

**+ 22843**      7 to 12 vertebral segments (List separately in addition to code for primary procedure)

▶(Use 22843 in conjunction with 22100-22102, 22110-22114, 22206, 22207, 22210-22214, 22220-22224, 22305-22327, 22532, 22533, 22548-22558, 22590-22612, 22630, 22633, 22634, 22800-22812, 63001-63030, 63040-63042, 63045-63047, 63050-63056, 63064, 63075, 63077, 63081, 63085, 63087, 63090, 63101, 63102, 63170-63290, 63300-63307)◀

**+ 22844**      13 or more vertebral segments (List separately in addition to code for primary procedure)

▶(Use 22844 in conjunction with 22100-22102, 22110-22114, 22206, 22207, 22210-22214, 22220-22224, 22305-22327, 22532, 22533, 22548-22558, 22590-22612, 22630, 22633, 22634, 22800-22812, 63001-63030, 63040-63042, 63045-63047, 63050-63056, 63064, 63075, 63077, 63081, 63085, 63087, 63090, 63101, 63102, 63170-63290, 63300-63307)◀

**+ 22845**  Anterior instrumentation; 2 to 3 vertebral segments (List separately in addition to code for primary procedure)

▶(Use 22845 in conjunction with 22100-22102, 22110-22114, 22206, 22207, 22210-22214, 22220-22224, 22305-22327, 22532, 22533, 22548-22558, 22590-22612, 22630, 22633, 22634, 22800-22812, 63001-63030, 63040-63042, 63045-63047, 63050-63056, 63064, 63075, 63077, 63081, 63085, 63087, 63090, 63101, 63102, 63170-63290, 63300-63307)◀

**+ 22846**      4 to 7 vertebral segments (List separately in addition to code for primary procedure)

▶(Use 22846 in conjunction with 22100-22102, 22110-22114, 22206, 22207, 22210-22214, 22220-22224, 22305-22327, 22532, 22533, 22548-22558, 22590-22612, 22630, 22633, 22634, 22800-22812, 63001-63030, 63040-63042, 63045-63047, 63050-63056, 63064, 63075, 63077, 63081, 63085, 63087, 63090, 63101, 63102, 63170-63290, 63300-63307)◀

**+ 22847**      8 or more vertebral segments (List separately in addition to code for primary procedure)

▶(Use 22847 in conjunction with 22100-22102, 22110-22114, 22206, 22207, 22210-22214, 22220-22224, 22305-22327, 22532, 22533, 22548-22558, 22590-22612, 22630, 22633, 22634, 22800-22812, 63001-63030, 63040-63042, 63045-63047, 63050-63056, 63064, 63075, 63077, 63081, 63085, 63087, 63090, 63101, 63102, 63170-63290, 63300-63307)◀

**+ 22848**  Pelvic fixation (attachment of caudal end of instrumentation to pelvic bony structures) other than sacrum (List separately in addition to code for primary procedure)

⊘=Modifier 51 Exempt   ⊙=Moderate Sedation   ✚=Add-on Code   ✗=FDA approval pending

▶(Use 22848 in conjunction with 22100-22102, 22110-22114, 22206, 22207, 22210-22214, 22220-22224, 22305-22327, 22532, 22533, 22548-22558, 22590-22612, 22630, 22633, 22634, 22800-22812, 63001-63030, 63040-63042, 63045-63047, 63050-63056, 63064, 63075, 63077, 63081, 63085, 63087, 63090, 63101, 63102, 63170-63290, 63300-63307)◀

**+ 22851** Application of intervertebral biomechanical device(s) (eg, synthetic cage(s), methylmethacrylate) to vertebral defect or interspace (List separately in addition to code for primary procedure)

▶(Use 22851 in conjunction with 22100-22102, 22110-22114, 22206, 22207, 22210-22214, 22220-22224, 22305-22327, 22532, 22533, 22548-22558, 22590-22612, 22630, 22633, 22634, 22800-22812, 63001-63030, 63040-63042, 63045-63047, 63050-63056, 63064, 63075, 63077, 63081, 63085, 63087, 63090, 63101, 63102, 63170-63290, 63300-63307)◀

### ✍ Rationale

Combined arthrodesis codes 22633 and 22634 have been added to the inclusionary parenthetical notes following codes 22840-22848 and 22851, indicating that 22633 and 22634 may be reported in conjunction with these codes.

## Shoulder

### INTRODUCTION OR REMOVAL

**23330** Removal of foreign body, shoulder; subcutaneous

**23331** deep (eg, Neer hemiarthroplasty removal)

**23332** complicated (eg, total shoulder)

▶(Do not report 23331, 23332 in conjunction with 23473, 23474 if a prosthesis [ie, humeral and/or glenoid component(s)] is being removed and replaced in the same shoulder)◀

### REPAIR, REVISION, AND/OR RECONSTRUCTION

**23470** Arthroplasty, glenohumeral joint; hemiarthroplasty

**23472** total shoulder (glenoid and proximal humeral replacement (eg, total shoulder))

(For removal of total shoulder implants, see 23331, 23332)

(For osteotomy, proximal humerus, use 24400)

**●23473** Revision of total shoulder arthroplasty, including allograft when performed; humeral **or** glenoid component

**●23474** humeral **and** glenoid component

▶(Do not report 23473, 23474 in conjunction with 23331, 23332 if a prosthesis [ie, humeral and/or glenoid component(s)] is being removed and replaced in the same shoulder)◀

### ✍ Rationale

As part of the RUC Relativity Assessment Workgroup (RAW) (formerly the Five-Year Review Identification Workgroup) analysis of codes, a need for additional codes to provide greater clarity for reporting the removal and replacement of an artificial implant placed in previous total shoulder arthroplasty was identified. Two new total shoulder revision codes, 23473 and 23474, were added for revision of a total shoulder arthroplasty that includes the removal of an artificial prosthesis (ie, humeral and/or glenoid component[s]) and replacement with a new prosthesis (artificial implant) in the same shoulder at the same time. Originally, the removal component of the shoulder revision procedure was reflected in codes 23331 and 23332 and was reported separately.

Because the removal of the prosthesis is included in codes 23473 and 23474, an exclusionary note has been added following codes 23331, 23332 and 23473, 23474 to indicate that codes 23331, 23332 and 23473, 23474 should not be reported together. The term "revision" in the new codes refers to removal of a prosthesis and replacement with a new prosthesis at the same time.

### Clinical Example (23473)

A 75-year-old female had a total shoulder arthroplasty 17 years ago has pain and limited motion with radiographic evidence of component loosening. She undergoes revision of the humeral component.

**Description of Procedure (23473)**

Under anesthesia, a deltopectoral incision is made from the mid-clavicle to the junction to the mid-third of the humerus. The deltopectoral interval is opened allowing identification of the conjoined tendon. Careful protection around neurovascular structures during the case, including the axillary and musculocutaneous nerve, is imperative. The subscapularis tendon is divided, tagged, and mobilized. A wide capsular release is performed for exposure and mobilization of the proximal humerus. Dislocation of the shoulder components is performed with intraoperative inspection and assessment of the humeral component. Extensive scar tissue is excised. Extraction instruments are used to remove the loose humeral component and loose glenoid component. Meticulous preparation and cleaning of the humeral canal, including removal of the fibrous membrane and all of the cement, is performed. The wound is irrigated with liters of antibiotic fluid. Cementing or a press-fit with or without a bone graft of the humeral component within the humeral shaft is performed. Judgment and technical skill are necessary to carefully align the humeral component in the proper height and degree of retroversion to prevent postoperative subluxation or dislocation. Reattachment of the subscapularis tendon is accomplished, followed by a reapproximation of the deltopectoral interval and closure of the subcutaneous tissue and skin.

### Clinical Example (23474)

A 75-year-old female had a total shoulder arthroplasty 17 years ago has pain and limited motion with radiographic evidence of component loosening. She undergoes revision of both the humeral and glenoid components.

**Description of Procedure (23474)**

Under anesthesia, a deltopectoral incision is made from the mid-clavicle to the junction to the mid-third of the humerus. The deltopectoral interval is opened allowing identification of the conjoined tendon. Careful protection around

⊘=Modifier 51 Exempt    ⊙=Moderate Sedation    ✚=Add-on Code    ✗=FDA approval pending

neurovascular structures during the case, including the axillary and musculocutaneous nerve, is imperative. The subscapularis tendon is divided, tagged, and mobilized. A wide capsular release is performed for exposure and mobilization of the proximal humerus. Dislocation of the shoulder components is performed with intraoperative inspection and assessment of the humeral and glenoid components. Extensive scar tissue is excised. Extraction instruments are used to remove the loose humeral component and loose glenoid component. Meticulous preparation and cleaning of the humeral canal, including removal of the fibrous membrane and all of the cement, is performed. Meticulous preparation and cleaning of the glenoid, including removal of the fibrous membrane and all of the cement, is performed. The wound is irrigated with liters of antibiotic fluid. The glenoid fossa is carefully prepared to accept a properly aligned glenoid component, with or without a bone graft. This component is fixed in place with cement or screws. Judgment and technical skill are necessary to carefully align the glenoid component in the proper position and version to prevent postoperative subluxation or dislocation. Cementing or a press-fit with or without a bone graft of the humeral component within the humeral shaft is performed. Judgment and technical skill are necessary to carefully align the humeral component in the proper height and degree of retroversion to prevent postoperative subluxation or dislocation. Reattachment of the subscapularis tendon is accomplished, followed by a reapproximation of the deltopectoral interval and closure of the subcutaneous tissue and skin.

## Humerus (Upper Arm) and Elbow

### INTRODUCTION OR REMOVAL

**24160**   Implant removal; elbow joint

▶(Do not report 24160 in conjunction with 24370 or 24371 if a prosthesis [ie, humeral and/or ulnar component(s)] is being removed and replaced in the same elbow)◀

**24164**      radial head

### ▶REPAIR, REVISION, AND/OR RECONSTRUCTION◀

**24360**   Arthroplasty, elbow; with membrane (eg, fascial)

**24361**      with distal humeral prosthetic replacement

**24362**      with implant and fascia lata ligament reconstruction

**24363**      with distal humerus and proximal ulnar prosthetic replacement (eg, total elbow)

▶(For revision of total elbow implant, see 24370, 24371)◀

**24365**   Arthroplasty, radial head;

**24366**      with implant

●**24370**   Revision of total elbow arthroplasty, including allograft when performed; humeral **or** ulnar component

►(Do not report 24370, 24371 in conjunction with 24160 if a prosthesis [ie, humeral and/or ulnar component(s)] is being removed and replaced in the same elbow)◄

##  Rationale

As part of the RUC Relativity Assessment Workgroup (RAW) (formerly the Five-Year Review Identification Workgroup) analysis of codes, a need for additional codes for reporting revision of a total elbow arthroplasty, including the removal of the prosthesis and replacement with a new prosthesis (artificial implant) was identified. Originally, the removal component of the elbow revision procedure (24363) was reported separately with code 24160, but codes 24363 and 24160 were not recognized when reported together and payment denials occurred. The new codes describe the revision of a total elbow arthroplasty that includes the removal of an artificial prosthesis (ie, humeral and/or ulnar component[s]) and replacement with a new prosthesis (artificial implant) in the same elbow. The term "revision" in the new codes refers to removal of a prosthesis and replacement with a new prosthesis at the same time. A series of instructional parenthetical notes have been added to disallow the use of 24160 in conjunction with 24370 or 24371 and to reference the new revision of elbow codes following the total elbow arthroplasty code 24363.

##  Clinical Example (24370)

A 68-year-old female had a total elbow arthroplasty 15 years ago has pain and limited motion with radiographic evidence of component loosening. She undergoes revision of the humeral component.

**Description of Procedure (24370)**

Under anesthesia, a posterior elbow incision is made. The ulnar nerve is identified for protection throughout the dissection. The triceps and extensor mechanism are released from their insertion on the ulna and then displaced in a radial direction. The elbow joint is exposed, scar tissue is excised, and contractures are released from the humerus for exposure and soft tissue balancing. Extraction instruments are used to remove the loose humeral component. Meticulous preparation and cleansing of the humeral canal, including fibrous membrane and cement removal, is necessary prior to the placement of the prosthetic humeral component. A burr and saw along with cutting guides are used to cut the proximal ulna or the distal humerus as necessary. After a trial component is inserted in a correct position, the final component is inserted using cement to complete the procedure. Judgment and technical skill are necessary to carefully align the component with the proper degree of rotation. The tourniquet is released, hemostasis is obtained, the collateral ligaments are repaired, and the triceps tendon/extensor mechanism is reapproximated to the proximal ulna. The subcutaneous tissue is approximated, and the skin is closed.

## Clinical Example (24371)

A 68-year-old female had a total elbow arthroplasty 15 years ago has pain and limited motion with radiographic evidence of component loosening. She undergoes revision of both the humeral and ulnar components.

**Description of Procedure (24371)**

Under anesthesia, a posterior elbow incision is made. The ulnar nerve is identified for protection throughout the dissection. The triceps and extensor mechanism are released from their insertion on the ulna and then displaced in a radial direction. The elbow joint is exposed, scar tissue is excised, and contractures are released from the humerus and ulna for exposure and soft tissue balancing. Extraction instruments are used to remove the loose humeral and ulnar components, along with all of the fibrous membrane and cement. The proximal ulna is carefully prepared to accept a properly aligned ulnar component, with or without a bone graft. Meticulous preparation and cleansing of the humeral canal, including cement removal, is necessary prior to the placement of the prosthetic humeral component. A burr and saw along with cutting guides are used to cut the proximal ulna and the distal humerus as necessary. After trial components are inserted in a correct position, the final components are inserted using cement to complete the procedure. Judgment and technical skill are necessary to carefully align the components with the proper degree of rotation. The tourniquet is released, hemostasis is obtained, the collateral ligaments are repaired, and the triceps tendon/extensor mechanism is reapproximated to the proximal ulna. The subcutaneous tissue is approximated, and the skin is closed.

## Foot and Toes

### OTHER PROCEDURES

▲28890    Extracorporeal shock wave, high energy, performed by a physician or other qualified health care professional, requiring anesthesia other than local, including ultrasound guidance, involving the plantar fascia

(For extracorporeal shock wave therapy involving musculoskeletal system not otherwise specified, see 0019T, 0101T, 0102T)

▶(For extracorporeal shock wave therapy involving integumentary system not otherwise specified, see 0299T, 0300T)◀

▶(Do not report 28890 in conjunction with 0299T, 0300T when treating the same area)◀

### ✍ Rationale

In support of the establishment of Category III codes 0299T and 0300T, an instructional parenthetical note has been added following 28890 directing the user to codes 0299T and 0300T for the reporting of extracorporeal shock wave therapy involving the integumentary system, not otherwise specified. An exclusionary parenthetical note has also been added precluding the reporting of extracorporeal shock wave involving the plantar fascia (28890), in addition to extracorporeal shock wave involving the integumentary system (Category III codes 0299T, 0300T) when treating the same area. See also discussion on CPT nomenclature reporting neutrality.

# Application of Casts and Strapping

LOWER EXTREMITY

**Strapping—Any Age**

**29520**     Strapping; hip

**29580**          Unna boot

**29581**     Application of multi-layer compression system; leg (below knee), including ankle and foot

▶(Do not report 29581 in conjunction with 29540, 29580, 29582, 36475, 36478)◀

**29582**          thigh and leg, including ankle and foot, when performed

▶(Do not report 29582 in conjunction with 29540, 29580, 29581, 36475, 36478)◀

**29583**          upper arm and forearm

▶(Do not report 29583 in conjunction with 29584)◀

**29584**          upper arm, forearm, hand, and fingers

▶(Do not report 29584 in conjunction with 29583)◀

▶(29590 has been deleted)◀

 **Rationale**

The manual therapy technique code 97140 is considered a separate and distinct procedure from the application of a multi-layer compression bandage codes 29581, 29582, 29583, and 29584. Therefore, code 97140 has been removed from the exclusionary parenthetical notes following codes 29581, 29582, 29583, and 29584. This revision will allow appropriate reporting of all distinct procedures performed on a patient.

As a result of AMA/Specialty Society RVS Update Committee (RUC) analysis, code 29590 was indentified as part of a family of casting/strapping codes that hit the high volume utilization. While code 29590 was not part of the screen, it was reviewed as part of the family and recommended for deletion. However, it was noted that the high utilization may have been partly due to inappropriate coding. Follow-up to information provided to the RUC indicated that this service is no longer provided. Therefore, code 29590 has been deleted with a parenthetical reference added, reflecting its deletion.

# Endoscopy/Arthroscopy

**29861**     Arthroscopy, hip, surgical; with removal of loose body or foreign body

**#29916**          with labral repair

▶(Do not report 29916 in conjunction with 29915, 29862, 29863)◀

⊘=Modifier 51 Exempt   ⊙=Moderate Sedation   ✚=Add-on Code   ✗=FDA approval pending

**Rationale**

The exclusionary parenthetical note following surgical hip arthroscopy code 29916 has been revised by simplifying the language and with the addition of code 29915. Code 29915 should not be reported in conjunction with code 29916.

## Respiratory System

### Larynx

#### INTRODUCTION

⊘**31500**    Intubation, endotracheal, emergency procedure

 **Rationale**

The cross-reference following code 31500 directing users to bronchography injection procedure code 31656 has been deleted, in concert with the deletion of the corresponding radiological supervision and interpretation codes 71040 and 71060. Bronchography has now been replaced by computed tomography (CT). If bronchography is performed, the unlisted code 76499 should be reported.

### Trachea and Bronchi

#### ENDOSCOPY

▶For endoscopy procedures, code appropriate endoscopy of each anatomic site examined. Surgical bronchoscopy always includes diagnostic bronchoscopy when performed by the same physician. Codes 31622-31649 include fluoroscopic guidance, when performed.◀

⊙**31622**    Bronchoscopy, rigid or flexible, including fluoroscopic guidance, when performed; diagnostic, with cell washing, when performed (separate procedure)

⊙**31634**        with balloon occlusion, with assessment of air leak, with administration of occlusive substance (eg, fibrin glue), if performed

▶(Do not report 31634 in conjunction with 31647, 31651 at the same session)◀

⊙**31635**        with removal of foreign body

▶(For removal of implanted bronchial valves, see 31648-31649)◀

⊙**31646**        with therapeutic aspiration of tracheobronchial tree, subsequent

(For catheter aspiration of tracheobronchial tree at bedside, use 31725)

⊙●**31647**        with balloon occlusion, when performed, assessment of air leak, airway sizing, and insertion of bronchial valve(s), initial lobe

⊙●**31648**        with removal of bronchial valve(s), initial lobe

▶(For removal and insertion of a bronchial valve at the same session, see 31647, 31648, and 31651)◀

---

⊙➕●**31649**        with removal of bronchial valve(s), each additional lobe (List separately in addition to code for primary procedure)

▶(Use 31649 in conjunction with 31648)◀

⊙➕●**31651**        with balloon occlusion, when performed, assessment of air leak, airway sizing, and insertion of bronchial valve(s), each additional lobe (List separately in addition to code for primary procedure[s])

▶(Use 31651 in conjunction with 31647)◀

▶(31656 has been deleted. To report, use 31899)◀

### 🖎 Rationale

Codes 31647, 31648, 31649, and 31651 have been added to report bronchoscopy services for the insertion and removal of bronchial valves. These codes are intended to replace Category III codes 0250T, 0251T, and 0252T when these services are performed. Each of the codes includes additional descriptor information that was formerly included as part of the Category III codes, which were used to identify these services.

Code 31647 is used to report bronchoscopy with airway sizing, assessment of air leak, balloon occlusion (when performed), and insertion of bronchial valve(s) for the initial lobe for which this service is provided. Code 31651 has been added to identify these procedures when performed for additional lobes. A parenthetical note listed after this code informs users to report code 31647 for the add-on procedure.

Code 31648 identifies the removal of bronchial valve(s) from the initial lobe. When an insertion and removal procedures is provided during the same session, users are directed to report code 31647, 31648, and 31651 according to the specific services provided (an instructional parenthetical note has been placed following code 31648 to note this).

If bronchial valves are removed from additional lobes, then code 31649 is used to report the additional service, as this code is intended to be used only when removal of bronchial valves is provided for additional lung lobes. Because this code is an add-on code, language within the descriptor and a parenthetical note listed after the code instructs users regarding the appropriate method of reporting this service.

To accommodate the changes made, additional parenthetical notes have been included following existing codes 31634 and 31635 to: (1) exclude report of the bronchial valve insertion codes in addition to code 31634 (which is inherently included as part of these services); and (2) to direct users to the correct codes to report for removal of implanted bronchial valves (31648-31649). In addition, bronchoscopy with injection of contrast material for segmental bronchography code 31656 has been deleted, as bronchography has now been replaced by use of computed tomography. A parenthetical note has been added directing users to unlisted code 31899 in the event that this procedure is performed.

Because many of these procedures inherently include moderate sedation, the moderate sedation symbol has been included for those codes.

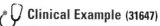 **Clinical Example** (31647)

A 64-year-old female with a persistent air leak after a surgical resection. Air leak (bronchopleural fistula) has not resolved with chest tube to suction for several days. During the bronchoscopy, the leak is identified in one lobe and bronchial valve(s) is inserted.

### Description of Procedure (31647)

After the air leak is localized, a sizing balloon is inflated in the target airway to measure the size of the airway and to determine the appropriate bronchial valve size for the selected airway. An appropriately sized bronchial valve is then loaded into a deployment catheter. The bronchoscope is advanced to the target bronchus, and the deployment catheter, which is introduced via the working channel, is positioned in the target airway orifice under direct vision. The valve is then deployed. The catheter is removed from the bronchoscope and correct positioning of the bronchial valve is confirmed. The sizing, loading, and insertion steps are repeated for additional valves inserted in the appropriate subsegments of a given lobe.

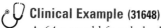 **Clinical Example** (31648)

A 64-year-old female had endobronchial valve(s) placed in a single lobe for control of a persistent air leak. Removal of the valve(s) is indicated from one lobe.

### Description of Procedure (31648)

Bronchoscopy is performed to identify the target valve(s) and conditions affecting removal. Removal is accomplished by clearing any obstruction and then using the appropriate forceps or other retrieval device introduced via the working channel of the bronchoscope and directed to the target valve. The removal rod on the bronchial valve is grasped using the forceps, and the valve is gently pulled until it dislodges from the airway wall. The valve is pulled as close as possible to the end of the bronchoscope. The bronchoscope and valve are carefully withdrawn from the patient, with care taken to navigate the valve within the endotracheal tube or rigid bronchoscope to prevent dislodgment. Intubation is strongly recommended to avoid potential valve dislodgement at the vocal cords or in the posterior oropharynx. Intraoperative fluoroscopy may also be required to facilitate valve removal in some cases

**Clinical Example** (31649)

A 59-year-old male had endobronchial valve(s) placed in more than one lobe for control of a persistent air leak. Removal of the valves from both lobes is indicated. The valve from the first lobe has been removed (reported separately) and now the second valve is removed..

### Description of Procedure (31649)

Bronchoscopy is performed to identify the target valve(s) and conditions affecting removal. Removal is accomplished by clearing any obstruction and then using the appropriate forceps or other retrieval device introduced via the working channel of the bronchoscope and directed to the target valve. The removal rod on the bronchial valve is grasped using the forceps, and the valve is gently pulled until it dislodges from the airway wall. The valve is pulled as close as possible to the end of the bronchoscope. The bronchoscope and valve are carefully withdrawn from the patient, with care taken to navigate the valve within the endotracheal tube or rigid bronchoscope to prevent dislodgment. Intubation is strongly recommended to avoid potential valve dislodgement at the vocal cords or in the posterior oropharynx. Intraoperative fluoroscopy may also be required to facilitate valve removal in some cases. The process is repeated until all target valves are removed.

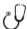

### Clinical Example (31651)

A 64-year-old female with a persistent air leak after a surgical resection. Air leak (bronchopleural fistula) has not resolved with chest tube to suction for several days. Leak has not resolved with bronchial valve(s) insertion into one lobe and a leak has been identified in an additional lobe, and bronchial valve(s) is inserted.

### Description of Procedure (31651)

Additional lobe(s) is also determined to be source of leak. A sizing balloon is inflated in the target airway to measure the size of the airway and to determine the appropriate bronchial valve size for the selected airway. An appropriately sized bronchial valve is loaded into a deployment catheter. The bronchoscope is advanced to the target bronchus, and the deployment catheter, which is introduced via the working channel, is positioned in the target airway orifice under direct vision. The valve is then deployed. The catheter is removed from the bronchoscope, and correct positioning of the bronchial valve is confirmed. The sizing, loading, and insertion steps are repeated for additional valves inserted in appropriate subsegments of a given lobe.

### ▶BRONCHIAL THERMOPLASTY◀

⊙●**31660**    Bronchoscopy, rigid or flexible, including fluoroscopic guidance, when performed; with bronchial thermoplasty, 1 lobe

⊙●**31661**        with bronchial thermoplasty, 2 or more lobes

 **Rationale**

Codes 31660 and 31661 have been added to report bronchial thermoplasty. These codes replace Category III codes 0276T and 0277T. To accommodate the placement for these codes and to allow better identification of these procedures, a new section heading has been added to the CPT code set to identify bronchial thermoplasty procedures.

For more information regarding the deletion of codes 0276T and 0277T, see the Rationale regarding these codes.

Asthma is traditionally treated with pharmaceuticals and the avoidance of asthma triggers. Bronchial thermoplasty is a stand-alone, therapeutic bronchoscopic procedure involving the use of a radiofrequency ablation device for the treatment of airway smooth muscle. Typically destructive procedures such as thermoplasty are used for the destruction of tissue such as for the removal of a tumor. This procedure differs, however, because it involves treatment of all central airways and is performed through a standard bronchoscope. The procedure is generally used

⃠=Modifier 51 Exempt   ⊙=Moderate Sedation   ✚=Add-on Code   ✗=FDA approval pending

to treat patients with severe asthma (ie, patients not well controlled on the best available medications).

 **Clinical Example (31660)**

A 40-year-old woman presents with a history of poorly controlled severe asthma. Bronchial thermoplasty is performed on either lower lobe.

### Description of Procedure (31660)

In this procedure, the physician uses the energy created from high-frequency radio waves to reduce airway smooth muscle tissue in the bronchial walls of the lung. The physician skilled in bronchoscopy, working with a skilled bronchoscopic assistant, directs the bronchoscope and operates the catheter. Effective treatment with the radiofrequency catheter requires appropriate patient sedation throughout the procedure. A standard patient return electrode is affixed to the patient to provide a complete circuit. After the attending physician or anesthesiologist administers the appropriate sedation, a standard flexible bronchoscope is inserted through the nose or mouth for access to the lung. A detailed inspection of the targeted lobe(s) of the lung is performed to plan the application of bronchial thermoplasty, thereby ensuring that the entire length of each and every accessible bronchial tube in the targeted lobe(s) is treated. A small radiofrequency catheter with an expandable electrode array is advanced through the accessory channel of a standard bronchoscope and positioned under direct bronchoscopic visualization into the first treatment area of the targeted lobe(s). The electrode array is then expanded and held in contact with the bronchial wall for up to 10 seconds while the radiofrequency controller delivers energy to the location. The bronchoscope and catheter are repositioned systematically approximately 55 times, such that the electrode array is brought into contact with the entire length of each and every accessible bronchial tube in the targeted lobe(s), thereby providing consistent and thorough thermal treatment throughout the targeted lung region.

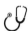 **Clinical Example (31661)**

A 40-year-old woman presents with a history of poorly controlled severe asthma, previously treated with bronchial thermoplasty on the lower lobes. Bronchial thermoplasty will be performed on both upper lobes.

### Description of Procedure (31661)

The procedure is similar to the procedure described for code 31660 but it is longer in scope, as it involves navigating the tortuous anatomy of the upper airways and covers more geography than either lower lobe. The bronchoscope and catheter are repositioned systematically approximately 75 times, such that the electrode array is brought into contact with the entire length of each and every accessible bronchial tube in the targeted lobe(s), thereby providing consistent and thorough thermal treatment throughout the targeted lung region.

## INTRODUCTION

▶(31715 has been deleted. To report, use 31899)◀

 **Rationale**

Transtracheal bronchography injection code 31715 has been deleted in concert with the deletion of the corresponding radiologic supervision and interpretation codes 71040 and 71060. Bronchography has now been replaced by use of computed tomography (CT). A parenthetical note has been added directing users to unlisted code 31899 in the event that transtracheal bronchography injection for bronchography is performed.

## Lungs and Pleura

### REMOVAL

▶(32420 has been deleted. To report, use 32405)◀

▶(32421 and 32422 have been deleted. To report, see 32554, 32555)◀

**32503** Resection of apical lung tumor (eg, Pancoast tumor), including chest wall resection, rib(s) resection(s), neurovascular dissection, when performed; without chest wall reconstruction(s)

**32504**      with chest wall reconstruction

▶(Do not report 32503, 32504 in conjunction with 19260, 19271, 19272, 32100, 32551, 32554, 32555)◀

### INTRODUCTION AND REMOVAL

⊙**32550** Insertion of indwelling tunneled pleural catheter with cuff

▶(Do not report 32550 in conjunction with 32554, 32555)◀

(If imaging guidance is performed, use 75989)

⊙▲**32551** Tube thoracostomy, includes connection to drainage system (eg, water seal), when performed, open (separate procedure)

⊙**32553** Placement of interstitial device(s) for radiation therapy guidance (eg, fiducial markers, dosimeter), percutaneous, intra-thoracic, single or multiple

(Report supply of device separately)

(For percutaneous placement of interstitial device[s] for intra-abdominal, intrapelvic, and/or retroperitoneal radiation therapy guidance, use 49411)

●**32554** Thoracentesis, needle or catheter, aspiration of the pleural space; without imaging guidance

●**32555**      with imaging guidance

●**32556** Pleural drainage, percutaneous, with insertion of indwelling catheter; without imaging guidance

●**32557**      with imaging guidance

▶(For insertion of indwelling tunneled pleural catheter with cuff, use 32550)◀

⊘=Modifier 51 Exempt   ⊙=Moderate Sedation   ✚=Add-on Code   𝒩=FDA approval pending

►(For open procedure, use 32551)◄

►(Do not report 32554-32557 in conjunction with 32550, 32551, 76942, 77002, 77012, 77021, 75989)◄

## 🖋 Rationale

Codes 32554-32557 have been developed to identify pleural fluid aspiration (32554, 32555) and percutaneous pleural drainage (32556, 32557) procedures. These codes were developed to more accurately identify the type of procedure being provided (thoracocentesis versus drainage). To accommodate the addition of the new codes, codes 32420-32422 have been deleted, and parenthetical notes placed to direct users to the appropriate codes to report: (1) biopsy of the lung or mediastinum using a percutaneous needle (32405); and (2) aspiration of the pleural space (using a needle or a catheter) without imaging (32554) or with imaging (32555). A parenthetical note following code 32557 also directs users to code 32550 to identify insertion of an indwelling tunneled pleural catheter. To provide further instruction, an additional note has been placed following code 32550 to restrict the use of this code in conjuction with any of the thoracocentesis procedures. An exclusionary parenthetical note has also been placed following code 32557 to restrict the use of these codes (ie, 32554-32557) in conjunction with the aforementioned codes used to indentify the insertion of an indwelling tunneled pleural catheter (32550), tube thoracostomy (32551), and imaging needed to complete the procedure (75989, 76942, 77002, 77012, 77021). Similar exclusionary notes have also been placed following codes 75989, 76942, 77002, 77012, and 77021 to note exclusion of the use of these codes in conjunction with codes 32554-32557. For more information regarding exclusionary notes included for imaging services, see the Rationale sections that follow the appropriate imaging code.

Tube thoracostomy code 32551 has been revised to identify that this is an open procedure by adding the term "open" to the descriptor language. The example language (eg, for abscess, hemothorax, empyema) in the descriptor has been revised with the removal of the abscess, hemothorax, and empyema examples and the addition of water seal as an example. Language was also added to note that "connection to drainage system" is inherently included as part of the service.

To further clarify the intent for use of this code, the diagram previously included to identify code 32551 in the CPT codebook has been deleted. In addition, an instructional parenthetical note has been included following code 32557 to direct users to this open procedure for pleural fluid drainage.

A number of factors precipitated the change to code 32551. Despite the fact that the descriptor included the word "thoracostomy", which inherently identifies the procedure as "open", intended use for this code may have been confusing due to the inclusion of the examples of "hemothorax" and "empyema." Removal of these examples makes the language consistent with current CPT terminology, as code descriptors identify physician work and do not imply use for a particular condition.

## 🩺 Clinical Example (32551)

A 24-year-old patient presents to the emergency room after a motor vehicle collision. Breath sounds are diminished and a large right hemothorax is diagnosed. Via a thoracostomy (ie, open cutdown incision), a chest tube is inserted.

**Description of Procedure (32551)**

An incision is made over the rib below the interspace of the intended tube placement. Blunt dissection is carried out through all layers from the skin down through the subcutaneous tissues with additional administration of local anesthesia. The chest wall muscles are bluntly dissected, including the deep intercostal muscles and pleura. The clinician's finger is inserted down into the pleural cavity, digitally sweeping the thoracic cavity. Any fluid or blood under pressure is evacuated. A large bore thoracostomy tube is inserted into the pleural cavity, directed superiorly and posteriorly. Layered closure of muscle and skin is performed. A drainage system is attached, and the tube is fixed to the skin with tape.

 **Clinical Example (32554)**

A 74-year-old male patient presents short of breath with a chest x-ray showing a large left pleural effusion. Bedside aspiration is performed for diagnosis.

**Description of Procedure (32554)**

Chest is prepped and draped in the usual sterile fashion. One percent subcutaneous lidocaine solution is instilled as a local anesthetic. Fluid is obtained via needle aspiration. Puncture site is sterilely dressed. A sample of the fluid is sent to the laboratory for analysis.

 **Clinical Example (32555)**

A 57-year-old male patient presents with pneumonia and persistent fever despite antibiotic therapy. Aspiration of his parapneumonic effusion is performed with real-time ultrasound guidance.

**Description of Procedure (32555)**

A preliminary ultrasound of the chest is performed to localize the pleural fluid and target the site for drainage. Images are recorded. The chest is then prepped and draped in the usual sterile fashion. The skin and deeper tissues down to the parietal pleura are infiltrated with a local anesthetic under ultrasound guidance, taking care to avoid vessels. A thoracentesis catheter is advanced into the pleural effusion under ultrasound guidance and secured in place temporarily. Through the catheter, a variable amount of fluid is drained. The catheter is removed. The puncture site is dressed appropriately. A sample of fluid is sent to the laboratory for analysis.

 **Clinical Example (32556)**

A 72-year-old male patient presents with acute shortness of breath. Chest x-ray shows a right pneumothorax. Bedside chest tube placement is performed.

**Description of Procedure (32556)**

Chest is prepped and draped in the usual sterile fashion. One percent subcutaneous lidocaine solution is instilled as a local anesthetic. Catheter is placed through the intercostal space, secured in place, and connected to the suction drainage. Puncture site is then sterilely dressed.

⊘=Modifier 51 Exempt  ⊙=Moderate Sedation  ✚=Add-on Code  ✗=FDA approval pending

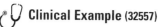

## Clinical Example (32557)

A 60-year-old male patient presents with fever and shortness of breath. CT scan shows a complex parapneumonic effusion. Concern is for an empyema. Image-guided pleural drainage tube placement is performed.

### Description of Procedure (32557)

Moderate sedation is administered. A preliminary CT scan of the chest is performed to confirm the presence of a pleural fluid collection (empyema) and target the site for drainage. Images are recorded. The chest is prepped and draped in the usual sterile fashion. The skin and deeper tissues down to the parietal pleura are infiltrated with a local anesthetic under CT guidance, taking care to avoid vessels. A needle is advanced into the pleural collection under CT guidance, and a guidewire is advanced through the needle. Tract to the pleural space is dilated using a series of fascial dilators. A multiside hole drainage catheter is advanced into the pleural collection under CT guidance and secured in place temporarily. The catheter is secured in place and connected to the suction drainage. Postprocedure CT images may be obtained (included in procedure code). The puncture site is dressed appropriately. A sample of fluid is sent to the laboratory for analysis.

### ►STEREOTACTIC RADIATION THERAPY ◄

►Thoracic stereotactic body radiation therapy (SRS/SBRT) is a distinct procedure which may involve collaboration between a surgeon and radiation oncologist. The surgeon identifies and delineates the target for therapy. The radiation oncologist reports the appropriate code(s) for clinical treatment planning, physics and dosimetry, treatment delivery and management from the Radiation Oncology section (see 77295, 77331, 77370, 77373, 77435). The same physician should not report target delineation services with radiation treatment management codes (77427-77499).

Target delineation involves specific determination of tumor borders to identify tumor volume and relationship with adjacent structures (eg, chest wall, intraparenchymal vasculature and atelectatic lung) and previously placed fiducial markers, when present. Target delineation also includes availability to identify and validate the thoracic target prior to treatment delivery when a fiducial-less tracking system is utilized.

Do not report target delineation more than once per entire course of treatment when the treatment requires greater than one session.◄

●32701    Thoracic target(s) delineation for stereotactic body radiation therapy (SRS/SBRT), (photon or particle beam), entire course of treatment

►(Do not report 32701 in conjunction with 77261-77799)◄

►(For placement of fiducial markers, see 31626, 32553)◄

### Rationale

Because current approved technology allows stereotactic body radiation (SRS/SBRT) to be performed in the thoracic region of the body, a new code (32701), guidelines, and a new heading have been added to the Respiratory System section for reporting thoracic target delineation for SRS/SBRT. Code 32701 is intended to describe noncranial or nonspinal stereotactic radiosurgery, or stereotactic body radiation therapy performed in the thoracic region of the body.

Thoracic stereotactic body radiation therapy is a distinct procedure that utilizes externally generated ionizing radiation to inactivate or eradicate defined target(s) in the body without the need to make an incision. The target is defined by, and the treatment is delivered using high-resolution stereotactic imaging.

The introductory guidelines describe the critical and nonduplicative physician work included in the process of care for SRS/SBRT. The guidelines indicate that the same physician should not report target delineation services (32701) with radiation treatment management codes (77427-77499).

The introductory language also describes each component of the service involved in target delineation. Target delineation code 32701 should not be reported more than once per entire course of treatment, when the treatment requires greater than one session.

Two parenthetical notes have been added following code 32701. The first note instructs that code 32701 should not be reported in conjunction with codes 77261-77799. The second note directs users to codes 31626 and 32553 for the placement of fiducial markers.

### Clinical Example (32701)

A 71-year-old female with a biopsy proven 2.5 cm stage 1A non-small cell lung cancer (T1N0M0) located in the periphery of the right lower lobe is felt to be a poor surgical candidate, because of advanced chronic obstructive pulmonary disease, and is scheduled for stereotactic body radiotherapy (SRS/SBRT).

### Description of Procedure (32701)

Stereotactic computerized imaging studies (computed tomography [CT]; magnetic resonance imaging [MRI]; and/or positron emission tomography [PET]; radiology reported separately) are obtained. A CT simulation +/- respiratory gating is performed separately in radiation oncology. The physician works with the radiation oncologist to verify that the target is optimally imaged. The treatment planning computer is utilized to process all of the stereotactic and simulation images in a planning program with image fusion. The physician collaborates with the radiation oncologist to outline the target volume throughout the fused data sets and/ or maximum intensity projection data set. This process includes the integration of all imaging and functional tests previously acquired and analyzed by the physician. The physician jointly prepares the dosimetry plan with the radiation oncologist and the radiation physicist. Multiple dosimetry plans may be necessary to achieve optimal dose coverage of the target lesion while minimizing the dose to the surrounding normal structures. The plan that achieves the greatest radiation dose to the target with the least radiation risk to critical surrounding tissues is ultimately selected. The patient is then brought to the linear accelerator and positioned on the treatment table. The physician is available to make changes in the treatment plan, if optimal positioning cannot be achieved. Correct positioning of the patient is radiographically verified and treatment is delivered.

## Heart and Pericardium

### PACEMAKER OR PACING CARDIOVERTER-DEFIBRILLATOR

| | System | |
|---|---|---|
| **Transvenous Procedure** | **Pacemaker** | **Implantable Cardioverter-Defibrillator** |
| Insert transvenous single lead only without pulse generator | 33216 | 33216 |
| Insert transvenous dual leads without pulse generator | 33217 | 33217 |
| Insert transvenous multiple leads without pulse generator | 33217 + 33224 | 33217 + 33224 |
| Initial pulse generator insertion only with existing single lead | 33212 | 33240 |
| Initial pulse generator insertion only with existing dual leads | 33213 | 33230 |
| Initial pulse generator insertion only with existing multiple leads | 33221 | 33231 |
| Initial pulse generator insertion or replacement plus insertion of transvenous single lead | 33206 (atrial) or 33207 (ventricular) | 33249 |
| Initial pulse generator insertion or replacement plus insertion of transvenous dual leads | 33208 | 33249 |
| Initial pulse generator insertion or replacement plus insertion of transvenous multiple leads | 33208 + 33225 | 33249 + 33225 |
| Upgrade single chamber system to dual chamber system | 33214 (includes removal of existing   pulse generator) | 33241 + 33249 |
| Removal pulse generator only (without replacement) | 33233 | 33241 |
| Removal pulse generator with replacement pulse generator only single lead system (transvenous) | 33227 | 33262 |
| Removal pulse generator with replacement pulse generator only dual lead system (transvenous) | 33228 | 33263 |
| Removal pulse generator with replacement pulse generator only multiple lead system (transvenous) | 33229 | 33264 |
| Removal transvenous electrode only single lead system | 33234 | 33244 |
| Removal transvenous electrode only dual lead system | 33235 | 33244 |
| Removal and replacement of pulse generator and transvenous electrodes | 33233 + (33234 or 33235) + (33206 or 33207 or 33208) and 33225, when appropriate | 33241 + 33244 + 33249 and 33225, when appropriate |
| Conversion of existing system to bi-ventricular system (addition of LV lead and removal of current pulse generator with insertion of new pulse generator with bi-ventricular pacing capabilities | 33225 + 33228 or 33229 | 33225 + 33263 or 33264 |

+ ▲33225   Insertion of pacing electrode, cardiac venous system, for left ventricular pacing, at time of insertion of pacing cardioverter-defibrillator or pacemaker pulse generator (eg, for upgrade to dual chamber system) (List separately in addition to code for primary procedure)

▶(Use 33225 in conjunction with 33206, 33207, 33208, 33212, 33213, 33214, 33216, 33217, 33221, 33228, 33229, 33230, 33231, 33233, 33234, 33235, 33240, 33249, 33263, 33264)◀

▶(Use 33225 in conjunction with 33222 only with pacemaker pulse generator pocket relocation and with 33223 only with pacing cardioverter-defibrillator [ICD] pocket relocation)◀

## Rationale

Code 33222 has been removed from the parenthetical note following add-code 33225 for left ventricular pacing electrode insertion. Code 33225 was revised in 2012 to indicate that pocket revision was included. However, code 33222, *Revision or relocation of skin pocket for pacemaker*, describes pocket revision. To avoid duplicate reporting of the skin pocket procedure, code 33222 has been removed from the parenthetical listing following add-on code 33225. Further, code 33223, *Revision of skin pocket for cardioverter-defibrillator*, was not listed in the parenthetical note as a primary code for 33225. The difference between codes 33223 and 33222 (other than one referring to a pacemaker and the other referring to a cardioverter-defibrillator) is that code 33223 is restricted to skin pocket revision, while code 33222 is skin pocket revision or relocation. The difference between codes 33223 and 33222 (other than one referring to a pacemaker and the other referring to a cardioverter-defibrillator) is that code 33223 is restricted to skin pocket revision, while code 33222 is skin pocket revision or relocation.

Codes 33228, 33229, 33263, and 33264 were added to the same parenthetical instruction to accurately depict the applicable stand-alone codes. The revised descriptor for code 33225 and additional parenthetical note appropriately define the condition under which code 33222 would be separately reported in addition to code 33225 at the time of pocket relocation.

The Transvenous Procedures table includes instructions for reporting combination codes for: (a) left ventricular pacing lead placement (33224 or 33225), and (b) removal or replacement of a previously placed pacemaker or ICD generator with left ventricular lead.

### ▶HEART (INCLUDING VALVES) AND GREAT VESSELS◀

▶Patients receiving major cardiac procedures may require simultaneous cardiopulmonary bypass insertion of cannulae into the venous and arterial vasculatures with support of circulation and oxygenation by a heart-lung machine. Most services are described by codes in dyad arrangements to allow distinct reporting of procedures with or without cardiopulmonary bypass. Cardiopulmonary bypass is distinct from support of cardiac output using devices (eg, ventricular assist or intra-aortic balloon). For cardiac assist services see 33960-33983, 33990-33993.◀

33300   Repair of cardiac wound; without bypass

Ⓢ=Modifier 51 Exempt   ⊙=Moderate Sedation   ✛=Add-on Code   𝒩=FDA approval pending

**Rationale**

The Wounds of the Heart and Great Vessels subsection has been revised to "Heart (Including Valves) and Great Vessels" in order to include the cardiac valve procedure codes. A new guideline has been added to distinguish cardiopulmonary bypass from support of cardiac output using cardiac assist services (33906-33983, 33990-33993).

## CARDIAC VALVES

### Aortic Valve

▶Codes 33361-33365, 0318T are used to report transcatheter aortic valve replacement (TAVR)/transcatheter aortic valve implantation (TAVI). TAVR/TAVI requires two physician operators and all components of the procedure are reported using modifier 62.

Codes 33361-33365, 0318T include the work, when performed, of percutaneous access, placing the access sheath, balloon aortic valvuloplasty, advancing the valve delivery system into position, repositioning the valve as needed, deploying the valve, temporary pacemaker insertion for rapid pacing (33210), and closure of the arteriotomy when performed. Codes 33361-33365, 0318T include open arterial or cardiac approach.

Angiography, radiological supervision, and interpretation performed to guide TAVR/TAVI (eg, guiding valve placement, documenting completion of the intervention, assessing the vascular access site for closure) are included in these codes.

Diagnostic left heart catheterization codes (93452, 93453, 93458-93461) and the supravalvular aortography code (93567) should **not** be used with TAVR/TAVI services (33361-33365, 0318T) to report:

1. Contrast injections, angiography, roadmapping, and/or fluoroscopic guidance for the TAVR/TAVI,

2. Aorta/left ventricular outflow tract measurement for the TAVR/TAVI, or

3. Post-TAVR/TAVI aortic or left ventricular angiography, as this work is captured in the TAVR/TAVI services codes (33361-33365, 0318T).

Diagnostic coronary angiography performed at the time of TAVR/TAVI may be separately reportable if:

1. No prior catheter-based coronary angiography study is available and a full diagnostic study is performed, or

2. A prior study is available, but as documented in the medical record:

   a. The patient's condition with respect to the clinical indication has changed since the prior study, or

b. There is inadequate visualization of the anatomy and/or pathology, or

c. There is a clinical change during the procedure that requires new evaluation.

d. For same session/same day diagnostic coronary angiography services, report the appropriate diagnostic cardiac catheterization code(s) appended with modifier 59 indicating separate and distinct procedural service from TAVR/TAVI.

Diagnostic coronary angiography performed at a separate session from an interventional procedure may be separately reportable.

Other cardiac catheterization services are reported separately when performed for diagnostic purposes not intrinsic to TAVR/TAVI.

Percutaneous coronary interventional procedures are reported separately, when performed.

When transcatheter ventricular support is required in conjunction with TAVR/TAVI, the appropriate code should be reported with the appropriate ventricular assist device (VAD) procedure code (33990-33993, 33975, 33976, 33999) or balloon pump insertion code (33967, 33970, 33973).

The TAVR/TAVI cardiovascular access and delivery procedures are reported with 33361-33365, 0318T. When cardiopulmonary bypass is performed in conjunction with TAVR/TAVI, codes 33361-33365, 0318T should be reported with the appropriate add-on code for percutaneous peripheral bypass (33367), open peripheral bypass (33368), or central bypass (33369).◄

● **33361**   Transcatheter aortic valve replacement (TAVR/TAVI) with prosthetic valve; percutaneous femoral artery approach

● **33362**      open femoral artery approach

● **33363**      open axillary artery approach

● **33364**      open iliac artery approach

● **33365**      transaortic approach (eg, median sternotomy, mediastinotomy)

►(Use 0318T for transapical approach [eg, left thoracotomy])◄

+ ● **33367**      cardiopulmonary bypass support with percutaneous peripheral arterial and venous cannulation (eg, femoral vessels) (List separately in addition to code for primary procedure)

►(Use 33367 in conjunction with 33361-33365, 0318T)◄

►(Do not report 33367 in conjunction with 33368, 33369)◄

+ ● **33368**      cardiopulmonary bypass support with open peripheral arterial and venous cannulation (eg, femoral, iliac, axillary vessels) (List separately in addition to code for primary procedure)

►(Use 33368 in conjunction with 33361-33365, 0318T)◄

►(Do not report 33368 in conjunction with 33367, 33369)◄

+ ● **33369**      cardiopulmonary bypass support with central arterial and venous cannulation (eg, aorta, right atrium, pulmonary artery) (List separately in addition to code for primary procedure)

►(Use 33369 in conjunction with 33361-33365, 0318T)◄

►(Do not report 33369 in conjunction with 33367, 33368)◄

⊘=Modifier 51 Exempt   ⊙=Moderate Sedation   ✚=Add-on Code   ⫫=FDA approval pending

**33400**    Valvuloplasty, aortic valve; open, with cardiopulmonary bypass

### ✍ Rationale

The Category III codes 0256T, 0258T, and 0259T for transcatheter aortic valve replacement procedures have been moved to Category I status, with new guidelines and parenthetical notes established to instruct users on the appropriate reporting of the new codes in the Surgery/Cardiovascular System/Cardiac Valves/Aortic Valve subsection. Category III code 0257T has been deleted and replaced with Category III code 0318T for the transapical approach for transcatheter aortic valve placement. When peripheral access is inadequate, cardiac procedures involving the placement of an intracardiac prosthesis (ie, stent or valve) can be achieved through transthoracic cardiac exposure via mediastinal, thoracotomy, or subxiphoid approach. The implantation of a prosthetic aortic heart valve through a transthoracic approach can be divided into an approach procedure and a therapeutic (valve implantation) procedure because two different physicians will often perform different parts of the procedure. Namely, a cardiothoracic surgeon will provide cardiac access, and an interventional cardiologist will manipulate the wire and valve under fluoroscopy.

Therefore, codes 33361-33365 and 0318T are used to report transcatheter aortic valve replacement (TAVR) or transcatheter aortic valve implantation (TAVI). TAVR or TAVI that requires two physician operators and all components of the procedure are reported using modifier 62, *Two Surgeons*. Codes 33361-33365 and 0318T include the work, when performed, of percutaneous access, placing the access sheath, balloon aortic valvuloplasty, advancing the valve delivery system into position, repositioning the valve as needed, deploying the valve, temporary pacemaker insertion for rapid pacing (33210), and closure of the arteriotomy when performed.

Codes 33362-33365 and 0318T also include open arterial or cardiac approach. Angiography, radiological supervision, and interpretation performed to guide TAVR or TAVI are included in these codes (eg, guiding valve placement, documenting completion of the intervention, and assessing the vascular access site for closure).

The guidelines denote the circumstances in which diagnostic left heart catheterization codes (93452, 93453, 93458-93461) and the supravalvular aortography code (93567) should not be reported in addition to TAVR or TAVI services (33361-33365, 0318T). Also denoted are those circumstances in which the same session or same day diagnostic coronary angiography services, other cardiac catheterization services, and percutaneous coronary interventional procedures are reported separately, when performed.

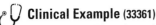

### Clinical Example (33361)

An 83-year-old male with aortic stenosis, coronary artery disease, and Class III-IV heart failure. The aortic stenosis is life-limiting and severely symptomatic, and is characterized as critical with a documented aortic valve orifice area of 0.6 cm². He has multiple additional co-morbidities that make his risk of mortality with conventional open heart aortic valve replacement greater than 10%, by objective predictive criteria. He is evaluated by the valve-team comprised of a cardiac surgeon and an interventional cardiologist, who agree that the operative risks outweigh the benefit. The team, therefore, recommends transcatheter aortic valve replacement.

### Description of Procedure (33361)

A temporary transvenous pacemaker electrode is advanced into the apex of the right ventricle and tested for proper electrical capture. Arterial access (eg, femoral, radial, or brachial) for the reference pigtail catheter is obtained by needle puncture (Seldinger technique), followed by passage of a standard guidewire and pigtail angiographic catheter. The catheter is positioned within the aortic root using fluoroscopy. A root aortogram(s) is/are obtained using power contrast injection and cineangiography to determine the optimal angiographic angle relative to the native aortic valve.

Femoral arterial access is obtained (Seldinger technique) for the valve delivery system. Angiography of the access vessel is performed to confirm anatomical suitability of the vessel for passage of the delivery catheter. Using fluoroscopic guidance, a standard guidewire is advanced to the descending aorta and exchanged for a stiff guidewire with an angiographic catheter. Over the stiff guidewire, the arteriotomy is progressively enlarged with dilators, and a large-bore vessel introducer sheath is inserted and advanced to a level that is inferior to the renal arteries. The guidewire is removed, and antithrombotic therapy is administered to achieve therapeutic anticoagulation levels.

Under fluoroscopic guidance, access across the native aortic valve is obtained using a guidewire and catheter of the physician's choice. This typically requires multiple attempts and multiple angiographic views due to the severe aortic valve stenosis. Once the guidewire is across the aortic valve and positioned in the left ventricle, a small catheter is advanced over the guidewire into the left ventricle, and the guidewire is exchanged for a stiff guidewire. Ventricular ectopy induced by the catheter/wire is frequent and may be sustained and require repositioning. A large balloon catheter is passed over the guidewire and positioned within the native aortic valve. Rapid pacing is initiated to minimize balloon movement and balloon aortic valvuloplasty is performed: the balloon is inflated by one physician while another physician continuously adjusts the balloon catheter position to minimize any potential movement and resultant left ventricular trauma or perforation. Typically, this results in hypotension and ventricular ectopy. The balloon is then rapidly deflated and the patient is monitored for hemodynamic recovery. Supravalvular aortography is performed to assess the aorta and ventricle for trauma and to assess for aortic insufficiency. Concurrently, the prosthetic valve is loaded into or onto the delivery catheter. Correct orientation of the valve on the delivery catheter is confirmed by the physician before inserting the valve-delivery catheter

⃠=Modifier 51 Exempt   ⊚=Moderate Sedation   ✚=Add-on Code   ⋏=FDA approval pending

system into the introducer sheath. The valvuloplasty catheter is exchanged for the prosthetic delivery catheter over the previously positioned stiff guidewire while maintaining access across the native aortic valve. The delivery catheter is advanced to the aortic root and positioned across the native aortic valve annulus under fluoroscopic guidance. In addition, transesophageal echocardiography may be used to position the prosthesis within the aortic annulus. (If performed, TEE is separately reported.) Multiple supravalvular aortograms may be performed to facilitate placement before a satisfactory valve position is chosen. The prosthesis is then deployed within the native aortic valve, typically during rapid ventricular pacing.

After confirming satisfactory position and function of the valve, as well as assessing the degree of any paravalvular regurgitation or presence of mechanical complications that might require open, urgent surgical intervention or coronary compromise requiring percutaneous coronary intervention, the delivery catheter, guidewire, and sheath are removed from the patient. The opening of the access artery is closed, typically via direct suture or with percutaneous suture. Percutaneous closure requires at least two separate suture delivery catheters due to the large size of the arteriotomy. The access site is monitored for adequate hemostasis. If heparin was administered, it may be reversed using protamine. A sterile dressing is applied to the entry site.

## Clinical Example (33362)

An 83-year-old male with aortic stenosis, coronary artery disease, and Class III-IV heart failure. The aortic stenosis is life-limiting and severely symptomatic, and is characterized as critical with a documented aortic valve orifice area of 0.6 cm$^2$. He has multiple additional co-morbidities that make his risk of mortality with conventional open heart aortic valve replacement greater than 10% by objective predictive criteria. He is evaluated by the valve-team comprised of a cardiac surgeon and an interventional cardiologist, who agree that the operative risks outweigh the benefit. The team therefore recommends transcatheter aortic valve replacement. The femoral vessels are found to be unsuitable for percutaneous cannulation, and an open femoral approach is utilized.

### Description of Procedure (33362)

A temporary transvenous pacemaker electrode is advanced into the apex of the right ventricle and tested for proper electrical capture. Arterial access (eg, femoral, radial, or brachial) for the reference pigtail catheter is obtained by needle puncture (Seldinger technique), followed by passage of a standard guidewire and pigtail angiographic catheter. The catheter is positioned within the aortic root using fluoroscopy. A root aortogram(s) is obtained using power contrast injection and cine angiography to determine the optimal angiographic angle relative to the native aortic valve. A skin incision is made in the inguinal region. The subcutaneous tissue is dissected until the common femoral artery is isolated. Care is taken to avoid injury to the femoral nerve and vein that lie in close proximity. The common, superficial, and deep femoral arteries are dissected and captured in vessel loops. The distal external iliac artery is typically included in the dissection. This approach facilitates introduction of the very large diameter sheath required for delivery of the transcatheter aortic valve. It also serves to apply countertraction and temporarily reduce tortuosity of the iliac arteries as the sheath is advanced. Intravenous antithrombotic therapy is begun. Angiography of the access vessel is performed to confirm anatomical suitability of the vessel for passage of the delivery catheter. A transverse arteriotomy is made in the anterior surface of the common femoral or distal-most external iliac artery. If necessary, an end-side prosthetic graft is sewn in place to facilitate catheter delivery and/or preserve distal leg perfusion. Using fluoroscopic guidance, a standard guidewire is advanced to the descending aorta and exchanged for a stiff guidewire with an angiographic catheter. Over the stiff guidewire, a large-bore vessel introducer sheath is inserted and advanced to a level that is inferior to the renal arteries.

Under fluoroscopic guidance, access across the native aortic valve is obtained using a guidewire and catheter of the physician's choice. This typically requires multiple attempts and multiple angiographic views due to the severe aortic valve stenosis. Once the guidewire is across the aortic valve and positioned in the left ventricle, a small catheter is advanced over the wire into the left ventricle, and the guidewire is exchanged for a stiff guidewire. Ventricular ectopy induced by the catheter/wire is frequent and may be sustained and require repositioning. A large balloon catheter is passed over the guidewire and positioned within the native aortic valve. Rapid pacing is initiated to minimize balloon movement and balloon aortic valvuloplasty is performed: the balloon is inflated by one physician while another physician continuously adjusts the balloon catheter position to minimize any potential movement and resultant left ventricular trauma or perforation. Typically, this results in hypotension and ventricular ectopy. The balloon is then rapidly deflated and the patient is monitored for hemodynamic recovery. Supravalvular aortography is performed to assess the aorta and ventricle for trauma and to assess for aortic insufficiency. Concurrently, the prosthetic valve is loaded into or onto the delivery catheter. Correct orientation of the valve on the delivery catheter is confirmed by the physician before inserting the valve-delivery catheter system into the introducer sheath. The valvuloplasty catheter is exchanged for the prosthetic delivery catheter over the previously positioned stiff guidewire while maintaining access across the native aortic valve. The delivery catheter is advanced to the aortic root and positioned across the native aortic valve annulus under fluoroscopic guidance. In addition, transesophageal echocardiography may be used to position the prosthesis within the aortic annulus. (If performed, TEE is separately reported.) Multiple supravalvular aortograms may be performed to facilitate placement before a satisfactory valve position is chosen. The prosthesis is then deployed within the native aortic valve, typically during rapid ventricular pacing.

After confirming satisfactory position and function of the valve, as well as assessing the degree of any paravalvular regurgitation or presence of mechanical complications that might require open, urgent surgical intervention or coronary compromise requiring percutaneous coronary intervention, the delivery catheter, guidewire, and sheath are removed from the patient. The femoral arteriotomy is repaired with very fine (eg, 6-0 polypropylene) sutures. Hemostasis is achieved, the wound is irrigated, and the soft tissue is reapproximated in several layers. Skin closure is performed with staples or sutures.

## Clinical Example (33363)

An 83-year-old male with aortic stenosis, coronary artery disease, and Class III-IV heart failure. The aortic stenosis is life-limiting and severely symptomatic, and is characterized as critical with a documented aortic valve orifice area of 0.6 cm$^2$. He has multiple additional co-morbidities that make his risk of mortality with conventional open heart aortic valve replacement greater than 10%, by objective predictive criteria. He is evaluated by the valve-team comprised of a cardiac surgeon and an interventional cardiologist, who agree that the operative risks outweigh the benefit. The team, therefore, recommends transcatheter aortic valve replacement. The patient has severe aortoiliac occlusive disease that precludes the femoral or iliac arterial approach for prosthesis delivery.

### Description of Procedure (33363)

A temporary transvenous pacemaker electrode is advanced into the apex of the right ventricle and tested for proper electrical capture. Arterial access (eg, femoral, radial, or brachial) for the reference pigtail catheter is obtained by needle puncture (Seldinger technique), followed by passage of a standard guidewire and pigtail angiographic catheter. The catheter is positioned within the aortic root using fluoroscopy. A root aortogram(s) is obtained using power contrast injection and cine angiography to determine the optimal angiographic angle relative to the native aortic valve. A subclavicular incision is made, and the subcutaneous tissue is dissected until the axillary artery is located. Care is taken to avoid injury to the axillary nerve and vein that lie in close proximity. Once adequate approach is achieved and intravenous antithrombotic therapy begun, proximal and distal vascular clamps are applied. A longitudinal arteriotomy is made. The conduit (a large diameter tubular segment of synthetic bypass graft) is brought onto the field, tailored to appropriate size, and an anastomosis of conduit to axillary artery is sutured with fine polypropylene. The conduit is clamped and vascular clamps are removed from the axillary artery. The suture line is checked for hemostasis and additional sutures are applied as required. A sheath is passed over a guidewire through the graft and a pigtail angiographic catheter is positioned within the aortic root using fluoroscopy. A root aortogram(s) is obtained using power contrast injection and cine angiography to determine the optimal angiographic angle relative to the native aortic valve. Typically, several aortograms in different angles are required.

Under fluoroscopic guidance, access across the native aortic valve is obtained using a guidewire and catheter of the physician's choice. This typically requires multiple attempts and multiple angiographic views due to the severe aortic valve stenosis. Once the guidewire is across the aortic valve and positioned in the left ventricle, a small catheter is advanced over the wire into the left ventricle, and the wire is exchanged for a stiff guidewire. Ventricular ectopy induced by the catheter/wire is frequent and may be sustained and require repositioning. A large balloon catheter is passed over the guidewire and positioned within the native aortic valve. Rapid pacing is initiated to minimize balloon movement and balloon aortic valvuloplasty is performed: the balloon is inflated by one physician while another physician continuously adjusts the balloon catheter position to minimize any potential movement and resultant left ventricular trauma or perforation. Typically, this results in hypotension and ventricular ectopy. The balloon is then rapidly deflated and the patient is monitored for hemodynamic recovery. Supravalvular aortography is performed to assess the aorta and ventricle for trauma and to assess for aortic insufficiency. Concurrently, the prosthetic valve is loaded into or onto the delivery catheter. Correct orientation of the valve on the delivery catheter is confirmed by the physician before inserting the valve-delivery catheter system into the introducer sheath. The valvuloplasty catheter is exchanged for the prosthetic delivery catheter over the previously positioned stiff guidewire while maintaining access across the native aortic valve. The delivery catheter is advanced to the aortic root and positioned across the native aortic valve annulus under fluoroscopic guidance. In addition, transesophageal echocardiography may be used to position the prosthesis within the aortic annulus. (If performed, TEE is separately reported.) Multiple supravalvular aortograms may be performed to facilitate placement before a satisfactory valve position is chosen. The prosthesis is then deployed within the native aortic valve, typically during rapid ventricular pacing.

After confirming satisfactory position and function of the valve, as well as assessing the degree of any paravalvular regurgitation or presence of mechanical complications that might require open, urgent surgical intervention or coronary compromise requiring percutaneous coronary intervention, the delivery catheter, guidewire, and sheath are removed from the patient. The axillary artery is then clamped with a partial occlusion clamp to isolate the graft, which is excised, leaving a 5- to 6-mm cuff. This is oversewn in two layers with polypropylene suture, de-aired, and the clamp removed. Hemostasis is achieved. The wound is irrigated and closed in layers.

 **Clinical Example (33364)**

An 83-year-old male with aortic stenosis, coronary artery disease, and Class III-IV heart failure. The aortic stenosis is life-limiting and severely symptomatic, and is characterized as critical with a documented aortic valve orifice area of 0.6 cm$^2$. He has multiple additional co-morbidities that make his risk of mortality with conventional open heart aortic valve replacement greater than 10%, by objective predictive criteria. He is evaluated by the valve-team comprised of a cardiac surgeon and an interventional cardiologist, who agree that the operative risks outweigh the benefit. The team, therefore, recommends transcatheter aortic valve replacement. Preoperative studies indicate that the femoral vessels are too small and diseased to permit either the percutaneous or open femoral arterial approach for prosthesis delivery and therefore an open iliac approach is selected.

**Description of Procedure (33364)**

A temporary transvenous pacemaker electrode is advanced into the apex of the right ventricle and tested for proper electrical capture. Arterial access (eg, femoral, radial, or brachial) for the reference pigtail catheter is obtained by needle puncture (Seldinger technique), followed by passage of a standard guidewire and pigtail angiographic catheter. The catheter is positioned within the aortic root using fluoroscopy. A root aortogram(s) is obtained using power contrast injection and cine angiography to determine the optimal angiographic angle relative to the native aortic valve.

$\bigcirc$=Modifier 51 Exempt  $\odot$=Moderate Sedation  ✚=Add-on Code  ⎈=FDA approval pending

A transverse suprainguinal skin incision is made and a retroperitoneal dissection plane is developed. The dissection is continued deep into the pelvis until the iliac artery is located. Care is taken to avoid injury to the nerves, veins, and ureter that lie in close proximity. The common, internal, and external iliac arteries are dissected and isolated with vessel loops. Intravenous antithrombotic therapy is administered. A longitudinal arteriotomy is made. A graft conduit (a large diameter tubular segment of synthetic bypass graft) is brought onto the field, tailored to appropriate size, and an end-to-side anastomosis of conduit to common iliac artery is sutured with fine polypropylene. The conduit is clamped and vascular clamps are removed. The suture line is checked for hemostasis and additional sutures are applied as required. A sheath is passed over a guidewire through the graft, and a pigtail angiographic catheter is positioned within the aortic root using fluoroscopy. A root aortogram(s) is obtained using power contrast injection and cine angiography to determine the optimal angiographic angle relative to the native aortic valve. Typically, several aortograms in different angles are required.

Under fluoroscopic guidance, access across the native aortic valve is obtained using a guidewire and catheter of the physician's choice. This typically requires multiple attempts and multiple angiographic views due to the severe aortic valve stenosis. Once the guidewire is across the aortic valve and positioned in the left ventricle, a small catheter is advanced over the wire into the left ventricle, and the wire is exchanged for a stiff guidewire. Ventricular ectopy induced by the catheter/wire is frequent and may be sustained and require repositioning. A large balloon catheter is passed over the guidewire and positioned within the native aortic valve. Rapid pacing is initiated to minimize balloon movement and balloon aortic valvuloplasty is performed: the balloon is inflated by one physician while another physician continuously adjusts the balloon catheter position to minimize any potential movement and resultant left ventricular trauma or perforation. Typically, this results in hypotension and ventricular ectopy. The balloon is then rapidly deflated and the patient is monitored for hemodynamic recovery. Supravalvular aortography is performed to assess the aorta and ventricle for trauma and to assess for aortic insufficiency. Concurrently, the prosthetic valve is loaded into or onto the delivery catheter. Correct orientation of the valve on the delivery catheter is confirmed by the physician before inserting the valve-delivery catheter system into the introducer sheath. The valvuloplasty catheter is exchanged for the prosthetic delivery catheter over the previously positioned stiff guidewire while maintaining access across the native aortic valve. The delivery catheter is advanced to the aortic root and positioned across the native aortic valve annulus under fluoroscopic guidance. In addition, transesophageal echocardiography may be used to position the prosthesis within the aortic annulus. (If performed, TEE is separately reported.) Multiple supravalvular aortograms may be performed to facilitate placement before a satisfactory valve position is chosen. The prosthesis is then deployed within the native aortic valve, typically during rapid ventricular pacing.

After confirming satisfactory position and function of the valve, as well as assessing the degree of any paravalvular regurgitation or presence of mechanical complications that might require open, urgent surgical intervention or coronary compromise requiring percutaneous coronary intervention, the delivery catheter, guidewire, and sheath are removed from the patient. The iliac arterial graft site is then clamped with a partial occlusion clamp to isolate the graft, which is excised, leaving a 5- to 6-mm cuff. This is oversewn in two layers with polypropylene suture, de-aired, and the clamp removed. Hemostasis is achieved. The wound is irrigated and closed in layers.

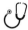 **Clinical Example (33365)**

An 83-year-old male with aortic stenosis, coronary artery disease, and Class III-IV heart failure. The aortic stenosis is life-limiting and severely symptomatic, and is characterized as critical with a documented aortic valve orifice area of 0.6 cm$^2$. He has multiple additional co-morbidities that make his risk of mortality with conventional open heart aortic valve replacement greater than 10%, by objective predictive criteria. He is evaluated by the valve-team comprised of a cardiac surgeon and an interventional cardiologist, who agree that the operative risks outweigh the benefit. The team, therefore, recommends transcatheter aortic valve replacement. Because of severe peripheral vascular disease, including severe aortoiliac, femoral and axillary artery disease, along with severe pulmonary disease that precludes a transapical approach, a direct aortic approach is recommended via either median sternotomy or mediastinotomy.

**Description of Procedure (33365)**

A temporary transvenous pacemaker electrode is advanced into the apex of the right ventricle and tested for proper electrical capture. Arterial access (eg, femoral, radial, or brachial) for the reference pigtail catheter is obtained by needle puncture (Seldinger technique), followed by passage of a standard guidewire and pigtail angiographic catheter. The catheter is positioned within the aortic root using fluoroscopy. A root aortogram(s) is obtained using power contrast injection and cine angiography to determine the optimal angiographic angle relative to the native aortic valve.

A full or partial median sternotomy incision is performed. Dissection of the thymic fat pad reveals the pericardium, which is opened vertically. Sutures are used to retract and expose the ascending aorta. Alternatively, an anterior mediastinotomy is performed to provide access to the ascending aorta. Antithromotic therapy is begun. Epiaortic ultrasonic scanning is performed to identify a disease-free site for sheath delivery. A pledgeted double pursestring suture is placed in the mid ascending aorta, and the adventia is locally dissected within the pursestring. The aorta is opened with a knife, the vascular sheath is introduced, and the pursestring suture is tightened to achieve hemostasis. A root aortogram(s) is/are obtained using power contrast injection and cine angiography to determine the optimal angiographic angle relative to the native aortic valve. Typically, several aortograms in different angles are required.

Under fluoroscopic guidance, access across the native aortic valve is obtained using a guidewire and catheter of the physician's choice. This typically requires multiple attempts and multiple angiographic views due to the severe aortic valve stenosis. Once the guidewire is across the aortic valve and positioned in the left ventricle, a small catheter is advanced over the wire into the left ventricle, and the wire is exchanged for a stiff guidewire. Ventricular ectopy induced by the catheter/

○=Modifier 51 Exempt   ◉=Moderate Sedation   ✦=Add-on Code   𝒩=FDA approval pending

wire is frequent and may be sustained and require repositioning. A large balloon catheter is passed over the guidewire and positioned within the native aortic valve. Rapid pacing is initiated to minimize balloon movement and balloon aortic valvuloplasty is performed: the balloon is inflated by one physician while another physician continuously adjusts the balloon catheter position to minimize any potential movement and resultant left ventricular trauma or perforation. Typically, this results in hypotension and ventricular ectopy. The balloon is then rapidly deflated and the patient is monitored for hemodynamic recovery. Supravalvular aortography is performed to assess the aorta and ventricle for trauma and to assess for aortic insufficiency. Concurrently, the prosthetic valve is loaded into or onto the delivery catheter. Correct orientation of the valve on the delivery catheter is confirmed by the physician before inserting the valve-delivery catheter system into the introducer sheath. The valvuloplasty catheter is exchanged for the prosthetic delivery catheter over the previously positioned stiff guidewire while maintaining access across the native aortic valve. The delivery catheter is advanced to the aortic root and positioned across the native aortic valve annulus under fluoroscopic guidance. In addition, transesophageal echocardiography may be used to position the prosthesis within the aortic annulus. (If performed, TEE is separately reported.) Multiple supravalvular aortograms may be performed to facilitate placement before a satisfactory valve position is chosen. The prosthesis is then deployed within the native aortic valve, typically during rapid ventricular pacing.

After confirming satisfactory position and function of the valve, as well as assessing the degree of any paravalvular regurgitation or presence of mechanical complications that might require open, urgent surgical intervention or coronary compromise requiring percutaneous coronary intervention, the delivery catheter and guidewire are removed from the patient. The sheath is removed from the ascending aorta and the aortic double pursestring suture is tied. Additional sutures may be required for hemostasis. The pericardium is closed over a single drain. Anticoagulation is reversed. After achieving satisfactory hemostasis, the sternum is reapproximated with stainless steel wires. The wound is irrigated and closed in layers.

###  Clinical Example (33367)

An 83-year-old male with aortic stenosis, coronary artery disease, and Class III-IV heart failure. The aortic stenosis is life-limiting and severely symptomatic, and is characterized as critical with a documented aortic valve orifice area of 0.6 cm². He has multiple additional co-morbidities that make his risk of mortality with conventional open heart aortic valve replacement greater than 10%, by objective predictive criteria. He is evaluated by the valve-team comprised of a cardiac surgeon and an interventional cardiologist, who agree that the operative risks outweigh the benefit. The team, therefore, recommends transcatheter aortic valve replacement. In the course of the procedure, the patient becomes unstable and full extracorporeal cardiopulmonary support is required. Note: This is an add-on service to the TAVR/TAVI, which is reported separately.

**Description of Procedure (33367)**

A patient undergoing transcatheter aortic valve replacement (TAVR) becomes hemodynamically unstable and cannot be stabilized with inotropic support or any standard medical means. The patient is anticoagulated. The artery and vein are cannulated with sheaths using direct percutaneous access. Guidewires are advanced into the distal abdominal aorta and into the superior vena cava. Dilators are employed to ultimately place a sufficient sized arterial cannula and a multiply ported venous drainage cannula across the right atrium into the superior vena cava. The cannulas are de-aired and connected to a cardiopulmonary bypass circuit. Cardiopulmonary bypass is initiated. Cardiopulmonary bypass with its attendant volume shifts and the activation of the inflammatory system is managed with volume replacement and alpha effector agents. Anticoagulation is maintained. Management continues while the TAVR procedure is completed. The patient's temperature, hematocrit, pH, and levels of oxygenation and electrolytes are normalized, and the patient is weaned from cardiopulmonary bypass. Anticoagulation is reversed. The cannulas are removed percutaneously. Hemostasis is achieved through percutaneous closure devices or, if necessary, open vascular repair (reported separately).

 **Clinical Example (33368)**

An 83-year-old male with aortic stenosis, coronary artery disease, and Class III-IV heart failure. The aortic stenosis is life-limiting and severely symptomatic, and is characterized as critical with a documented aortic valve orifice area of 0.6 cm². He has multiple additional co-morbidities that make his risk of mortality with conventional open heart aortic valve replacement greater than 10%, by objective predictive criteria. He is evaluated by the valve-team comprised of a cardiac surgeon and an interventional cardiologist, who agree that the operative risks outweigh the benefit. The team, therefore, recommends transcatheter aortic valve replacement. In the course of the procedure, the patient becomes unstable and full extracorporeal cardiopulmonary support is required. However, the femoral vessels are not suitable for percutaneous cannulation, therefore an open approach is utilized. In the course of the procedure, the patient becomes unstable and full extracorporeal cardiopulmonary support is required. Note: This is an add-on service to the TAVR/TAVI, which is reported separately.

**Description of Procedure (33368)**

A patient undergoing transcatheter aortic valve replacement (TAVR) becomes hemodynamically unstable and cannot be stabilized with inotropic support or any standard medical means. The patient is anticoagulated. A new incision is made and the artery and vein are exposed and controlled with vessel loops. The artery is clamped and a transverse arteriotomy is performed. A suitably sized arterial cannula is advanced over a guidewire. A pursestring polypropylene suture is place in the vein, and a guidewire is inserted through a needle placed within it and advanced into the vena cava under fluoroscopic guidance. A multiple-port venous drainage cannula is passed over the guidewire, across the right atrium, and into the vena cava. The cannulas are de-aired and connected to a cardiopulmonary bypass circuit. Cardiopulmonary bypass is initiated. Cardiopulmonary bypass with its attendant volume shifts and the activation of the inflammatory system is managed with volume replacement and alpha effector agents. Anticoagulation is maintained. Management continues while the TAVR procedure is completed. The patient's temperature, hematocrit, pH, and levels of oxygenation and electrolytes are normalized, and the patient is weaned from cardiopulmonary bypass. The venous cannula is removed, and bleeding is controlled by tying the previously placed pursestring suture. The arterial cannula is removed, and the arteriotomy is repaired with 6-0 polypropylene sutures. Anticoagulation is reversed, and after assuring hemostasis, the wound is closed in layers.

 **Clinical Example** (33369)

An 83-year-old male with aortic stenosis, coronary artery disease, and Class III-IV heart failure. The aortic stenosis is life-limiting and severely symptomatic, and is characterized as critical with a documented aortic valve orifice area of 0.6 cm$^2$. He has multiple additional co-morbidities that make his risk of mortality with conventional open heart aortic valve replacement greater than 10%, by objective predictive criteria. He is evaluated by the valve-team comprised of a cardiac surgeon and an interventional cardiologist, who agree that the operative risks outweigh the benefit. The team, therefore, recommends transcatheter aortic valve replacement. In the course of the procedure, the patient becomes unstable and full extracorporeal cardiopulmonary support is required. However, because of severe aortoiliac disease, central arterial and venous access is required for institution of safe cardiopulmonary bypass. In the course of the procedure, the patient becomes unstable and full extracorporeal cardiopulmonary support is required. Note: This is an add-on service to the TAVR/TAVI, which is reported separately.

**Description of Procedure** (33369)

A patient undergoing transcatheter aortic valve replacement (TAVR) becomes hemodynamically unstable and cannot be stabilized with inotropic support or any standard medical means. The patient is anticoagulated. If not already achieved by the TAVR approach, exposure of the great vessels is obtained by rapid median sternotomy and the creation of a pericardial well. The aorta is directly cannulated for arterial inflow and a dual stage venous return cannula is placed through a right atrial incision. Cardiopulmonary bypass is initiated. Pursestring sutures are then placed about both cannulae and secured. Cardiopulmonary bypass with its attendant volume shifts and the activation of the inflammatory system is managed with volume replacement and alpha effector agents. Anticoagulation is maintained. Management continues while the TAVR procedure is completed. The patient's temperature, hematocrit, pH, and levels of oxygenation and electrolytes are normalized, and the patient is weaned from cardiopulmonary bypass. Anticoagulation is reversed, the cannulae are removed, and hemostasis is achieved by tying the previously placed pursestring sutures. Additional sutures may be required. After assuring hemostasis, the sternum is reapproximated with stainless steel wires over mediastinal drains. The wound is then irrigated and closed in layers.

## VENOUS GRAFTING ONLY FOR CORONARY ARTERY BYPASS

The following codes are used to report coronary artery bypass procedures using venous grafts only. These codes should NOT be used to report the performance of coronary artery bypass procedures using arterial grafts and venous grafts during the same procedure. See 33517-33523 and 33533-33536 for reporting combined arterial-venous grafts.

▶Procurement of the saphenous vein graft is included in the description of the work for 33510-33516 and should not be reported as a separate service or co-surgery. To report harvesting of an upper extremity vein, use 35500 in addition to the bypass procedure. To report harvesting of a femoropopliteal vein segment, report 35572 in addition to the bypass procedure. When surgical assistant performs graft procurement, add modifier 80 to 33510-33516. For percutaneous ventricular assist device insertion, removal, repositioning, see 33990-33993.◀

**33510**   Coronary artery bypass, vein only; single coronary venous graft

## COMBINED ARTERIAL-VENOUS GRAFTING FOR CORONARY BYPASS

The following codes are used to report coronary artery bypass procedures using venous grafts and arterial grafts during the same procedure. These codes may NOT be used alone.

To report combined arterial-venous grafts it is necessary to report two codes: (1) the appropriate combined arterial-venous graft code (33517-33523); and (2) the appropriate arterial graft code (33533-33536).

▶Procurement of the saphenous vein graft is included in the description of the work for 33517-33523 and should not be reported as a separate service or co-surgery. Procurement of the artery for grafting is included in the description of the work for 33533-33536 and should not be reported as a separate service or co-surgery, except when an upper extremity artery (eg, radial artery) is procured. To report harvesting of an upper extremity artery, use 35600 in addition to the bypass procedure. To report harvesting of an upper extremity vein, use 35500 in addition to the bypass procedure. To report harvesting of a femoropopliteal vein segment, report 35572 in addition to the bypass procedure. When surgical assistant performs arterial and/or venous graft procurement, add modifier 80 to 33517-33523, 33533-33536, as appropriate. For percutaneous ventricular assist device insertion, removal, repositioning, see 33990-33993.◀

**+33517**   Coronary artery bypass, using venous graft(s) and arterial graft(s); single vein graft (List separately in addition to code for primary procedure)

## ARTERIAL GRAFTING FOR CORONARY ARTERY BYPASS

The following codes are used to report coronary artery bypass procedures using either arterial grafts only or a combination of arterial-venous grafts. The codes include the use of the internal mammary artery, gastroepiploic artery, epigastric artery, radial artery, and arterial conduits procured from other sites.

To report combined arterial-venous grafts it is necessary to report two codes: (1) the appropriate arterial graft code (33533-33536); and (2) the appropriate combined arterial-venous graft code (33517-33523).

▶Procurement of the artery for grafting is included in the description of the work for 33533-33536 and should not be reported as a separate service or co-surgery, except when an upper extremity artery (eg, radial artery) is procured. To report harvesting of an upper extremity artery, use 35600 in addition to the bypass procedure. To report harvesting of an upper extremity vein, use 35500 in addition to the bypass procedure. To report harvesting of a femoropopliteal vein segment, report 35572 in addition to the bypass procedure. When surgical assistant performs arterial and/or venous graft procurement, add modifier 80 to 33517-33523, 33533-33536, as appropriate. For percutaneous ventricular assist device insertion, removal, repositioning, see 33990-33993.◀

**33533**  Coronary artery bypass, using arterial graft(s); single arterial graft

### 🖎 Rationale

In concert with the new percutaneous ventricular assist device codes 33990-33993, instructions have been added to the Venous Grafting Only for Coronary Artery Bypass, Combined Arterial-Venous Grafting for Coronary Bypass, and Arterial Grafting for Coronary Artery Bypass sections directing users to codes 33990-33993 for percutaneous ventricular assist device insertion, removal, and repositioning, when performed at the same session as coronary artery bypass procedures using venous grafts and arterial grafts.

## SEPTAL DEFECT

**33675**  Closure of multiple ventricular septal defects;

**33676**  with pulmonary valvotomy or infundibular resection (acyanotic)

**33677**  with removal of pulmonary artery band, with or without gusset

▶(Do not report 33675-33677 in conjunction with 32100, 32551, 32554, 32555, 33210, 33681, 33684, 33688)◀

### 🖎 Rationale

In support of the changes to the thoracentesis and pleural drainage code changes in the Respiratory System section, the exclusionary parenthetical note following code 33677 has been revised with the removal of deleted code 32422, and the addition of new codes 32554 and 32555.

## CARDIAC ASSIST

▶The insertion of a ventricular assist device (VAD) can be performed via percutaneous (33990, 33991) or transthoracic (33975, 33976, 33979) approach. The location of the ventricular assist device may be intracorporeal or extracorporeal.

For surgical insertion of cannula(s) for prolonged extracorporeal circulation for cardiopulmonary insufficiency (ECMO), use 36822.

Open arterial exposure when necessary to facilitate percutaneous ventricular assist device insertion (33990, 33991), may be reported separately (34812). Extensive repair or replacement of an artery may be additionally reported (eg, 35226 or 35286).

Removal of a ventricular assist device (33977, 33978, 33980, 33992) includes removal of the entire device, including the cannulas. Removal of a percutaneous ventricular assist device at the same session as insertion is not separately reportable. For removal of a percutaneous ventricular assist device at a separate and distinct session, but on the same day as insertion, report 33992 appended with modifier 59 indicating a distinct procedural service.

Repositioning of a percutaneous ventricular assist device at the same session as insertion is not separately reportable. Repositioning of percutaneous ventricular assist device not necessitating imaging guidance is not a reportable service. For repositioning of a percutaneous ventricular assist device necessitating imaging guidance at a separate and distinct session, but on the same day as insertion, report 33993 with modifier 59 indicating a distinct procedural service◄.

Replacement of a ventricular assist device pump (ie, 33981-33983) includes the removal of the pump and insertion of a new pump, connection, de-airing, and initiation of the new pump.

►Replacement of the entire implantable ventricular assist device system, ie, pump(s) and cannulas, is reported using the insertion codes (ie, 33975, 33976, 33979). Removal (ie, 33977, 33978, 33980) of the ventricular assist device system being replaced is not separately reported. Replacement of a percutaneous ventricular assist device is reported using implantation codes (ie, 33990, 33991). Removal (ie, 33992) is not reported separately.◄

**33960** Prolonged extracorporeal circulation for cardiopulmonary insufficiency; initial day

⊘**33961** each subsequent day

(Do not report modifier 63 in conjunction with 33960, 33961)

(For insertion of cannula for prolonged extracorporeal circulation, use 36822)

**33967** Insertion of intra-aortic balloon assist device, percutaneous

**33968** Removal of intra-aortic balloon assist device, percutaneous

**33970** Insertion of intra-aortic balloon assist device through the femoral artery, open approach

**33971** Removal of intra-aortic balloon assist device including repair of femoral artery, with or without graft

**33973** Insertion of intra-aortic balloon assist device through the ascending aorta

**33974** Removal of intra-aortic balloon assist device from the ascending aorta, including repair of the ascending aorta, with or without graft

**33975** Insertion of ventricular assist device; extracorporeal, single ventricle

**33976** extracorporeal, biventricular

**33977** Removal of ventricular assist device; extracorporeal, single ventricle

**33978** extracorporeal, biventricular

**33979** Insertion of ventricular assist device, implantable intracorporeal, single ventricle

**33980** Removal of ventricular assist device, implantable intracorporeal, single ventricle

**33981** Replacement of extracorporeal ventricular assist device, single or biventricular, pump(s), single or each pump

**33982** Replacement of ventricular assist device pump(s); implantable intracorporeal, single ventricle, without cardiopulmonary bypass

**33983** implantable intracorporeal, single ventricle, with cardiopulmonary bypass

⊙●**33990** Insertion of ventricular assist device, percutaneous including radiological supervision and interpretation; arterial access only

⊙●**33991** both arterial and venous access, with transseptal puncture

⊙●**33992** Removal of percutaneous ventricular assist device at separate and distinct session from insertion

⊙●**33993** Repositioning of percutaneous ventricular assist device with imaging guidance at separate and distinct session from insertion

### ✐ Rationale

A new subsection has been established with a new heading, guidelines, and family of codes pertaining to percutaneous ventricular assist device procedures. The percutaneous ventricular assist device insertion Category III codes 0048T and 0050T have been moved to Category I status, two new subsection headings have been added distinguish transthoracic cardiac assist procedures from percutaneous cardiac assist procedures, with new guidelines and parenthetical notes established to instruct users on the appropriate reporting of the four new codes in the Surgery/Cardiovascular System/Cardiac Assist subsection. Instructions have also been added to the Bypass Grafting subsections directing users to codes 33990-33993 for percutaneous ventricular assist device insertion, removal, and repositioning.

A percutaneous ventricular assist device (pVAD) is a mechanical pump that helps a weakened heart eject blood to the body. The pVAD device does not replace the heart. It assists the patient's own heart to pump blood, decreasing the work of the weakened ventricle. These devices are commonly utilized in patients with impaired ventricular function undergoing high-risk procedures (eg, complex endovascular coronary intervention, high-risk arrhythmia ablation, valvuloplasty, percutaneous valve repair, or replacement, such as transcatheter aortic valve replacement). In other instances, pVAD may be utilized in critically ill patients with severe ventricular dysfunction for medical stabilization. PVAD is most commonly reported in conjunction with complex endovascular, percutaneous coronary, or valvular interventions. However, the vast majority of endovascular, percutaneous coronary, or valvular interventions are done without the assistance of pVAD.

Open arterial exposure, when necessary to facilitate percutaneous ventricular assist device (VAD) insertion (33991, 33992), may be reported separately (34812). Because VAD removal of the entire device, including the cannulas, is inherent in codes 33977, 33978, and 33980, a new code (33992) has been added for removal of a percutaneous ventricular assist device at a separate and distinct session, but on the same day as insertion. In this circumstance, code 33992 should be reported with modifier 59 appended indicating a distinct procedural service has been performed.

Repositioning of a VAD is not separately reportable when performed at the same session or when the repositioning does not require imaging guidance. However, code 33993 may be reported with modifier 59 appended when repositioning of a VAD is performed at a separate and distinct session.

## Clinical Example (33990)

A 68-year-old obese male with oxygen dependent obstructive pulmonary disease, diabetes mellitus, hypertension, and dyslipidemia presents with signs of acute systolic heart failure and unstable angina. Cardiac catheterization demonstrates a left ventricular ejection fraction of 25%, down from 60% one year ago. Coronary angiography shows a long, heavily calcified 90% stenosis in the left anterior descending artery (LAD), a long, heavily calcified 80% stenosis in the left circumflex artery (LCX), and a 50% focal right coronary stenosis. Cardiac surgery consult deems him too high risk for surgical revascularization due to severe pulmonary disease and comorbidities. Rotational atherectomy of the calcified LAD and LCX lesions is planned with placement of arterial pVAD due to the severely impaired left ventricular function and large myocardial territories at risk.

### Description of Procedure (33990)

A "time out" occurs during which confirmation of critical information is ensured, such as the patient's identity, planned procedure, access route, allergies, signed consent, availability of proper equipment, and any unusual circumstances that might influence the procedure.

A peripheral intravenous (IV) access site is obtained. If general anesthesia is induced, the patient is intubated and connected to a mechanical ventilator. If conscious sedation is used, oxygen saturation monitoring is secured. A radial artery catheter may be inserted for hemodynamic monitoring. The heart rate and rhythm are monitored throughout the procedure. Transesophageal echocardiography (TEE) or transthoracic echocardiography (TTE) may be used by an echocardiographer to confirm the ejection fraction and to rule out ventricular thrombus. (If performed, TTE/TEE is reported separately.) The patient is prepped and draped.

Femoral arterial access for the reference pigtail catheter is obtained by needle puncture (modified Seldinger technique). After arterial access is obtained, serial dilation of the femoral artery is performed up to 11Fr. A 13 French peel-away sheath or a 14F indwelling sheath is then positioned in the femoral artery over a standard guidewire. (Note: the device is available in both 13F and 21F versions.) A catheter is then advanced over a wire from the femoral artery up to the ascending aorta and then used to cross the aortic valve into the left ventricle. The standard guidewire is exchanged out through the catheter for the transcatheter percutaneous ventricular assist device (pVAD) guidewire, which is then positioned in the ventricle toward the apex. The catheter is withdrawn over the wire, leaving the wire alone in the ventricle. This typically generates significant ventricular ectopy and repositioning of the wire. Using fluoroscopic guidance, the pVAD device is backloaded onto the guidewire and then advanced over the wire into the aortoiliac system, around the aortic arch, through the aortic valve, and into the ventricle. The wire is then removed. Under fluoroscopic guidance, the pVAD catheter is positioned so that the inflow of the cannula is properly positioned below the aortic valve. The pVAD transcatheter/transvalvular catheter is then activated to counteract the passive flow through the catheter from the aorta. In this manner, the pump is in a transvalvular position with uptake placed in the ventricle and arterial delivery into the aorta. The other end of the pVAD catheter exits through the arterial access site and is fixed externally to prevent untoward inward migration (ie, too much catheter inside the heart). The external end of the device is connected to the control console, and the pump is adjusted as needed to optimize its output.

During the interventional procedure, the transcatheter/transvalvular assist device is adjusted as necessary to achieve an optimal performance level to maintain systolic pressure during long inflations of the coronaries and to provide unloading of the ventricle during the entire procedure. If device removal is appropriate at the conclusion of the case, weaning of the pump is gradually performed. The patient's temperature, hematocrit, and oxygenation and electrolytes are normalized as necessary. Once the transcatheter device is set at a low, or a neutral setting (no forward flow), the pump is withdrawn to the iliac artery and turned off. Once the activated clotting time (ACT) is reduced to less than 150 seconds, the pump is withdrawn through the sheath and removed. Arterial hemostasis is achieved with prolonged manual pressure or via an arterial closure system. The patient's vital signs are recorded every hour until release to the step-down unit with checks of the groin by the nursing staff every hour for the next 4 hours, then every 2 hours as directed.

## Clinical Example (33991)

A 75-year-old obese male with oxygen dependent obstructive pulmonary disease, diabetes mellitus, hypertension, and dyslipidemia presents with signs of acute systolic heart failure and unstable angina. Cardiac catheterization demonstrates a left ventricular ejection fraction of 15%, down from 60% one year ago. Coronary angiography shows a long, heavily calcified 90% stenosis in the left anterior descending artery (LAD), a long, heavily calcified 80% stenosis in the left circumflex artery (LCX), and a 50% focal right coronary stenosis. Cardiac surgery consult deems him too high risk for surgical revascularization due to severe pulmonary disease and comorbidities. Rotational atherectomy of the calcified LAD and LCX lesions is planned with placement of arterial-venous pVAD with transseptal puncture due to the severely impaired left ventricular function and large myocardial territories at risk.

### Description of Procedure (33991)

A peripheral intravenous (IV) access site is obtained. If general anesthesia is induced, the patient is intubated and connected to a mechanical ventilator. If conscious sedation is used, oxygen saturation monitoring is secured. Pulmonary and radial artery catheters may be inserted for hemodynamic monitoring. The heart rate and rhythm are monitored throughout the procedure. Transesophageal echocardiography (TEE) or transthoracic echocardiography (TTE) may be used by an echocardiographer to confirm ejection fraction and to rule out left atrial thrombus. (If performed, TEE is reported separately.) The patient is prepped and draped.

The femoral artery and femoral vein are accessed percutaneously or by cutdown. An appropriate catheter is inserted over a wire through the venous sheath into the venous system under fluoroscopic guidance up to the superior vena cava. The guidewire is removed. A rigid transeptal puncture needle is carefully advanced through the catheter stopping just short of the end of the catheter. The needle-catheter unit is flushed and attached to a second pressure manifold and then withdrawn to the level of the fossa ovalis in the interatrial septum under fluoroscopic guidance. The imaging system is rotated in both the anterior and lateral positions to confirm proper positioning with respect to the arterial catheter positioned just above the aortic valve. The needle-catheter unit is then advanced several millimeters while observing the pressure waveform. The transeptal puncture is achieved. Left atrial position is confirmed by pressure waveform analysis, oxygen saturation measurement, and contrast injection through the system. If the needle-catheter unit has not traversed the septum properly, complications are first excluded and then the device is repositioned and a repeat attempt is performed until successful. The transseptal procedure typically requires more than one attempt to achieve success. The transseptal needle is removed, the catheter is flushed, and a guidewire is advanced through the catheter into the left atrium. The catheter is removed and a dilating catheter is advanced over the guidewire across the interatrial septum into the left atrium in order to dilate the septum. The venous access site is progressively dilated over a guidewire to allow the placement of a large bore cannula. The large bore 21F venous percutaneous ventricular assist device (pVAD) cannula is flushed and then advanced over the guidewire into the left atrium under fluoroscopic guidance. The femoral artery is progressively dilated over the previously placed guidewire to allow placement of a large bore 16F pVAD arterial return catheter, which is advanced over the wire into the proximal iliac artery or distal aorta for arterial return. The pVAD cannulas are de-aired and connected to the external pump. The pump is activated and proper flows are ensured. If flows are inadequate, suggesting malpositioning of the left atrial cannula, the cannula is repositioned under fluoroscopic guidance. During the interventional procedure, the pump is running at high performance level and thus maintains delivery of oxygenated blood to the body while the heart is compromised and unloads the heart during the entire procedure.

If device removal is appropriate at the conclusion of the case, weaning of the pump is gradually performed. The patient's temperature, hematocrit, pH, and oxygenation and electrolytes are normalized as necessary, and the patient is weaned. The heart pump console is turned off. The left atrial catheter is withdrawn from the atrium, into the inferior vena cava, and once the activated clotting time (ACT) is reduced to less than 150 seconds, the device is ultimately withdrawn from the femoral vein under direct fluoroscopic or echocardiographic guidance. Prolonged manual compression is applied to the exit site to achieve hemostasis, and a deep skin suture may also be applied to the area around the cannulation site to enhance hemostasis. The arterial catheter(s) is usually removed, and arterial hemostasis is achieved with prolonged manual compression, with an arterial closure system, or by surgical closure. The patient's vital signs are recorded every hour until release to the step-down unit with checks of the groin by the nursing staff every hour for the next 4 hours, then every 2 hours as directed.

## Clinical Example (33992)

A 68-year-old male presents with a large anterior STEMI and progresses rapidly to cardiogenic shock. An arterial-venous pVAD is implanted emergently. Despite successful stent placement to the occluded proximal left anterior descending artery, he manifests persistent hypotension, pulmonary edema, and EF 25%. The pVAD is maintained in place for prolonged hemodynamic support post procedure. Two days later, he has clinically improved with ejection fraction up to 35%. He remains stable during weaning of the pVAD and the device is now removed successfully.

### Description of Procedure (33992)

For arterial approach devices, the device flow is reduced to minimal flow (or neutral setting), and withdrawn from the ventricle into the aorta under fluoroscopic or echocardiographic guidance. Once it approaches the iliac artery, the device is turned off and with the activated clotting time (ACT) less than 150 seconds, the device is removed. The arterial catheter(s) is removed and arterial hemostasis is achieved with prolonged manual compression, with an arterial closure system, or by surgical closure. The patient's vital signs are recorded every hour until release to the step-down unit with checks of the groin by the nursing staff every hour for the next 4 hours, then every 2 hours as directed.

For arterial-venous approach devices, the heart pump console is turned off. The left atrial catheter is withdrawn from the left atrium, across the right atrium, into the inferior vena cava and, once the ACT is reduced to less than 150 seconds, the device is ultimately withdrawn from the femoral vein under direct fluoroscopic or echocardiographic guidance. Prolonged manual compression is applied to the exit site to achieve hemostasis, and a deep skin suture may also be applied to the area around the cannulation site to enhance hemostasis. The arterial catheter(s) is/are removed and manual pressure applied, or the artery is closed surgically with prolonged manual compression, with an arterial closure system, or by surgical closure. The patient's vital signs are recorded every hour until release to the step-down unit with checks of the groin by the nursing staff every hour for the next 4 hours, then every 2 hours as directed.

## Clinical Example (33993)

A 75-year-old male presents with a large anterior STEMI and progresses rapidly to cardiogenic shock. An arterial pVAD is implanted emergently. Despite successful stent placement to the occluded proximal left anterior descending artery, he manifests persistent hypotension, pulmonary edema, and EF 25%. The pVAD is maintained in place for prolonged hemodynamic support post procedure. Upon transfer to the coronary care unit, the patient's oxygen saturation and blood pressure drop, and an alarm sounds on the device console. Vasopressors are started to augment blood pressure. Echocardiogram confirms the pVAD has come back from the desired left ventricular position to a position now completely in the ascending aorta, indicating the need to reposition the device. The patient is brought back to the catheterization laboratory, where the device is repositioned into the left ventricular under fluoroscopic guidance.

## Description of Procedure (33993)

For venous approach devices, the devices are visualized and repositioned as necessary with respect to the right atrium and pulmonary artery as needed. For arterial approach devices, the pump is visualized and the device is repositioned with respect to the aortic valve as needed. For combined arterial and venous devices, the venous and arterial cannulas are visualized and repositioned as necessary with respect to the right atrium and aortoiliac system. For combined arterial and venous devices with transeptal access, the venous and arterial cannulas are visualized and repositioned as necessary with respect to the right and left atria and the aortoiliac system. Once back in position, the pump is restarted to maintain adequate cardiac support.

## Arteries and Veins

### TRANSLUMINAL ANGIOPLASTY

(35480 has been deleted. To report, see 0234T, 0235T)

(35481 has been deleted. To report, use 0236T)

(35482 has been deleted. To report, use 0238T)

(35483 has been deleted. To report, see 37225, 37227)

(35484 has been deleted. To report, use 0237T)

(35485 has been deleted. To report, see 37229, 37231, 37233, 37235)

(35490 has been deleted. To report, see 0234T, 0235T)

(35491 has been deleted. To report, use 0236T)

(35492 has been deleted. To report, use 0238T)

(35493 has been deleted. To report, see 37225, 37227)

(35494 has been deleted. To report, use 0237T)

(35495 has been deleted. To report, see 37229, 37231, 37233, 37235)

### VASCULAR INJECTION PROCEDURES

#### Intravenous

⊙▲**36010**  Introduction of catheter, superior or inferior vena cava

#### Intra-Arterial—Intra-Aortic

**36120**  Introduction of needle or intracatheter; retrograde brachial artery

⊙▲**36140**  extremity artery

⊘=Modifier 51 Exempt  ⊙=Moderate Sedation  ✚=Add-on Code  ⋀=FDA approval pending

***Diagnostic Studies of Arteriovenous (AV) Shunts for Dialysis:*** For diagnostic studies, the arteriovenous (AV) dialysis shunt (AV shunt) is defined as beginning with the arterial anastomosis and extending to the right atrium. This definition includes all upper and lower extremity AV shunts (arteriovenous fistulae [AVF] and arteriovenous grafts [AVG]). Code 36147 includes the work of directly accessing and imaging the entire AV shunt. Antegrade and/or retrograde punctures of the AV shunt are typically used for imaging, and contrast may be injected directly through a needle or through a catheter placed into the AV shunt. Occasionally the catheter needs to be advanced further into the shunt to adequately visualize the arterial anastomosis or the central veins, and all manipulation of the catheter for diagnostic imaging of the AV shunt is included in 36147. Advancement of the catheter to the vena cava to adequately image that segment of the AV shunt is included in 36147 and is not separately reported. Advancement of the catheter tip through the arterial anastomosis to adequately visualize the anastomosis is also considered integral to the work of 36147 and is not separately reported.

***Interventions for Arteriovenous (AV) Shunts Created for Dialysis (AV Grafts and AV Fistulae):*** For the purposes of coding interventional procedures in arteriovenous (AV) shunts created for dialysis (both arteriovenous fistulae [AVF] and arteriovenous grafts [AVG]), the AV shunt is artificially divided into two vessel segments. The first segment is peripheral and extends from the peri-arterial anastomosis through the axillary vein (or entire cephalic vein in the case of cephalic venous outflow). The second segment includes the veins central to the axillary and cephalic veins, including the subclavian and innominate veins through the vena cava. Interventions performed in a single segment, regardless of the number of lesions treated, are coded as a single intervention.

**36160**    Introduction of needle or intracatheter, aortic, translumbar

▶***Diagnostic Studies of Cervicocerebral Arteries:*** Codes 36221-36228 describe non-selective and selective arterial catheter placement and diagnostic imaging of the aortic arch, carotid, and vertebral arteries. Codes 36221-36226 include the work of accessing the vessel, placement of catheter(s), contrast injection(s), fluoroscopy, radiological supervision and interpretation, and closure of the arteriotomy by pressure, or application of an arterial closure device. Codes 36221-36228 describe arterial contrast injections with arterial, capillary, and venous phase imaging, when performed.

Code 36227 is an add-on code to report unilateral selective arterial catheter placement and diagnostic imaging of the ipsilateral external carotid circulation and includes all the work of accessing the additional vessel, placement of catheter(s), contrast injection(s), fluoroscopy, radiological supervision and interpretation. Code 36227 is reported in conjunction with 36222, 36223, or 36224.

Code 36228 is an add-on code to report unilateral selective arterial catheter placement and diagnostic imaging of the initial and each additional intracranial branch of the internal carotid or vertebral arteries. Code 36228 is reported in conjunction with 36224 or 36226. This includes any additional second or third order catheter selective placement in the same primary branch of the internal carotid, vertebral, or basilar artery and includes all the work of accessing the additional vessel, placement of catheter(s), contrast injection(s), fluoroscopy, radiological supervision and interpretation. It is not reported more than twice per side regardless of the number of additional branches selectively catheterized.

Codes 36221-36226 are built on progressive hierarchies with more intensive services inclusive of less intensive services. The code inclusive of all of the services provided for that vessel should be reported (ie, use the code inclusive of the most intensive services provided).
Only one code in the range 36222-36224 may be reported for each ipsilateral carotid territory. Only one code in the range 36225-36226 may be reported for each ipsilateral vertebral territory.

Code 36221 is reported for non-selective arterial catheter placement in the thoracic aorta and diagnostic imaging of the aortic arch and great vessel origins. Codes 36222-36228 are reported for unilateral artery catheterization. Do not report 36221 in conjunction with 36222-36226 as these selective codes include the work of 36221 when performed.

Do not report 36222, 36223, or 36224 together for ipsilateral angiography. Instead, select the code that represents the most comprehensive service using the following hierarchy of complexity (listed in descending order of complexity): 36224>36223>36222.

Do not report 36225 and 36226 together for ipsilateral angiography. Select the code that represents the more comprehensive service using the following hierarchy of complexity (listed in descending order of complexity): 36226>36225.

When bilateral carotid and/or vertebral arterial catheterization and imaging is performed, add modifier 50 to codes 36222-36228 if the same procedure is performed on both sides. For example, bilateral extracranial carotid angiography with selective catheterization of each common carotid artery would be reported with 36222 and modifier 50. However, when different territory(ies) is studied in the same session on both sides of the body, modifiers may be required to report the imaging performed. Use modifier 59 to denote that different carotid and/or vertebral arteries are being studied. For example, when selective right internal carotid artery catheterization accompanied by right extracranial and intracranial carotid angiography is followed by selective left common carotid artery catheterization with left extracranial carotid angiography, use 36224 to report the right side and 36222-59 to report the left side.

Diagnostic angiography of the cervicocerebral vessels may be followed by an interventional procedure at the same session. Interventional procedures may be separately reportable using standard coding conventions.

Do not report 75774 as part of diagnostic angiography of the extracranial and intracranial cervicocerebral vessels. It may be appropriate to report 75774 for diagnostic angiography of upper extremities and other vascular beds performed in the same session.

Report 76376 or 76377 for 3D rendering when performed in conjunction with 36221-36228.

Report 76937 for ultrasound guidance for vascular access, when performed in conjunction with 36221-36228. ◄

⊙**36200**    Introduction of catheter, aorta

▶(For non-selective angiography of the extracranial carotid and/or cerebral vessels and cervicocerebral arch, when performed, use 36221)◄

**36215**    Selective catheter placement, arterial system; each first order thoracic or brachiocephalic branch, within a vascular family

**+36218**    additional second order, third order, and beyond, thoracic or brachiocephalic branch, within a vascular family (List in addition to code for initial second or third order vessel as appropriate)

(Use 36218 in conjunction with 36216, 36217)

▶(For angiography, see 36147, 36222-36228, 75600-75774, 75791)◄

▶(For angioplasty, see 35471, 35472, 35475)◀

(For transcatheter therapies, see 37200-37208, 61624, 61626)

▶(When coronary artery, arterial conduit [eg, internal mammary, inferior epigastric or free radical artery] or venous bypass graft angiography is performed in conjunction with cardiac catheterization, see the appropriate cardiac catheterization, injection procedure, and imaging supervision code[s] [93455, 93457, 93459, 93461, 93530-93533, 93564] in the **Medicine** section. When internal mammary artery angiography only is performed without a concomitant cardiac catheterization, use 36216 or 36217 as appropriate)◀

⊙●**36221**   Non-selective catheter placement, thoracic aorta, with angiography of the extracranial carotid, vertebral, and/or intracranial vessels, unilateral or bilateral, and all associated radiological supervision and interpretation, includes angiography of the cervicocerebral arch, when performed

▶(Do not report 36221 with 36222-36226)◀

⊙●**36222**   Selective catheter placement, common carotid or innominate artery, unilateral, any approach, with angiography of the ipsilateral extracranial carotid circulation and all associated radiological supervision and interpretation, includes angiography of the cervicocerebral arch, when performed

⊙●**36223**   Selective catheter placement, common carotid or innominate artery, unilateral, any approach, with angiography of the ipsilateral intracranial carotid circulation and all associated radiological supervision and interpretation, includes angiography of the extracranial carotid and cervicocerebral arch, when performed

⊙●**36224**   Selective catheter placement, internal carotid artery, unilateral, with angiography of the ipsilateral intracranial carotid circulation and all associated radiological supervision and interpretation, includes angiography of the extracranial carotid and cervicocerebral arch, when performed

⊙●**36225**   Selective catheter placement, subclavian or innominate artery, unilateral, with angiography of the ipsilateral vertebral circulation and all associated radiological supervision and interpretation, includes angiography of the cervicocerebral arch, when performed

⊙●**36226**   Selective catheter placement, vertebral artery, unilateral, with angiography of the ipsilateral vertebral circulation and all associated radiological supervision and interpretation, includes angiography of the cervicocerebral arch, when performed

⊙✛●**36227**   Selective catheter placement, external carotid artery, unilateral, with angiography of the ipsilateral external carotid circulation and all associated radiological supervision and interpretation (List separately in addition to code for primary procedure)

▶(Use 36227 in conjunction with 36222, 36223, or 36224)◀

⊙✛●**36228**   Selective catheter placement, each intracranial branch of the internal carotid or vertebral arteries, unilateral, with angiography of the selected vessel circulation and all associated radiological supervision and interpretation (eg, middle cerebral artery, posterior inferior cerebellar artery) (List separately in addition to code for primary procedure)

▶(Use 36228 in conjunction with 36224 or 36226)◀

▶(Do not report 36228 more than twice per side)◀

## ✍️ Rationale

In response to the AMA/Specialty Society RVS Update Committee (RUC) analyses for procedure codes in the "Codes Reported together 75% or More" screen, the workgroup determined that there was duplication of work among the carotid angiography codes when various carotid angiography services were provided together. As a result of these findings, 8 new codes (36221-36228) were created to address the duplication of work among the carotid angiography codes. In addition, angiography supervision and interpretation codes 75650, 75660, 75662, 75665, 75671, 75676, 75680, and 75685 were deleted because the work in these codes were also combined or bundled into codes 36221-36228. For a discussion related to these deletions, see the Radiology/Diagnostic Radiology (Diagnostic Imaging)/Vascular Procedures/Aorta and Arteries subsection. Other corresponding changes to the CPT code set include a new subsection in the Vascular Injection Procedures section, titled Diagnostic Studies of Cervicocerebral Arteries, along with introductory guidelines that clarify the intent and use of codes 36221-36228.

In addition to providing specific guidance regarding intended use and appropriate reporting instructions for codes 36221-36228, the guidelines also convey instructions for appropriate use of modifiers 50 and 59 with codes 36221-36228. The guidelines also offer guidance on how to appropriately report diagnostic angiography code 75774, 3-dimensional rendering codes 76376 or 76377, and ultrasound guidance code 76937 with codes 36221-36228.

Codes 36221-36228 describe services such as nonselective or selective arterial catheter placement, including diagnostic imaging of the aortic arch, carotid, or vertebral arteries.

Code 36221 describes nonselective arterial catheter placement in the thoracic aorta and diagnostic imaging of the aortic arch and great vessel origins. Do not report 36221 in conjunction with 36222-36226, as these selective codes include the work of 36221 when performed.

Code 36222 describes unilateral selective catheter placement in the common carotid or innominate artery and diagnostic imaging of the ipsilateral extracranial cartoid circulation and all associated radiological supervision and interpretation, including the cervicocerebral arch, when performed.

Code 36223 describes unilateral selective catheter placement in the common carotid or innominate artery and diagnostic imaging of the ipsilateral intracranial carotid circulation and all associated radiological supervision and interpretation, including angiography of the extracranial carotid and cervicocerebral arch, when performed.

Code 36224 describes unilateral selective catheter placement in the internal carotid artery and diagnostic imaging of the ipsilateral intracranial carotid circulation and all associated radiological supervision and interpretation, including angiography of the extracranial carotid and cervicocerebral arch, when performed.

Code 36225 describes unilateral selective catheter placement in the subclavian or innominate artery and diagnostic imaging of the ipsilateral vertebral circulation and all associated radiological supervision and interpretation, including angiography of the cervicocerebral arch, when performed.

Code 36226 describes unilateral selective catheter placement in the vertebral artery and diagnostic imaging of the ipsilateral vertebral circulation and all associated radiological supervision and interpretation, including angiography of the cervicocerebral arch, when performed.

Add-on code 36227 describes unilateral selective catheter placement in the external carotid artery and diagnostic imaging of the ipsilateral external carotid circulation and all associated radiological supervision and interpretation. Code 36227 should be reported in conjunction with 36222, 36223, or 36224.

Add-on code 36228 describes unilateral selective catheter placement of each intracranial branch of the internal carotid or vertebral arteries and diagnostic imaging of the selected vessel circulation (eg, middle cerebral artery, posterior inferior cerebellar artery) and all associated radiological supervision and interpretation. Code 36228 should be reported in conjunction with 36224 or 36226. Code 36228 should not be reported more than twice per side.

To maintain consistency and uniformity throughout the CPT code set, a parenthetical note was added following code 36200 directing users to report 36221 for nonselective angiography of the extracranial carotid and/or cerebral vessels and cervicocerebral arch, when performed. The second parenthetical note following code 36218 was also updated by adding codes 36222-36228 to the list of codes to see for angiography procedures. The third parenthetical note was also updated by eliminating reference to codes 37228-37235. In addition, the second parenthetical note following code 37216 was updated to exclude reporting codes 37215 and 37216 with codes 36222-36224 for the treated carotid artery.

The Angiography, Carotid Artery illustration, which previously followed deleted code 75660, has been relocated to precede code 36222.

New codes 36227-36228 are identified with a ⊘ symbol, which indicates that these codes are exempt from the use of modifier 51.

### Clinical Example (36221)

A 72-year-old male with extensive smoking history and family history of aortic aneurysmal disease presents with a six-month history of intermittent symptoms of cerebral ischemia. Ultrasound demonstrates bilateral <30% internal carotid artery stenoses, but increased velocity is noted in the left common carotid artery. A diagnostic cervicocerebral arch arteriogram is requested.

### Description of Procedure (36221)

Right common femoral arterial access is obtained and an arterial sheath is placed. A wire is inserted, and a pigtail catheter is advanced over the wire retrograde into the ascending aorta. Test injection of contrast is performed. After all tubing is checked to ensure that no air bubbles or blood products are present, contrast is injected through the catheter with digital subtraction imaging over the area of interest in multiple projections to evaluate the aortic arch, great vessel origins, and extracranial carotid arteries. The wire is reinserted, and the pigtail catheter is removed. Contrast material is injected with imaging over the common femoral artery to ensure that no vessel injury, dissection, pseudoaneurysm, or significant iatrogenic vasospasm has occurred. The sheath is removed. The arteriotomy is closed by the application of pressure or an arterial closure device, as appropriate.

### Clinical Example (36222)

A 75-year-old male with a prior right carotid endarterectomy three years ago presents with ultrasound evidence for a >80% asymptomatic internal carotid artery restenosis. A diagnostic carotid arteriogram is requested.

#### Description of Procedure (36222)

Right common femoral arterial access is obtained and an arterial sheath is placed. A wire is inserted, and a pigtail catheter is advanced over the wire retrograde into the ascending aorta. Test injection of contrast is performed. After all tubing is checked to ensure that no air bubbles or blood products are present, contrast is injected through the catheter with digital subtraction imaging over the area of interest in multiple projections to evaluate the aortic arch, great vessel origins, and extracranial carotid arteries. A guidewire is placed into the indwelling diagnostic pigtail catheter. This catheter is removed over a guidewire. The guidewire and catheter combination are advanced selectively under real-time fluoroscopic guidance as well as roadmap imaging first into the innominate artery followed by the right common carotid artery. The guidewire is removed. A test injection of contrast is performed. After all tubing is checked to ensure that no air bubbles or blood products are present, contrast is injected through the catheter with digital subtraction imaging over the area of interest in the extracranial carotid territory using multiple projections. The selective catheter is removed. Contrast material is injected with imaging over the common femoral artery to ensure that no vessel injury, dissection, pseudoaneurysm, or significant iatrogenic vasospasm has occurred. The sheath is removed. The arteriotomy is closed with pressure or the application of an arterial closure device, as appropriate.

### Clinical Example (36223)

A 66-year-old female presents with complaints of left upper extremity numbness and weakness, symptoms of right cerebral TIA, and ultrasound documentation of right internal carotid artery 70% stenosis. A diagnostic cerebral arteriogram is requested.

#### Description of Procedure (36223)

Right common femoral arterial access is obtained and an arterial sheath is placed. A wire is inserted, and a pigtail catheter is advanced over the wire retrograde into the ascending aorta. Test injection of contrast is performed. After all tubing is checked to ensure that no air bubbles or blood products are present, contrast is injected through the catheter with digital subtraction imaging over the area of interest in multiple projections to evaluate the aortic arch, great vessel origins, and extracranial carotid arteries. A guidewire is introduced through the pigtail catheter, and the catheter is exchanged for a selective catheter. The selective catheter is guided into the right common carotid artery under real-time fluoroscopic guidance and/or roadmap imaging guidance using either the guidewire technique or contrast puff technique. A test injection of contrast is performed. After all tubing is checked to ensure that no air bubbles or blood products are present contrast is injected through the catheter with digital subtraction imaging over the areas of interest. Multiple contrast injections are made, and digital subtraction imaging of the extracranial and intracranial carotid distributions is acquired in anteroposterior (AP), oblique, and lateral projections. If necessary, oblique views are obtained to profile the carotid bifurcation and the intracranial pathology. The selective catheter is removed. Contrast material is injected with imaging over the common femoral artery to ensure that no vessel injury, dissection, pseudoaneurysm, or significant iatrogenic vasospasm has occurred. The sheath is removed. The arteriotomy is closed with pressure or the application of an arterial closure device, as appropriate.

## Clinical Example (36224)

A 55-year-old male has sudden onset of severe headache with a brief period of unconsciousness. A CT scan shows diffuse subarachnoid hemorrhage in the basal cisterns suspicious for an anterior communicating artery aneurysm. A diagnostic cerebral arteriogram is requested.

### Description of Procedure (36224)

Right common femoral arterial access is obtained and an arterial sheath is placed. A wire is inserted, and a pigtail catheter is advanced over the wire retrograde into the ascending aorta. Contrast is injected through the catheter with digital subtraction imaging over the area of interest in multiple projections to evaluate the aortic arch, great vessel origins, and extracranial carotid arteries. A guidewire is introduced through the pigtail catheter, and the catheter is exchanged for a selective catheter. The selective catheter is guided into the right common carotid artery under fluoroscopic guidance. Multiple contrast material injections are made and digital imaging of the extracranial carotid distribution is acquired in anteroposterior (AP), oblique, and lateral projections. A steerable guidewire is inserted, and the catheter is advanced into the internal carotid artery over the guidewire under fluoroscopic guidance. Multiple contrast material injections are made and digital imaging of the intracranial carotid distribution is acquired in AP, oblique, and lateral projections into the arterial, capillary, and venous phases. Contrast material is injected with imaging over the common femoral artery to ensure that no vessel injury, dissection, pseudoaneurysm, or significant iatrogenic vasospasm has occurred. The sheath is removed. The arteriotomy is closed with pressure or the application of an arterial closure device, as appropriate.

## Clinical Example (36225)

A 68-year-old male presents with a recent posterior circulation stroke. A diagnostic vertebral arteriogram is requested.

### Description of Procedure (36225)

Right common femoral arterial access is obtained and an arterial sheath is placed. A wire is inserted, and a pigtail catheter is advanced over the wire retrograde into the ascending aorta. Test injection of contrast is performed. After all tubing is checked to ensure that no air bubbles or blood products are present, contrast is injected through the catheter with digital subtraction imaging over the area of interest in multiple projections to evaluate the aortic arch, great vessel origins, and extracranial carotid arteries. A guidewire is introduced through the pigtail catheter, and the catheter is exchanged for a selective catheter. The selective catheter is guided into the right subclavian artery under real-time fluoroscopic guidance and/or roadmap imaging guidance using either the guidewire technique or contrast puff technique. A test injection of contrast is performed. After all tubing is checked to ensure that no air bubbles or blood products are present, contrast is injected through the catheter with digital subtraction imaging over the areas of interest. Multiple contrast injections are made, and digital subtraction imaging of the extracranial and intracranial vertebrobasilar distributions is acquired in anteroposterior (AP), oblique, and lateral projections. If necessary, oblique views are obtained to profile the vertebral origin and the intracranial pathology. The selective catheter is removed. Contrast material is injected with imaging over the common femoral artery to ensure that no vessel injury, dissection, pseudoaneurysm, or significant iatrogenic vasospasm has occurred. The sheath is removed. The arteriotomy is closed with pressure or the application of an arterial closure device, as appropriate.

### Clinical Example (36226)

A 42-year-old female has sudden onset of severe headache with a brief period of unconsciousness. A CT scan shows third ventricular hemorrhage and subarachnoid hemorrhage. A diagnostic vertebral arteriogram is requested.

### Description of Procedure (36226)

Right common femoral arterial access is obtained and an arterial sheath is placed. A wire is inserted, and a pigtail catheter is advanced over the wire retrograde into the ascending aorta. Contrast is injected through the catheter with digital subtraction imaging over the area of interest in multiple projections to evaluate the aortic arch, great vessel origins, and extracranial carotid arteries. A guidewire is introduced through the pigtail catheter, and the catheter is exchanged for a selective catheter. The selective catheter and guidewire combination are guided into the right subclavian artery under fluoroscopic guidance. Multiple contrast material injections are made, and digital imaging of the extracranial vertebral artery distribution is acquired in multiple projections. A steerable guidewire is inserted, and the catheter is advanced into the right vertebral artery over the guidewire under fluoroscopic guidance. Multiple contrast material injections are made, and digital imaging of the intracranial vertebral artery distribution is acquired in anteroposterior (AP), oblique, and lateral projections in arterial, capillary, and venous phases. The selective catheter is removed. Contrast material is injected with imaging over the common femoral artery to ensure that no vessel injury, dissection, pseudoaneurysm, or significant iatrogenic vasospasm has occurred. The sheath is removed. The arteriotomy is closed with pressure or the application of an arterial closure device, as appropriate.

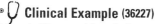

## Clinical Example (36227)

A 55-year-old male has sudden onset of severe headache with a brief period of unconsciousness. A noncontrast CT scan demonstrates diffuse subarachnoid hemorrhage. Angiography of the intracranial circulation fails to demonstrate etiology of hemorrhage. A diagnostic external carotid arteriogram is performed.

### Description of Procedure (36227)

A steerable guidewire is inserted, and the catheter is advanced into the external carotid artery over the guidewire under fluoroscopic guidance. Multiple contrast material injections are made, and digital imaging of the extracranial carotid distribution is acquired in anteroposterior (AP), oblique, and lateral projections. The selective catheter is removed. A formal report that includes image interpretation of the external carotid is dictated, transcribed, edited, and authenticated for archival in the permanent medical record.

## Clinical Example (36228)

A 45-year-old female presents with sudden onset of severe headache with a brief period of unconsciousness. A CT scan demonstrates a right frontal hemorrhage and findings suspicious of a 4-cm arteriovenous malformation. A diagnostic cerebral arteriogram is requested. Initial angiography confirms an anterior circulation arteriovenous malformation supplied by the right middle cerebral artery. Selective angiography of right middle cerebral artery is performed.

### Description of Procedure (36228)

Under fluoroscopic guidance, an exchange length guidewire is navigated into the distal internal carotid artery, and the selective catheter is exchanged for a guide catheter. The guide catheter is attached to a Touhy-Borst adapter and a heparinized flush. A baseline activated clotting time is obtained. Heparin, based on the patient's weight, is administered intravenously, and a repeat activated clotting time is obtained to ensure that adequate anticoagulation has been established. If necessary, additional heparin is administered, and subsequent activated clotting times are obtained. A microcatheter over a microguidewire is inserted into the guide catheter and navigated into a distal branch of the middle cerebral artery under roadmap fluoroscopic guidance. Multiple roadmaps may be required. The microwire is removed, and the microcatheter is flushed with normal saline. Contrast material is injected, and digital imaging of the distal middle cerebral artery territory in at least two projections into the arterial, capillary, and venous phases is performed. If necessary, additional oblique views are obtained to delineate the pathology. Contrast material is injected manually or with a power injector into the guide catheter, and digital imaging of the intracranial carotid distribution is acquired in anteroposterior (AP) and lateral projections into the arterial, capillary, and venous phases to rule out thromboembolic complications, contrast extravasation, or vascular injury. A postprocedure activated clotting time is obtained. A formal report that includes image interpretation of the right middle cerebral artery is dictated, transcribed, edited, and authenticated for archival in the permanent medical record.

## TRANSCATHETER PROCEDURES

Codes for catheter placement and the radiologic supervision and interpretation should also be reported, in addition to the code(s) for the therapeutic aspect of the procedure.

### Mechanical Thrombectomy

Code(s) for catheter placement(s), diagnostic studies, and other percutaneous interventions (eg, transluminal balloon angioplasty, stent placement) provided are separately reportable.

Codes 37184-37188 specifically include intraprocedural fluoroscopic radiological supervision and interpretation services for guidance of the procedure.

▶Intraprocedural injection(s) of a thrombolytic agent is an included service and not separately reportable in conjunction with mechanical thrombectomy. However, subsequent or prior continuous infusion of a thrombolytic is not an included service and is separately reportable (see 37211-37214).◀

For coronary mechanical thrombectomy, use 92973.

For mechanical thrombectomy for dialysis fistula, use 36870.

### ▶Transcatheter Thrombolytic Infusion◀

▶Codes 37211 or 37212 are used to report the initial day of transcatheter thrombolytic infusion(s) including follow-up arteriography/venography, and catheter position change or exchange, when performed. To report bilateral thrombolytic infusion through a separate access site(s), use modifier 50 in conjunction with 37211, 37212. Code 37213 is used to report continued transcatheter thrombolytic infusion(s) on subsequent day(s), other than initial day and final day of treatment. Code 37214 is used to report final day of transcatheter thrombolytic infusion(s). When initiation and completion of thrombolysis occur on the same day, report only 37211 or 37212.

Code(s) for catheter placement(s), diagnostic studies, and other percutaneous interventions (eg, transluminal balloon angioplasty, stent placement) provided may be separately reportable.

Codes 37211-37214 include fluoroscopic guidance and associated radiological supervision and interpretation.

Ongoing evaluation and management services on the day of the procedure related to thrombolysis are included in 37211-37214. If a significant, separately identifiable E/M service is performed by the same physician on the same day of the procedure, report the appropriate level of E/M service and append modifier 25.

Ultrasound guidance for vascular access is not included in 37211-37214. Code 76937 may be reported separately when performed if all the required elements are performed.◀

## OTHER PROCEDURES

⊙37191 Insertion of intravascular vena cava filter, endovascular approach including vascular access, vessel selection, and radiological supervision and interpretation, intraprocedural roadmapping, and imaging guidance (ultrasound and fluoroscopy), when performed;

(For open surgical interruption of the inferior vena cava through a laparotomy or retroperitoneal exposure, use 37619)

 ⊘=Modifier 51 Exempt ⊙=Moderate Sedation ✚=Add-on Code 𝒩=FDA approval pending

⊙**37193**  Retrieval (removal) of intravascular vena cava filter, endovascular approach including vascular access, vessel selection, and radiological supervision and interpretation, intraprocedural roadmapping, and imaging guidance (ultrasound and fluoroscopy), when performed

►(Do not report 37193 in conjunction with 37197)◄

**37195**  Thrombolysis, cerebral, by intravenous infusion

⊙●**37197**  Transcatheter retrieval, percutaneous, of intravascular foreign body (eg, fractured venous or arterial catheter), includes radiological supervision and interpretation, and imaging guidance (ultrasound or fluoroscopy), when performed

►(For percutaneous retrieval of a vena cava filter, use 37193)◄

**37200**  Transcatheter biopsy

(For radiological supervision and interpretation, use 75970)

►(37201 has been deleted. To report see 37211-37214)◄

\#⊙●**37211**  Transcatheter therapy, arterial infusion for thrombolysis other than coronary, any method, including radiological supervision and interpretation, initial treatment day

\#⊙●**37212**  Transcatheter therapy, venous infusion for thrombolysis, any method, including radiological supervision and interpretation, initial treatment day

\#⊙●**37213**  Transcatheter therapy, arterial or venous infusion for thrombolysis other than coronary, any method, including radiological supervision and interpretation, continued treatment on subsequent day during course of thrombolytic therapy, including follow-up catheter contrast injection, position change, or exchange, when performed;

\#⊙●**37214**  cessation of thrombolysis including removal of catheter and vessel closure by any method

►(Report 37211-37214 once per date of treatment)◄

►(For declotting by thrombolytic agent of implanted vascular access device or catheter, use 36593)◄

**37202**  Transcatheter therapy, infusion other than for thrombolysis, any type (eg, spasmolytic, vasoconstrictive)

(For thrombolysis of coronary vessels, see 92975, 92977)

(For radiological supervision and interpretation, use 75896)

►(37203 has been deleted. To report, use 37197)◄

(For removal of a vena cava filter, use 37193)

**37205**  Transcatheter placement of an intravascular stent(s) (except coronary, carotid, vertebral, iliac, and lower extremity arteries), percutaneous; initial vessel

(For radiological supervision and interpretation, use 75960)

(For transcatheter placement of intravascular cervical carotid artery stent(s), see 37215, 37216)

(For transcatheter placement of intracranial stents, use 61635)

►(For transcatherter coronary stent placement, see 92928-92944)◄

(For transcatheter stent placement of extracranial vertebral or intrathoracic carotid artery stent(s), see Category III codes 0075T, 0076T)

(For stent placement in iliac, femoral, popliteal, and tibial/peroneal arteries, see 37221, 37223, 37226, 37227, 37230, 37231, 37234, 37235)

**37207**    Transcatheter placement of an intravascular stent(s) (except coronary, carotid, vertebral, iliac and lower extremity arteries), open; initial vessel

**+37208**        each additional vessel (List separately in addition to code for primary procedure)

(Use 37208 in conjunction with 37207)

(For radiological supervision and interpretation, use 75960)

(For catheterizations, see 36215-36248)

▶(For transcatheter placement of intracoronary stent[s], see 92928-92944)◄

▶(37209 has been deleted. For exchange of a previously placed intravascular catheter during thrombolytic therapy, see 37211-37214)◄

**37211**    ▶Code is out of numerical sequence. See 37191-37216◄

**37212**    ▶Code is out of numerical sequence. See 37191-37216◄

**37213**    ▶Code is out of numerical sequence. See 37191-37216◄

**37214**    ▶Code is out of numerical sequence. See 37191-37216◄

⊙**37215**    Transcatheter placement of intravascular stent(s), cervical carotid artery, percutaneous; with distal embolic protection

⊙**37216**        without distal embolic protection

▶(Do not report 37215, 37216 in conjunction with 36222-36224 for the treated carotid artery)◄

### ✍ Rationale

In response to the AMA RUC Five-Year Review Identification Workgroup analysis to combine codes that are frequently reported together, thrombolytic infusion codes 37201 and 37209 have been deleted from the code set. In support of these deletions, radiology codes 75896 and 75898 have been revised. The services previously reported with codes 37201 and 37209 and components of 75896 and 75898 are now combined and reported with new transcatheter thrombolytic codes 37211-37214. To accommodate these changes, the CPT code set now includes a new Transcatheter Thrombolytic Infusion subsection, four new transcatheter thrombolytic infusion procedure codes (37211-37214), and introductory guidelines that explain the intent and appropriate use of these new codes.

For consistency and uniformity, the existing Mechanical Thrombectomy guidelines have also been updated to include reference to the new combined transcatheter thrombolytic therapy codes 37211-37214. References to codes 37201, 75896, and 75898 have been deleted. Similarly, changes have also been made in the Radiology Transcatheter Procedures and Medicine subsections to reflect the

⊘=Modifier 51 Exempt    ⊙=Moderate Sedation    +=Add-on Code    𝒩=FDA approval pending

addition of the new combined transcatheter thrombolytic infusion procedures to the CPT code set.

The new Transcatheter Thrombolytic Infusion guidelines instruct and clarify that: (1) 37211 or 37212 is used to report the initial day of transcatheter thrombolytic infusion(s), including when the follow-up arteriography or venography, and catheter position change or exchange is performed; (2) modifier 50 is reported in conjunction with codes 37211, 37212 when bilateral thrombolytic infusion is performed through a separate access site(s); (3) code 37213 is reported when continued transcatheter thrombolytic infusion(s) on subsequent day(s), other than initial day and final day of treatment, is performed; and (4) code 37214 is reported on the final day of transcatheter thrombolytic infusion(s).

When initiation and completion of thrombolysis occur on the same day, only report codes 37211 or 37212. Catheter placement(s), diagnostic studies, and other percutaneous interventions provided may be reported separately. All fluoroscopic guidance and associated radiological supervision and interpretation is now included in codes 37211-37214. Codes 37211-37214 do not include ultrasound guidance for vascular access. However, code 76937 may be reported separately if all the required elements are performed.

The guidelines also include a clarifying statement to allow reporting of distinctly separate E/M services in addition to the thrombolytic service when required. Codes 37211-37214 are only reported once per date of treatment.

Another result of the AMA RUC Five-Year Review Identification Workgroup analysis is the deletion of code 37203 along with the radiological supervision and interpretation code 75961 and their associated cross-references. The services previously reported with codes 37203 and 75961 are now combined into code 37197 for reporting percutaneous transcatheter retrieval of intravascular foreign body with radiological supervision and interpretation. The cross-reference note following code 37193 has been revised by removing codes 37203 and 75961 and adding new code 37197.

In addition, code 37209 has been deleted, as this exchange of a previously placed intravascular catheter during thrombolytic therapy is now an inclusive component of the new transcatheter therapy procedures (37211-37214). Cross-reference notes have been added to direct users to report the new codes.

The symbol (⊙) has been appended to codes 37197, 37211-37214 to indicate that these services include moderate sedation, and these codes are also included in Appendix G of the codebook. In addition, the resequencing symbol (#) has also been appended to codes 37211-37214 to indicate that these codes are out of numerical sequence. Four reference notes have been added to instruct the user to the appropriate code range of 37191-37216 for the placement of codes 37211-37214.

In support of the changes to the Vascular Injection Procedures section, the exclusionary parenthetical note following code 37216 has been revised with the removal of deleted codes 75671 and 75680 and the addition of new codes 36222-36224.

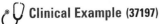 **Clinical Example (37197)**

A 59-year-old female with metastatic breast cancer has a fractured venous catheter related to her indwelling venous port. The catheter fragment has migrated to the right ventricle, and the distal tip is in the main pulmonary artery. Catheter fragment retrieval is performed from a percutaneous femoral vein approach.

**Description of Procedure (37197)**

Administration or supervision of administration of conscious sedation. The location of the access vessel (common femoral vein) is determined with palpation of the adjacent common femoral artery. Superficial and deep local anesthesia is administered. Using Seldinger technique, the access vessel is punctured and a guidewire is advanced. Serial 4 and 5 French dilators are passed, and an 8 French vascular sheath is placed into the accessed common femoral vein. A second guidewire is placed, the 8 French sheath is removed, and the sheath is replaced over one of the guidewires (leaving the second wire external to the sheath). A guide catheter is manipulated centrally into the heart adjacent to the foreign body fragment. The coaxial wire is removed, and a snare is placed through the guide catheter. The guide catheter and snare combination are used to capture the foreign body fragment in the snare under fluoroscopic guidance. When captured, the fragment is firmly gripped in the snare/guide catheter system. The fragment and guide/snare system are retracted to the sheath. The sheath and fragment/guide/snare are removed as a unit, leaving the safety wire in position. The fragment is inspected to judge completeness of removal. The chest is fluoroscopically evaluated to assure no remaining catheter fragments are present. The safety guidewire is removed. Manual compression is utilized for closure of the venotomy to achieve hemostasis.

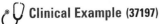 **Clinical Example (37211)**

A 76-year-old male with a right femoral-popliteal bypass presents to the emergency room with a painful, ischemic leg. Physical exam shows absent graft and distal pulses. Motor/sensory exam shows mild sensory deficit, but no motor deficit. The patient is taken to the procedure room where aortogram and runoff angiography exams are performed. (Diagnostic angiography reported separately). Acute thrombosis of the graft is shown, as well as thrombosis of the popliteal artery. Arterial thrombolysis is performed.

**Description of Procedure (37211)**

The patient is monitored for moderate sedation. An exchange length guidewire is inserted into the diagnostic catheter, and the diagnostic catheter is removed under fluoroscopic guidance. Under fluoroscopic guidance, a coaxial infusion catheter system is introduced over the guidewire and positioned with the distal tip in the popliteal artery and with the proximal sideholes in the thrombosed fem-pop graft. Angiography is performed to document the location of the catheter and the status of the runoff vessels. The catheters and access sheath are sutured into position at the skin entrance site. A bolus injection of thrombolytic agent is performed. Thrombolysis infusion is initiated.

⃠=Modifier 51 Exempt   ⊙=Moderate Sedation   ✚=Add-on Code   �=FDA approval pending

## Clinical Example (37212)

A 45-year-old female presents with sudden onset of a severely swollen and painful left leg. Duplex ultrasound shows acute left leg deep vein thrombosis affecting the femoral vein. Diagnostic venography confirms thrombosis and also demonstrates thrombosis extending to the common iliac vein (venography reported separately). Venous thrombolysis is performed using a popliteal vein approach.

### Description of Procedure (37212)

The patient is monitored for moderate sedation. An exchange length guidewire is inserted into the diagnostic catheter, and the diagnostic catheter is removed under fluoroscopic guidance. Under fluoroscopic guidance, a coaxial infusion catheter system is introduced over the guidewire and positioned with the distal tip in the inferior vena cava and with the proximal sideholes in the thrombosed vein. Angiography is performed to document the location of the catheter. The catheters and access sheath are sutured into position at the skin entrance site. A bolus injection of thrombolytic agent is performed. Thrombolysis infusion is initiated.

## Clinical Example (37213)

A 76-year-old male with an occluded right femoral-popliteal bypass had thrombolysis infusion started the prior day. He has been managed in the intensive care unit overnight. He undergoes follow-up angiography which demonstrates a residual thrombus. A catheter exchange is performed and thrombolytic infusion is resumed.

### Description of Procedure (37213)

The patient is monitored for moderate sedation. Thrombolytic infusion is temporarily stopped. Contrast is injected through the infusion catheter and angiography is performed, studying the area that is being infused. Angiography shows partial success in clot dissolution. The decision is made to exchange the infusion catheter and advance the tip further down the graft. The dressings at the catheter site are removed, and the area is prepped and draped. Over a guidewire, the existing catheter is removed and exchanged for a replacement. Angiography is performed to confirm the correct catheter tip position, and to ensure that the catheter exchange has not altered the clot position. The catheter and access sheath are resutured into position at the skin entrance site. The catheter and access sheath side-arm are connected to the infusion pumps. Thrombolysis infusion is re-started.

## Clinical Example (37214)

A 76-year-old male with an occluded right femoral-popliteal bypass has been treated by continuous infusion of thrombolysis for 2 days. He is clinically improved, and there is no longer evidence of leg ischemia. He undergoes follow-up angiography which demonstrates successful thrombolysis. The catheter is removed and vessel closed.

### Description of Procedure (37214)

Moderate sedation is monitored. Thrombolytic infusion is temporarily stopped. Contrast is injected through the infusion catheter and angiography is performed, studying the area that is being infused. Angiography shows completed therapy. The infusion catheter is removed. Hemostasis obtained with manual compression, closure device, or standard closure of the arteriotomy.

## ENDOVASCULAR REVASCULARIZATION (OPEN OR PERCUTANEOUS, TRANSCATHETER)

Codes 37220-37235 are to be used to describe lower extremity endovascular revascularization services performed for occlusive disease. These lower extremity codes are built on progressive hierarchies with more intensive services inclusive of lesser intensive services. The code inclusive of all of the services provided for that vessel should be reported (ie, use the code inclusive of the most intensive services provided). Only one code from this family (37220-37235) should be reported for each lower extremity vessel treated.

These lower extremity endovascular revascularization codes all include the work of accessing and selectively catheterizing the vessel, traversing the lesion, radiological supervision and interpretation directly related to the intervention(s) performed, embolic protection if used, closure of the arteriotomy by pressure and application of an arterial closure device or standard closure of the puncture by suture, and imaging performed to document completion of the intervention in addition to the intervention(s) performed. Extensive repair or replacement of an artery may be additionally reported (eg, 35226 or 35286). These codes describe endovascular procedures performed percutaneously and/or through an open surgical exposure. These codes include balloon angioplasty (eg, low-profile, cutting balloon, cryoplasty), atherectomy (eg, directional, rotational, laser), and stenting (eg, balloon-expandable, self-expanding, bare metal, covered, drug-eluting). Each code in this family (37220-37235) includes balloon angioplasty, when performed.

These codes describe revascularization therapies (ie, transluminal angioplasty, atherectomy, and stent placement) provided in three arterial vascular territories: iliac, femoral/popliteal, and tibial/peroneal.

►When treating multiple vessels within a territory, report each additional vessel using an add-on code, as applicable. Select the base code that represents the most complex service using the following hierarchy of complexity (in descending order of complexity): atherectomy and stent> atherectomy>stent>angioplasty. When treating multiple lesions within the same vessel, report one service that reflects the combined procedures, whether done on one lesion or different lesions, using the same hierarchy.◄

### 🖎 Rationale

In 2011, the CPT code set was expanded to include lower extremity endovascular revascularization services performed for occlusive disease (37220-37235) and guidelines that provide guidance for use of these codes.

In 2012, the introductory guidelines were updated to: (1) clarify the specific types of closure procedures that are included for these lower extremity endovascular procedures; (2) inform users that pressure application of the arterial closure device or standard closure of the puncture site by suture is inherently included as part of the procedure; and (3) specify services that should be separately reported (including extensive repair or replacement of an artery, ie, code 35226 or 35286).

In an effort to continue to provide greater clarity regarding the appropriate use and intent of these procedures, CPT 2013's introductory guidelines have been expanded. Language has been added to inform users about various aspects of appropriate code selection and assignment, including:

- When treating multiple vessels within a territory, an add-on code is reported for each additional vessel, as applicable.

- Procedures are reported according to a hierarchy in descending order of complexity.

- Users should select the base code that represents the most complex service using the following hierarchy of complexity (in descending order of complexity): atherectomy and stent>atherectomy>stent>angioplasty.

- When treating multiple lesions within the same vessel, report one service that reflects the combined procedures, whether done on one lesion or different lesions, using the same hierarchy.

# Hemic and Lymphatic Systems

## General

### BONE MARROW OR STEM CELL SERVICES/PROCEDURES

**38220**  Bone marrow; aspiration only

▶(For needle aspiration of bone marrow for the purpose of bone grafting, use 38220)◀

▶(Do not report 38220-38230 for bone marrow aspiration for platelet rich stem cell injection. For bone marrow aspiration for platelet rich stem cell injection, use 0232T)◀

**38230**  Bone marrow harvesting for transplantation; allogeneic

**38232**      autologous

(For autologous and allogeneic blood-derived peripheral stem cell harvesting for transplantation, see 38205-38206)

▶(For bone marrow aspiration, use 38220)◀

### Rationale

Three parenthetical notes have been added to the Bone Marrow or Stem Cell Services/Procedures section to provide further clarification on the appropriate reporting of codes 38220-38230. The first note follows code 38220 and instructs users to report code 38220 for needle aspiration of bone marrow for the purposes of bone grafting. The second note also follows code 38220 and instructs users not to report codes 38220-38230 for bone marrow aspiration for platelet-rich stem cell injections, but to report code 0232T instead. The third and final note follows code 38232 and directs users to code 38220 for bone marrow aspiration.

To differentiate, code 38220 may be used for needle aspiration of bone marrow for the purpose of bone grafting or aspiration of bone marrow for diagnostic purposes. Although the parenthetical instruction following code 20938 directs users to code 38220, in this instance code 38220 involves aspiration of bone marrow for grafting in an arthrodesis procedure. When the bone marrow is obtained prior to the arthrodesis, the placement of the bone marrow aspirate is included as part of the arthrodesis procedure and is not reported separately.

▶Hematopoietic cell transplantation (HCT) refers to the infusion of hematopoietic progenitor cells (HPC) obtained from bone marrow, peripheral blood apheresis, and/or umbilical cord blood. These procedure codes (38240-38243) include physician monitoring of multiple physiologic parameters, physician verification of cell processing, evaluation of the patient during as well as immediately before and after the HPC/lymphocyte infusion, physician presence during the HPC/lymphocyte infusion with associated direct physician supervision of clinical staff, and management of uncomplicated adverse events (eg, nausea, urticaria) during the infusion, which is not separately reportable.

HCT may be autologous (when the HPC donor and recipient are the same person) or allogeneic (when the HPC donor and recipient are not the same person). Code 38241 is used to report any autologous transplant while 38240 is used to report an allogeneic transplant. In some cases allogeneic transplants involve more than one donor and cells from each donor are infused sequentially whereby one unit of 38240 is reported for each donor infused. Code 38242 is used to report a donor lymphocyte infusion. Code 38243 is used to report a HPC boost from the original allogeneic HPC donor. A lymphocyte infusion or HPC boost can occur days, months or even years after the initial hematopoietic cell transplant. The lymphocyte infusion is used to treat relapse, infection, or post-transplant lymphoproliferative syndrome. HPC boost represents an infusion of hematopoietic progenitor cells from the original donor that is being used to treat a relapse or post-transplant cytopenia(s). Codes 38240, 38242, and 38243 should not be reported together on the same date of service.

If a separately identifiable evaluation and management service is performed on the same date of service, the appropriate E/M service code, including office or other outpatient services, established (99211-99215), hospital observation services (99217-99220, 99224-99226), hospital inpatient services (99221-99223, 99231-99239), and inpatient neonatal and pediatric critical care (99471, 99472, 99475, 99476) may be reported, using modifier 25, in addition to 38240, 38242 or 38243. Post-transplant infusion management of adverse reactions is reported separately using the appropriate E/M, prolonged service or critical care code(s). In accordance with place of service and facility reporting guidelines, the fluid used to administer the cells and other infusions for incidental hydration (eg, 96360, 96361) are not separately reportable. Similarly, infusion(s) of any medication(s) concurrently with the transplant infusion are not separately reportable. However, hydration or administration of medications (eg, antibiotics, narcotics) unrelated to the transplant are separately reportable using modifier 59.◀

▲38240   Hematopoietic progenitor cell (HPC); allogeneic transplantation per donor

▲38241       autologous transplantation

#●38243       HPC boost

▲38242   Allogeneic lymphocyte infusions

(For bone marrow aspiration, use 38220)

▶(For modification, treatment, and processing of hematopoietic progenitor cell specimens for transplantation, see 38210-38215)◀

▶(For cryopreservation, freezing, and storage of hematopoietic progenitor cells for transplantation, use 38207)◀

▶(For thawing and expansion of hematopoietic progenitor cells for transplantation, see 38208, 38209)◀

       ⊘=Modifier 51 Exempt   ⊙=Moderate Sedation   ✚=Add-on Code   𝒩=FDA approval pending

▶(For compatibility studies, see 81379-81383, 86812-86822)◀

**38243**    ▶Code is out of numerical sequence. See 38240-38242◀

### ✍️ Rationale

In response to concerns regarding valuation and work represented in the family of codes 38240-38242, several changes and additions have been made to the CPT code set to clarify appropriate use of these services. First, a new subsection heading in the Hemic and Lymphatic Systems section for Transplantation and Post-Transplantation Cellular Infusions has been added along with introductory language and guidelines for appropriate reporting of these services. Second, codes 38240, 38241, and 38242 have been editorially revised. Third, code 38243 has been established to report HPC boost. Fourth, the parenthetical notes following code 38242 have been revised to provide direction for appropriate reporting of these services. Last, a cross-reference has been added in the Pathology and Laboratory/Transfusion Medicine section of the CPT code set following code 86950 directing users to the appropriate code for reporting allogeneic lymphocyte infusion (38242).

### 🩺 Clinical Example (38240)

The patient is a 40-year old female with acute myelogenous leukemia who has relapsed after obtaining a remission. An allogeneic HPC transplant is performed.

#### Description of Procedure (38240)

The physician supervises the initiation of the product infusion and is present for the first 15 to 30 minutes. The physician remains immediately available to manage toxicities and complications occurring during the infusion. The physician evaluates the patient at the end of the infusion.

### 🩺 Clinical Example (38241)

The patient is a 68-year-old male with non-Hodgkins lymphoma in second remission. Patient has co-morbidities of ischemic heart disease, diabetes and a recently treated aspergilloma. An autologous HPC transplant is performed.

#### Description of Procedure (38241)

The physician supervises the initiation of the product infusion and is present for the first 15 to 30 minutes. The physician remains immediately available to manage toxicities and complications occurring during the infusion. The physician evaluates the patient at the end of the infusion.

### 🩺 Clinical Example (38242)

The patient is a 67-year-old female who had a prior allogeneic transplant for B-cell chronic lymphocytic leukemia. She has recently relapsed. Her T-cell lymphocytes are 50% donor and 50% host. A T-lymphocyte infusion using lymphocytes from the original donor is performed.

**Description of Procedure (38242)**

The physician supervises the initiation of the product infusion and is present for the first 15 to 30 minutes. The physician remains immediately available to manage toxicities and complications occurring during the infusion. The physician evaluates the patient at the end of the infusion.

## Clinical Example (38243)

The patient is a 68-year-old female who received an allogeneic (unrelated donor) transplant for acute myeloid leukemia (AML). Three months after transplant, the recipient is pancytopenic and transfusion dependent for red cells and platelets. The blood cells are of donor origin. The remaining peripheral blood progenitor cells from the original transplant donor are infused to treat the pancytopenia.

**Description of Procedure (38243)**

The physician supervises the initiation of the product infusion and is present for the first 15 to 30 minutes. The physician remains immediately available to manage toxicities and complications occurring during the infusion. The physician evaluates the patient at the end of the infusion.

# Digestive System

## Esophagus

### ENDOSCOPY

⊙**43200**    Esophagoscopy, rigid or flexible; diagnostic, with or without collection of specimen(s) by brushing or washing (separate procedure)

⊙**43205**    with band ligation of esophageal varices

⊙●**43206**    with optical endomicroscopy

▶(Report supply of contrast agent separately)◀

▶(Do not report 43206 in conjunction with 88375)◀

▶(43234 has been deleted. To report, use 43235)◀

⊙**43235**    Upper gastrointestinal endoscopy including esophagus, stomach, and either the duodenum and/or jejunum as appropriate; diagnostic, with or without collection of specimen(s) by brushing or washing (separate procedure)

⊙**43251**    with removal of tumor(s), polyp(s), or other lesion(s) by snare technique

⊙●**43252**    with optical endomicroscopy

▶(Report supply of contrast agent separately)◀

▶Do not report 43252 in conjunction with 88375)◀

▶(For biopsy specimen pathology, use 88305)◀

⊘=Modifier 51 Exempt  ⊙=Moderate Sedation  ✚=Add-on Code  ✗=FDA approval pending

## Rationale

Code 43234 has been deleted. This code was originally established for reporting upper gastrointestinal panendoscopy using a small-diameter endoscope. However, this approach is not highly utilized, with most patients receiving the service identified by code 43235, *(Upper gastrointestinal endoscopy including esophagus, stomach, and either the duodenum and/or jejunum as appropriate; diagnostic, with or without collection of specimen[s] by brushing or washing (separate procedure), using a standard endoscope).* As a result, a parenthetical note has been added to direct users to report code 43235 to identify upper gastrointestinal endoscopy.

Codes 43206, 43252, and Pathology Laboratory code 88375 have been established to identify real-time cellular observation of mucosal tissue (intestinal) during an endoscopy procedure. Code 43206 is used to identify optical endomicroscopy when performed with esophagoscopy and code 43252 is used to identify optical endomiscroscopy when performed with upper gastrointestinal endoscopy (EGD). Both services inherently include moderate sedation. These procedures also include diagnostic injection procedures required for administration of the contrast agent for the procedure. The supply of the contrast agent itself, however, is not included as part of the procedure. Therefore, a parenthetical note has been included to direct that the agent should be reported separately. Provision of either service includes the interpretation and report for the service and code 88375 should not be reported in conjunction with these codes. As a result, a parenthetical note has been included following both codes to exclude the use of these codes with code 88375. For more information regarding the use of code 88375, see the Rationale for this code.

Optical endomicroscopy uses in vivo microscopic imaging to facilitate real-time cellular observation of mucosal tissue during an endoscopy procedure. It is used selectively when there is suspicion of early stage pre-neoplastic/dysplasia disease in patients undergoing endoscopy procedures. Optical endomicroscopy allows the physician to better identify anatomical sites where a targeted biopsy is warranted to establish a diagnosis. Therefore, by avoiding random biopsies, which has a high likelihood of missing abnormal tissue, optical endomicroscopy allows the physician to make real-time therapeutic decisions that would otherwise require multiple biopsy procedures.

## Clinical Example (43206)

A 63-year-old female with reflux symptoms non-responsive to pharmacologic measures is referred for examination.

### Description of Procedure (43206)

An esophagoscopy examination is performed, which identifies abnormal tissue in the distal esophagus suspicious for Barrett's esophagus. Optical endomicroscopic examination of the tissue is performed and images are reviewed, identifying areas that are suspicious for pre-malignant and/or malignant tissue, facilitating performance of biopsy (separate procedure). At the conclusion of the procedure, the endoscope is withdrawn.

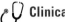 **Clinical Example (43252)**

A 53-year-old first generation male of Hispanic descent with a history of abdominal discomfort and early satiety unresponsive to pharmacological measures is referred for examination.

**Description of Procedure (43252)**

An esophagogastroduodenoscopy (EGD) examination is performed, which identifies abnormal mucosa at the esophagogastric junction. Optical endomicroscopic examination of the tissue is performed and images are reviewed, identifying areas that are suspicious for pre-malignant and/or malignant tissue, facilitating performance of biopsy (separate procedure). At the conclusion of the procedure, the endoscope is withdrawn.

## Stomach

### EXCISION

**43640**   Vagotomy including pyloroplasty, with or without gastrostomy; truncal or selective

(For pyloroplasty, use 43800)

(For vagotomy, see 64752-64760)

**43641**      parietal cell (highly selective)

▶(For upper gastrointestinal endoscopy, see 43235-43259)◀

 **Rationale**

In support of the deletion of simple upper gastrointestinal endoscopy code 43234, the cross-reference note following code 43641 has been revised to direct users to code 43235-43259 for upper gastrointestinal endoscopy.

### LAPAROSCOPY

**43647**   Laparoscopy, surgical; implantation or replacement of gastric neurostimulator electrodes, antrum

**43648**      revision or removal of gastric neurostimulator electrodes, antrum

(For open approach, see 43881, 43882)

(For insertion of gastric neurostimulator pulse generator, use 64590)

(For revision or removal of gastric neurostimulator pulse generator, use 64595)

(For electronic analysis and programming of gastric neurostimulator pulse generator, see 95980-95982)

(For laparoscopic implantation, revision, or removal of gastric neurostimulator electrodes, lesser curvature [morbid obesity], use 43659)

▶(For laparoscopic implantation, revision, replacement, or removal of vagus nerve blocking neurostimulator electrode array and/or pulse generator at the esophagogastric junction, see 0312T-0317T)◀

○=Modifier 51 Exempt   ⊙=Moderate Sedation   ✛=Add-on Code   𝒩=FDA approval pending

## BARIATRIC SURGERY

### Laparoscopy

**43770**    Laparoscopy, surgical, gastric restrictive procedure; placement of adjustable gastric restrictive device (eg, gastric band and subcutaneous port components)

**43775**        longitudinal gastrectomy (ie, sleeve gastrectomy)

(For open gastric restrictive procedure, without gastric bypass, for morbid obesity, other than vertical-banded gastroplasty, use 43843)

▶(For laparoscopic implantation, revision, replacement, removal or reprogramming of vagus nerve blocking neurostimulator electrode array and/or pulse generator at the esophagogastric junction, see 0312T-0317T)◀

## OTHER PROCEDURES

**43882**    Revision or removal of gastric neurostimulator electrodes, antrum, open

(For laparoscopic approach, see 43647, 43648)

(For insertion of gastric neurostimulator pulse generator, use 64590)

(For revision or removal of gastric neurostimulator pulse generator, use 64595)

(For electronic analysis and programming of gastric neurostimulator pulse generator, see 95980-95982)

(For open implantation, revision, or removal of gastric neurostimulator electrodes, lesser curvature [morbid obesity], use 43999)

▶(For laparoscopic implantation, revision, replacement, removal or reprogramming of vagus nerve blocking neurostimulator electrode array and/or pulse generator at the esophagogastric junction, see 0312T-0317T)◀

▶(For open implantation, revision, or removal of gastric lesser curvature or vagal trunk (EGJ) neurostimulator electrodes, [morbid obesity], use 43999)◀

### 🖊 Rationale

To provide users with appropriate instructions regarding appropriate codes to use to identify vagus nerve stimulation procedures for weight loss, parenthetical cross-references have been placed following codes 43648, 43775, and 43882. For additional information regarding the use of codes 0312T-0317T, see the Rationale for these codes.

An additional parenthetical note has been added following code 43882, directing users to unlisted code 43999 for open implantation, revision, or removal of gastric lesser curvature, or vagal trunk (EGJ) neurostimulator electrodes (morbid obesity).

# Intestines (Except Rectum)

## ENDOSCOPY, SMALL INTESTINE AND STOMAL

▶(For upper gastrointestinal endoscopy, see 43235-43258)◀

⊙**44360**  Small intestinal endoscopy, enteroscopy beyond second portion of duodenum, not including ileum; diagnostic, with or without collection of specimen(s) by brushing or washing (separate procedure)

### 🖎 Rationale

In support of the deletion of simple upper gastrointestinal endoscopy code 43234, the cross-reference above code 44360 has been revised to direct users to codes 43235-43258 for upper gastrointestinal endoscopy.

## OTHER PROCEDURES

**✚44701**  Intraoperative colonic lavage (List separately in addition to code for primary procedure)

(Use 44701 in conjunction with 44140, 44145, 44150, or 44604 as appropriate)

(Do not report 44701 in conjunction with 44300, 44950-44960)

**●44705**  Preparation of fecal microbiota for instillation, including assessment of donor specimen

▶(Do not report 44705 in conjunction with 74283)◀

▶(For fecal instillation by oro-nasogastric tube or enema, use 44799)◀

**44715**  Backbench standard preparation of cadaver or living donor intestine allograft prior to transplantation, including mobilization and fashioning of the superior mesenteric artery and vein

### 🖎 Rationale

Code 44705 has been established for reporting physician work provided for assessing donors and overseeing preparation of fecal microbiota. The service inherently includes: (1) development of the slurry that will be instilled into the recipient digestive tract, and (2) assessment of the donor specimen, including physician review of the results of testing for Clostridium difficile toxins in the donor stool as well as serologic testing of the donor's specimen for hepatitis A, B, and C viruses, HIV-1, HIV-2, and syphilis. Parenthetical notes have been added indicating that code 44705 should not be reported with therapeutic anemia code 74283. A cross-reference has also been added to direct users to unlisted code 44799 for fecal instillation via oro-nasogastric tube or enema. Donor education on specific procedures to follow on the day prior to and on the day of the instillation is completed by the clinical staff. In addition, laboratory testing provided for the patient is reported separately.

Fecal microbiota therapy is used to treat Clostridium difficile infection (CDI), which has become epidemic, with increased incidence, morbidity, and mortality, since newer, more virulent, and more antibiotic-resistant strains have emerged. CDI still occurs most commonly in health care facilities among elderly, inflammatory bowel disease, immunocompromised, or peripartum patients but is

⊘=Modifier 51 Exempt   ⊙=Moderate Sedation   ✚=Add-on Code   𝒩=FDA approval pending

increasingly identified in the community among healthy individuals without prior health care exposure.

###  Clinical Example (44705)

A 73-year-old female with refractory, relapsing C. difficile diarrhea despite multiple courses of antibiotic treatment, is referred for evaluation and consideration of treatment options. After assessment (reported separately as E/M), it is elected to utilize fecal microbiota therapy. The physician has selected the potential donor, and oversees evaluation and preparation of the specimen.

### Description of Procedure (44705)

The physician conducts a detailed review of the donor's past medical and surgical history and current health status pertaining to recent antibiotic use, travel, immunodeficiency disease, and related issues. The physician reviews the donor's medication list to determine whether the patient has used medications that are contraindicated for a transfaunal donation. The physician conducts a focused physical examination for conditions that may contraindicate donation. The physician reviews the laboratory tests with the donor. The physician makes a final determination of whether the donor is suitable. In the event that pathological conditions are identified by history, physical examination, or laboratory testing, the physician arranges referral of the donor to the donor's primary health care provider or emergency evaluation, if appropriate. Following collection of the fecal specimen, the physician oversees the preparation of the filtered material to be infused into the recipient. A "time out" relative to the infusion specimen is performed.

## Urinary System

## Bladder

### TRANSURETHRAL SURGERY

#### Urethra and Bladder

**52285** Cystourethroscopy for treatment of the female urethral syndrome with any or all of the following: urethral meatotomy, urethral dilation, internal urethrotomy, lysis of urethrovaginal septal fibrosis, lateral incisions of the bladder neck, and fulguration of polyp(s) of urethra, bladder neck, and/or trigone

●**52287** Cystourethroscopy, with injection(s) for chemodenervation of the bladder

▶(The supply of the chemodenervation agent is reported separately)◀

### 🖎 Rationale

Code 52287 has been established for reporting chemodenervation of the bladder for neurogenic incontinence. Existing codes 64614 and 64640 are specific to the chemodenervation of the internal anal sphincter, parotid and submandibular salivary glands, muscle innervated by facial nerve, neck muscles, extremity and/or trunk muscles, eccrine glands, and extraocular muscle. A code for chemodenervation of the smooth muscles of the bladder was not available, which necessitated the establishment of code 52287.

A parenthetical note was added following code 52287 indicating that supply of the chemodenervation agent is reported separately.

 ## Clinical Example (52287)

A 46-year-old female presents with urinary incontinence due to neurogenic detrusor overactivity. The patient is experiencing urinary urgency, frequency and urgency incontinence several times daily. Prior evaluation has consisted of a negative urine culture and cytology, diagnostic cystoscopy that was consistent with evidence of detrusor hyperactivity, and urodynamics that demonstrated uninhibited detrusor contractions in the absence of anatomical obstruction. The patient has failed oral anticholinergic/antimuscarinic medications, and is scheduled for treatment with chemodenervation of the bladder by intravesical injection of a neurotoxic agent.

### Description of Procedure (52287)

Prior to injection, the syringe containing the reconstituted drug is attached to the cystoscopic injection needle, which is then primed with approximately 1 mL of the diluted drug to remove any air. On the sterile field, the cystoscopic injection needle is loaded into the working channel of the cystoscope. The cystoscope is inserted through the patient's urethra into the bladder under direct visualization. The procedure is documented with still photographs from the video unit, and images are transferred to the medical record. The urinary bladder is distended to near capacity with approximately 300 cc cystoscopic irrigant using sterile normal saline. Under direct vision, the surgeon places the cystoscopic needle at 2 mm to 4 mm of depth into the bladder detrussor muscle, assuring the needle-depth has not perforated the bladder. The surgeon holds steady positioning of the needle in the bladder muscle. The surgeon directs the assistant to press 0.5 cc to 1 cc of drug from the syringe, as the surgeon observes the injection bleb of drug delivered to the bladder muscle. (This is a four-handed maneuver that requires an assistant; the surgeon cannot watch the bladder and the syringe at the same time.) This injection maneuver is repeated 10 to 60 times, spacing injections 1 cm apart and dispersing injections evenly throughout the bladder muscle, taking care to avoid critical landmarks and vascular structures. For the final injection, approximately 1 mL of sterile saline is injected so that the full dose is delivered. At the end of the injection procedure, the bladder is drained, and the cystoscope is reinserted to refill the bladder to observe for any bleeding and to assure that no perforations or injuries have occurred. The bladder is redrained at the end of the procedure.

## Extracranial Nerves, Peripheral Nerves, and Autonomic Nervous System

### NEUROSTIMULATORS (PERIPHERAL NERVE)

**64553**   Percutaneous implantation of neurostimulator electrode array; cranial nerve

**▲64561**       sacral nerve (transforaminal placement) including image guidance, if performed

**64570**   Removal of cranial nerve (eg, vagus nerve) neurostimulator electrode array and pulse generator

(Do not report 64570 in conjunction with 61888)

▶(For laparoscopic implantation, revision, replacement, or removal of vagus nerve blocking neurostimulator electrode array and/or pulse generator at the esophagogastric junction, see 0312T-0317T)◀

### ✏️ Rationale

Code 64561 was editorially revised to state "including image guidance, if performed" to clarify that image guidance is included in this procedure and should not be reported separately when performed.

To provide users with appropriate instructions regarding appropriate codes to use to identify vagus nerve stimulation procedures for weight loss, a parenthetical cross-reference has been placed following code 64570, directing users to Category III codes 0312T-0317T. For additional information regarding the use for codes 0312T-0317T, see the Rationale for these codes.

### ▶DESTRUCTION BY NEUROLYTIC AGENT (EG, CHEMICAL, THERMAL, ELECTRICAL OR RADIOFREQUENCY), CHEMODENERVATION◀

▶Codes 64600-64681 include the injection of other therapeutic agents (eg, corticosteroids). Do not report diagnostic/therapeutic injections separately. Do not report a code labeled as destruction when using therapies that are not destructive of the target nerve (eg, pulsed radiofrequency), use 64999. For codes labeled as chemodenervation, the supply of the chemodenervation agent is reported separately.◀

▶(For chemodenervation of internal anal sphincter, use 46505)◀

▶(For chemodenervation of the bladder, use 52287)◀

▶(For chemodenervation for strabismus involving the extraocular muscles, use 67345)◀

▶(For chemodenervation guided by needle electromyography or muscle electrical stimulation, see 95873, 95874)◀

### ✏️ Rationale

The heading for destruction by neurolytic agent has been revised to include "chemodenervation." The introductory guidelines pertaining to codes 64600-64681 have been revised to instruct the use of a separate supply code for reporting the chemodenervation agent. Also, instructions have been added to not use a destruction code when utilizing therapies that do not destroy a target nerve (eg, pulsed radiofrequency); instead, the unlisted nervous system procedure code 64999 should be used. The three parenthetical notes following code 64614 that direct users to other chemodenervation codes in the Surgery and Medicine sections have been relocated to follow the guidelines at the beginning of the Destruction by Neurolytic agent section. An additional note was added to this group of notes instructing users to report code 52287 for chemodenervation of the bladders listed in other subsections of Surgery and Medicine.

### Somatic Nerves

▲64612   Chemodenervation of muscle(s); muscle(s) innervated by facial nerve, unilateral (eg, for blepharospasm, hemifacial spasm)

▶(To report a bilateral procedure, use modifier 50)◀

64613       neck muscle(s) (eg, for spasmodic torticollis, spasmodic dysphonia)

▶(Report 64613 only once per session)◀

▶(Do not report 64613 with modifier 50)◀

▲64614       extremity and/or trunk muscle(s) (eg, for dystonia, cerebral palsy, multiple sclerosis)

▶(Report 64614 only once per session)◀

●64615       muscle(s) innervated by facial, trigeminal, cervical spinal and accessory nerves, bilateral (eg, for chronic migraine)

▶(Report 64615 only once per session)◀

▶(Do not report 64615 in conjunction with 64612, 64613, 64614)◀

### ✒ Rationale

Code 64615 has been established to report chemodenervation of muscle(s) innervated by facial, trigeminal, cervical spinal, and accessory nerves, bilateral (eg, for chronic migraine). Code 64615 is used to report a chemodenervation injection procedure for the treatment of chronic migraine. For the treatment, a patient must meet these criteria for migraine: 15 or more days of headache or a headache that lasts 4 hours or more per day. Prior to treatment, 31 injection sites over 7 muscle groups are typically identified on the face, head, neck, and upper back (the frontalis, corrugatore, procerus, occipatlis, temporalis, trapezius, and cervial paraspinal muscle groups). Code 64615 is reported only once per session. An exclusionary parenthetical note has been added following code 64615, to preclude reporting code 64615 with chemodenervation codes 64612, 64613, and 64614.

Code 64612 has been revised to include the term "unilateral," and code 64614 has been revised by removing "s" from the term extremity. Instructional parenthetical notes were added following this family of codes, instructing users that codes 64612-64614 are used only once per session.

A clarification has been added to the Destruction of Neurolytic Agent guidelines indicating that when reporting chemodenervation codes, the supply of the chemodenervation agent is reported separately. The instructional notes following code 64614 were moved to the introductory guidelines for Destruction of Neurolytic Agent, as they relate to the entire family of codes, and the term "Chemodenervation" has been added to the Destruction of Neurolytic Agent subheading.

###  Clinical Example (64612)

A 62-year-old male presents with nearly constant spasms of the left side of his face including the orbicularis oculi. Chemodenervation is recommended.

### Description of Procedure (64612)

The facial muscles are injected in 6 to 8 locations: three in the brow, one in the lateral canthus, one or two in the lower lid, one in the lateral aspect of the upper lid, and when needed, one in the nasal aspect of the upper lid. More muscles may be injected such as platysma and zygomaticus.

###  Clinical Example (64615)

A 46-year-old female presents with 19 headache days per month, of which 15 or more meet the criteria for migraine (headache lasting 4 hours or more per day). The decision is made to chemodenervate muscles innervated by the facial, trigeminal, cervical spinal and accessory nerves.

### Description of Procedure (64615)

The physician identifies 31 injection sites over 7 muscle groups on each side of the face, head, neck, and upper back (eg, the frontalis, corrugator, procerus, occipitalis, temporalis, trapezius, and cervical paraspinal muscle groups). The physician prepares each of the injection sites by cleaning with alcohol. The physician injects, controls bleeding, and ensures the patient is stable.

**Sympathetic Nerves**

**64650**    Chemodenervation of eccrine glands; both axillae

**64653**        other area(s) (eg, scalp, face, neck), per day

(Report the specific service in conjunction with code(s) for the specific substance(s) or drug(s) provided)

(For chemodenervation of extremities (eg, hands or feet), use 64999)

▶(For chemodenervation of bladder, use 52287)◀

 **Rationale**

A cross-reference was added following chemodenervation of the eccrine glands code 64653 to reference code 52287 for chemodenervation of the bladder. This instruction was also added to the introductory notes for codes 64600-64681.

# Eye and Ocular Adnexa

## Anterior Segment

### ANTERIOR CHAMBER

**Incision**

▲**65800**    Paracentesis of anterior chamber of eye (separate procedure); with removal of aqueous

▶(65805 has been deleted. To report, use 65800)◀

 **Rationale**

As part of the RUC Relativity Assessment Workgroup (RAW) (formerly the Five-Year Review Identification Workgroup) analysis of codes, it was determined that code 65805 was a high-volume frequently reported code, but it was never valued by the RUC, as it was Harvard-valued. In preparation for review of code 65805 to undergo RUC valuation, the involved societies from ophthalmology discovered that the service described in code 65805, *Paracentesis of anterior chamber of eye with therapeutic release of aqueous*, was very similar to the services described in 65800, *Paracentesis of anterior chamber of eye with diagnostic aspiration of aqueous*. Thus, it was recommended that code 65805 be deleted and combined into code 65800, with a change in terminology to state "with removal of aqueous," which adequately encompasses both the diagnostic aspiration of aqueous and therapeutic release of aqueous.

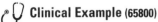 **Clinical Example** (65800)

A 70-year-old female presents six months after trabeculectomy with a hypopyon.

⊘=Modifier 51 Exempt    ⊙=Moderate Sedation    ✚=Add-on Code    ✗=FDA approval pending

**Description of Procedure (65800)**

The slit lamp is positioned to identify the operative field. The globe is grasped with micro-forceps and a 25-gauge needle on a syringe is positioned at the limbus, parallel to the iris plane. The needle is advanced through the cornea with the bevel oriented up, entering the anterior chamber, while remaining above the iris. A sample of aqueous is aspirated from the eye. The needle is removed. The physician plates samples onto 3 to 4 prepared culture media and a glass microscope slide.

## INTRAOCULAR LENS PROCEDURES

**66982** Extracapsular cataract removal with insertion of intraocular lens prosthesis (1-stage procedure), manual or mechanical technique (eg, irrigation and aspiration or phacoemulsification), complex, requiring devices or techniques not generally used in routine cataract surgery (eg, iris expansion device, suture support for intraocular lens, or primary posterior capsulorrhexis) or performed on patients in the amblyogenic developmental stage

▶(For insertion of ocular telescope prosthesis including removal of crystalline lens, use 0308T)◀

**66983** Intracapsular cataract extraction with insertion of intraocular lens prosthesis (1 stage procedure)

▶(Do not report 66983 in conjunction with 0308T)◀

**66984** Extracapsular cataract removal with insertion of intraocular lens prosthesis (1 stage procedure), manual or mechanical technique (eg, irrigation and aspiration or phacoemulsification)

(For complex extracapsular cataract removal, use 66982)

▶(For insertion of ocular telescope prosthesis including removal of crystalline lens, use 0308T)◀

**66985** Insertion of intraocular lens prosthesis (secondary implant), not associated with concurrent cataract removal

(To code implant at time of concurrent cataract surgery, see 66982, 66983, 66984)

 **Rationale**

In support of the establishment of a new Category III code 0308T, which is used for the insertion of an ocular telescope prosthesis, cross-reference notes have been added following codes 66982 and 66984 to direct users to new code 0308T. A parenthetical note was added following code 66983 to indicate that this code should not be reported in conjunction with 0308T.

# Ocular Adnexa

## EXTRAOCULAR MUSCLES

(Use 67320 in conjunction with 67311-67318)

## EYELIDS

### Incision

**67715**    Canthotomy (separate procedure)

(For canthoplasty, use 67950)

(For division of symblepharon, use 68340)

**# ▲67810**    Incisional biopsy of eyelid skin including lid margin

▶(For biopsy of skin of the eyelid, see 11100, 11101, 11310-11313)◀

### Excision, Destruction

**67800**    Excision of chalazion; single

**67808**         under general anesthesia and/or requiring hospitalization, single or multiple

**67810**    Code is out of numerical sequence. See 67700-67810

 **Rationale**

Code 67810 was editorially revised to clarify the depth and type of biopsy required for eyelid skin lesions when malignancy is suspected. This type of biopsy is classified as incisional biopsy, and it involves incision of the top and bottom layers of the lid margin. Code 67810 was also revised to distinguish it from biopsy codes 11100 and 11101 listed in the Integumentary System section for biopsy of skin and adjacent subcutaneous tissue, which is more commonly performed when biopsy of lesions are suspected to be benign. The placement of code 67810 was also changed so that it correctly appears under the Incision subheading instead of the Excision, Destruction subheading of the Eyelids subsection. A parenthetical note following code 67810 directs users to codes 11100 and 11101 for biopsy involving the skin and subcutaneous layer, and codes 11310-11313 for shaving of epidermal or dermal lesions was also added.

 **Clinical Example (67810)**

A 66-year-old female presents with a new lesion at the eyelid margin. Malignancy is suspected.

⊘=Modifier 51 Exempt   ⊙=Moderate Sedation   ✚=Add-on Code   ✗=FDA approval pending

**Description of Procedure (67810)**

The lesion is inspected and palpitated to assess depth, and to select the most representative site to obtain a specimen. The lesion is identified and a surgical "time out" is performed. The biopsy site is cleansed with a suitable antiseptic. Local anesthesia is achieved using lidocaine with epinephrine, which is drawn with a new needle infiltrated around the lesion for anesthesia and hemostasis. A drop of topical proparacaine is placed in the involved eye. An eye-shield is inserted. Sterile drapes are applied. The lesion is sharply removed, depending on its depth and the amount of tissue needed. The specimen is collected in a labeled formalin container. Hemostasis is achieved with cautery. The eye-shield is removed. The adequacy of eyelid closure and blink are determined. Antibiotic ointment and a sterile dressing are applied.

## Operating Microscope

▶The surgical microscope is employed when the surgical services are performed using the techniques of microsurgery. Code 69990 should be reported (without modifier 51 appended) in addition to the code for the primary procedure performed. Do not use 69990 for visualization with magnifying loupes or corrected vision. Do not report 69990 in addition to procedures where use of the operating microscope is an inclusive component (15756-15758, 15842, 19364, 19368, 20955-20962, 20969-20973, 22551, 22552, 22856-22861, 26551-26554, 26556, 31526, 31531, 31536, 31541, 31545, 31546, 31561, 31571, 43116, 43496, 49906, 61548, 63075-63078, 64727, 64820-64823, 65091-68850, 0184T, 0226T, 0227T, 0308T).◀

**+69990** Microsurgical techniques, requiring use of operating microscope (List separately in addition to code for primary procedure)

 **Rationale**

The note following code 69990 has been updated to include new Category III code 0308T, *Insertion of ocular telescope prosthesis including removal of crystalline lens*, as the operating microscope code should not be reported in addition to code 0308T.

# Radiology

A few revisions have been made in the Radiology section, some of which include: (1) deletion of the bronchography codes 71040 and 71060; (2) editorial revisions to the spine radiologic examination codes 72040, 72050, and 72052; (3) deletion of angiography codes 75650, 75660, 75662, 75665, 75671, 75676, 75680, and 75685; (4) revision of codes 75896 and 75898 to clarify that thrombolytic infusion is not an inclusive service and is separately reportable with the new combined transcatheter services 37211-37214; and (5) addition of instructional parenthetical notes added (for codes 72275, 77003 and 77012) throughout the Radiology subsections to instruct the appropriate reporting of the pre-sacral spinal fusion procedure codes, 22586, 0309T, 0195T, and 0196T.

Numerous revisions have been made to the Nuclear Medicine/Diagnostic Endocrine System subsection, which include: (1) deletion of the thyroid imaging codes 78000-78011; (2) addition of three new bundled thyroid imaging codes 78012-78014, which describe thyroid uptake and imaging procedures, and revision of the parenthetical notes following codes 76376 and 76377; (3) the revision of the parathyroid code 78070; and (4) the addition of SPECT and SPECT/CT parathyroid codes 78071 and 78072.

# Radiology

## Diagnostic Radiology (Diagnostic Imaging)

### Chest

**71035**   Radiologic examination, chest, special views (eg, lateral decubitus, Bucky studies)

▶(71040, 71060 have been deleted. To report, use 76499)◀

 **Rationale**

Bronchography has now been replaced by use of computed tomography (CT). As a result, bronchography codes 71040 and 71060 have been deleted. A cross-reference has been added to direct users to report Unlisted diagnostic radiographic procedure code 76499.

### Spine and Pelvis

▲**72040**   Radiologic examination, spine, cervical; 3 views or less

▲**72050**        4 or 5 views

▲**72052**        6 or more views

 **Rationale**

In an effort to more clearly define the work performed, and to reflect current clinical practice, Radiology codes 72040, 72050, and 72052 have been editorially revised.

When imaging studies of the spine or cervical region involve 3 views or less, code 72040 should be reported. Previously, code 72040 described imaging studies involving two or 3 views of the spine or cervical region.

When imaging studies of the spine or cervical region involve four or five views, code 72050 should be reported. Previously, code 72050 was reported when a minimum of 4 or 5 views were performed.

Finally, if imaging studies of six or more views of the spine or cervical region are performed, code 72052 should be reported. Previously, code 72052 was reported when a complete, including oblique and flexion and/or extension study was performed.

 **Clinical Example (72040)**

A 55-year-old female with cervical pain and no history of trauma. Rule out arthritis.

**Description of Procedure (72040)**

Supervise the technologist performing the examination. Radiographs of the cervical spine are interpreted and compared with prior studies, if applicable. A report is dictated for the medical record.

**Clinical Example (72050)**

A 43-year-old male presents with trauma to the cervical spine from auto accident. Clinical concern for instability.

**Description of Procedure (72050)**

Supervise the technologist performing the examination. Radiographs of the cervical spine are interpreted and compared with prior studies, if applicable. A report is dictated for the medical record.

**Clinical Example (72052)**

A 43-year-old male presents with trauma to the cervical spine from auto accident. There is clinical concern for instability.

**Description of Procedure (72052)**

Supervise the technologist performing the examination. Interpret the radiographs of the cervical spine. Compare the radiographs with prior studies, if applicable, and dictate a report for the patient's medical record.

72275    Epidurography, radiological supervision and interpretation

(72275 includes 77003)

(For injection procedure, see 62280-62282, 62310-62319, 64479-64484)

(Use 72275 only when an epidurogram is performed, images documented, and a formal radiologic report is issued)

▶(Do not report 72275 in conjunction with 22586, 0195T, 0196T, 0309T)◀

**Rationale**

A parenthetical note has been included following code 72275 to exclude use of this code in conjunction with any of the pre-sacral spinal fusion procedures (22586, 0195T, 0196T, 0309T). For more information regarding intended use for these codes, see the Rationale section for these codes.

## Vascular Procedures

### AORTA AND ARTERIES

75600    Aortography, thoracic, without serialography, radiological supervision and interpretation

▶(For supravalvular aortography performed at the time of cardiac catheterization, use 93567, which includes imaging supervision, interpretation, and report)◀

75605    Aortography, thoracic, by serialography, radiological supervision and interpretation

⃝=Modifier 51 Exempt    ⊙=Moderate Sedation    ✚=Add-on Code    ⫫=FDA approval pending

►(For supravalvular aortography performed at the time of cardiac catheterization, use 93567, which includes imaging supervision, interpretation, and report)◄

**75625** Aortography, abdominal, by serialography, radiological supervision and interpretation

►(75650 has been deleted. To report, see 36221-36226)◄

►(75660 has been deleted. To report, use 36227)◄

►(75662 has been deleted. To report, use 36227 and append modifier 50)◄

►(75665 has been deleted. To report, see 36223, 36224)◄

►(75671 has been deleted. To report, see 36223 and 36224 and append modifier 50 as appropriate)◄

►(75676 has been deleted. To report, see 36222-36224)◄

►(75680 has been deleted. To report, see 36222-36224 and append modifier 50 as appropriate)◄

►(75685 has been deleted. To report, see 36225, 36226)◄

**75741** Angiography, pulmonary, unilateral, selective, radiological supervision and interpretation

**75743** Angiography, pulmonary, bilateral, selective, radiological supervision and interpretation

**75746** Angiography, pulmonary, by nonselective catheter or venous injection, radiological supervision and interpretation

►(For pulmonary angiography by nonselective catheter or venous injection performed at the time of cardiac catheterization, use 93568, which includes imaging supervision, interpretation, and report)◄

**75756** Angiography, internal mammary, radiological supervision and interpretation

►(For internal mammary angiography performed at the time of cardiac catheterization, see 93455, 93457, 93459, 93461, 93564, which include imaging supervision, interpretation, and report)◄

**+75774** Angiography, selective, each additional vessel studied after basic examination, radiological supervision and interpretation (List separately in addition to code for primary procedure)

(Use 75774 in addition to code for specific initial vessel studied)

►(Do not report 75774 as part of diagnostic angiography of the extracranial and intracranial cervicocerebral vessels. It may be appropriate to report 75774 for diagnostic angiography of upper extremities and other vascular beds performed in the same session)◄

(For angiography, see 36147, 75600-75756, 75791)

(For catheterizations, see codes 36215-36248)

►(For cardiac catheterization procedures, see 93452-93462, 93531-93533, 93563-93568)◄

### 🖎 Rationale

To support the establishment of new codes (36221-36228), angiography supervision and interpretation codes 75650, 75660, 75662, 75665, 75671, 75676, 75680, and 75685 were deleted, since the work in these codes was combined or bundled into codes 36221-36228. Parenthetical notes associated with the deletion of these codes have been established to direct users to the appropriate arterial catheter placement codes to report.

A new instructional note has been added following code 75774 indicating that this code should not be reported as part of diagnostic angiography of the extracranial and intracranial cervicocerebral vessels. Instead, it may be appropriate to report code 75774 for diagnostic angiography of upper extremities and other vascular beds performed in the same session.

The cross-reference note following code 75774 related to introduction of catheter has been updated with new code ranges for cardiac catheter procedures. For more information regarding the intended use for these codes, see the Rationale following these codes.

In support of the changes implemented in the Medicine section, the notes following codes 75600 and 75605 have been revised to direct users to report code 93567 for supravalvular aortography performed at the time of cardiac catheterization. The notes following codes 75625, 75741, and 75743 that directed users to code 93567 for injection procedures have been deleted. The note following code 75746 has been revised to direct users to report code 93568 for pulmonary angiography by nonselective catheter or venous injection performed at the time of cardiac catheterization. The second note following code 75746, which directed users to codes 93451, 93453-93461, 93530-93533, 93563, 93564, and 93568 for the introduction of catheter and injection procedure has been deleted. The note following code 75756 has been revised to direct users to codes 93455, 93457, 93459, 93461, 93564 for internal mammary angiography performed at the time of cardiac catheterization.

## TRANSCATHETER PROCEDURES

▲75896    Transcatheter therapy, infusion, other than for thrombolysis, radiological supervision and interpretation

▶(For radiological supervision and interpretation for thrombolysis other than coronary, see 37211-37214)◀

▶(Do not report 75896 in conjunction with 37211-37214)◀

(For infusion for coronary disease, see 92975, 92977)

▲75898    Angiography through existing catheter for follow-up study for transcatheter therapy, embolization or infusion, other than for thrombolysis

▶(For thrombolysis infusion management other than coronary, see 37211-37214)◀

▶(Do not report 75898 in conjunction with 37211-37214)◀

▶(75900 has been deleted. For exchange of a previously placed intravascular catheter during thrombolytic therapy with contrast monitoring, radiological supervision and interpretation, see 37211-37214)◀

▶(75961 has been deleted. To report, use 37197)◀

(For removal of a vena cava filter, use 37193)

⊘=Modifier 51 Exempt    ⊙=Moderate Sedation    ✚=Add-on Code    𝒩=FDA approval pending

### ✐ Rationale

Codes 75896 and 75898 were both revised to clarify that thrombolytic infusion is not an inclusive service and is separately reportable with the new combined transcatheter services 37211-37214. Two parenthetical notes have been added following 75896 to direct user to codes 37211-37214 for radiological supervision and interpretation for thrombolysis other than coronary and to instruct that this code 75896 should not be reported in conjunction with thrombolytic infusion codes 37211-37214. Two parenthetical notes have been added following 75898 to direct the users to codes 37197-37214 for thrombolysis infusion management other than coronary, and to instruct that code 75898 should not be reported in conjunction with codes 37197-37214.

Code 75900 has been deleted. Previously, this code was reported when a previously placed intravascular catheter was exchanged during thrombolytic therapy. This service is now included in codes 37211-37214 and is not separately reportable. An instructional note has been added to indicate this change. Finally, code 75961, which was previously used to report transcatheter retrieval, percutaneous, of intravascular foreign body, radiological supervision and interpretation has been deleted. These transcatheter procedures that were reported with code 75961 should now be reported with the new combined transcatheter service code 37211.

**+ 75968** Transluminal balloon angioplasty, each additional visceral artery, radiological supervision and interpretation (List separately in addition to code for primary procedure)

(Use 75968 in conjunction with 75966)

▶(For percutaneous transluminal coronary angioplasty, see 92920-92944)◀

### ✐ Rationale

In support of the changes to the percutaneous coronary intervention codes in the Medicine subsection, the parenthetical note following transluminal balloon angioplasty radiological supervision and interpretation code 75968 has been revised with the replacement of codes 92982 and 92984 with new codes 92920-92944.

**75989** Radiological guidance (ie, fluoroscopy, ultrasound, or computed tomography), for percutaneous drainage (eg, abscess, specimen collection), with placement of catheter, radiological supervision and interpretation

▶(Do not report 75989 in conjunction with 32554, 32555, 32556, 32557, 47490)◀

### ✐ Rationale

An exclusionary parenthetical note has been added following code 75989 to restrict use of this code in conjunction with codes for thoracocentesis procedures (32554 and 32555) and pleural fluid drainage (32556 and 32557). For more information regarding the intended use of these codes, see the Rationale for these codes.

## Other Procedures

▲**76376**    3D rendering with interpretation and reporting of computed tomography, magnetic resonance imaging, ultrasound, or other tomographic modality with image postprocessing under concurrent supervision; not requiring image postprocessing on an independent workstation

(Use 76376 in conjunction with code[s] for base imaging procedure[s])

▶(Do not report 76376 in conjunction with 31627, 70496, 70498, 70544-70549, 71275, 71555, 72159, 72191, 72198, 73206, 73225, 73706, 73725, 74174, 74175, 74185, 74261-74263, 75557, 75559, 75561, 75563, 75565, 75571-75574, 75635, 76377, 78012-78999, 0159T)◀

▲**76377**          requiring image postprocessing on an independent workstation

(Use 76377 in conjunction with code[s] for base imaging procedure[s])

▶(Do not report 76377 in conjunction with 70496, 70498, 70544-70549, 71275, 71555, 72159, 72191, 72198, 73206, 73225, 73706, 73725, 74174, 74175, 74185, 74261-74263, 75557, 75559, 75561, 75563, 75565, 75571-75574, 75635, 76376, 78012-78999, 0159T)◀

(To report computer-aided detection, including computer algorithm analysis of MRI data for lesion detection/characterization, pharmacokinetic analysis, breast MRI, use Category III code 0159T)

▶(76376, 76377 require concurrent supervision of image postprocessing 3D manipulation of volumetric data set and image rendering)◀

### 🖉 Rationale

The exclusionary parenthetical notes following codes 76376 and 76377 were revised to reflect changes in the nuclear medicine codes. See also discussion on CPT nomenclature reporting neutrality.

## Diagnostic Ultrasound

### Chest

**76645**    Ultrasound, breast(s) (unilateral or bilateral), real time with image documentation

▶(Do not report 76645 in conjunction with 0301T)◀

### 🖉 Rationale

An exclusionary parenthetical note was added following 76645 to designate that a breast ultrasound should not be reported in conjunction with externally applied focused microwave code 0301T.

⊘=Modifier 51 Exempt   ⊙=Moderate Sedation   ✦=Add-on Code   ⊮=FDA approval pending

## Ultrasonic Guidance Procedures

**76942**   Ultrasonic guidance for needle placement (eg, biopsy, aspiration, injection, localization device), imaging supervision and interpretation

▶(Do not report 76942 in conjunction with 27096, 32554, 32555, 32556, 32557, 37760, 37761, 43232, 43237, 43242, 45341, 45342, 64479-64484, 64490-64495, 76975, 0213T-0218T, 0228T-0231T, 0232T, 0249T, 0301T)◀

(For injection(s) of platelet rich plasma, use 0232T)

 **Rationale**

The exclusionary parenthetical note following code 76942 was updated to include new codes for tube thoracostomy, thoracentesis, pleural drainage, paravertebral facet joint injections using ultrasound and applied focused microwave. For more information regarding the intended use for these services, see the Rationale for these codes.

## Other Procedures

**76998**   Ultrasonic guidance, intraoperative

▶(Do not report 76998 in conjunction with 36475-36479, 37760, 37761, 47370-47382, 0249T, 0301T)◀

 **Rationale**

The exclusionary parenthetical note following 76998 was revised to designate that intraoperative ultrasound guidance should not be reported in conjunction with codes for endovenous ablation therapy, ligation of perforated veins, laparoscopy, surgical, ablation of liver tumor, endovascular repair of iliac artery bifurcation, and applied focused microwave.

# Radiologic Guidance

## Fluoroscopic Guidance

**77002**   Fluoroscopic guidance for needle placement (eg, biopsy, aspiration, injection, localization device)

(See appropriate surgical code for procedure and anatomic location)

(77002 includes all radiographic arthrography with the exception of supervision and interpretation for CT and MR arthrography)

▶(Do not report 77002 in conjunction with 32554, 32555, 32556, 32557, 70332, 73040, 73085, 73115, 73525, 73580, 73615, 0232T)◀

(For injection(s) of platelet rich plasma, use 0232T)

(77002 is included in the organ/anatomic specific radiological supervision and interpretation procedures 49440, 74320, 74355, 74445, 74470, 74475, 75809, 75810, 75885, 75887, 75980, 75982, 75989)

## ✍ Rationale

The exclusionary parenthetical note following code 77002 has been revised to restrict use of this code in conjunction with codes for thoracocentesis procedures (32554 and 32555) and pleural fluid drainage (32556 and 32557). For more information regarding the intended use for these codes, see the Rationale following these codes.

**77003**   Fluoroscopic guidance and localization of needle or catheter tip for spine or paraspinous diagnostic or therapeutic injection procedures (epidural or subarachnoid)

(Injection of contrast during fluoroscopic guidance and localization [77003] is included in 22526, 22527, 27096, 62263, 62264, 62267, 62270-62282, 62310-62319)

(Fluoroscopic guidance for subarachnoid puncture for diagnostic radiographic myelography is included in supervision and interpretation codes 72240-72270)

(For epidural or subarachnoid needle or catheter placement and injection, see 62270-62282, 62310-62319)

(For sacroiliac joint arthrography, see 27096)

(For paravertebral facet joint injection, see 64490-64495. For paravertebral facet joint nerve destruction by neurolysis, see 64633-64636. For transforaminal epidural needle placement and injection, see 64479-64484)

▶(Do not report 77002, 77003 in conjunction with 22586, 27096, 64479–64484, 64490-64495, 64633-64636, 0195T, 0196T, 0309T)◀

## ✍ Rationale

A parenthetical note following code 77003 has been revised to exclude the use of this code in conjunction with any of the pre-sacral spinal fusion procedure codes 22586, 0309T, 0195T, and 0196T. For more information regarding intended use for these codes, see the Rationale following these codes.

## Computed Tomography Guidance

**77011**   Computed tomography guidance for stereotactic localization

**77012**   Computed tomography guidance for needle placement (eg, biopsy, aspiration, injection, localization device), radiological supervision and interpretation

▶(Do not report 77011, 77012 in conjunction with 22586, 0195T, 0196T, 0309T)◀

▶(Do not report 77012 in conjunction with 27096, 32554, 32555, 32556, 32557, 64479-64484, 64490-64495, 64633-64636, 0232T)◀

## ✍ Rationale

An exclusionary parenthetical note has been added following code 77012 to exclude use of codes 77011 and 77012 in conjunction with any of the procedure codes used to identify pre-sacral spinal fusion procedures (22586, 0309T, 0195T, and 0196T).

    ⊘=Modifier 51 Exempt   ⊙=Moderate Sedation   ✚=Add-on Code   ✗=FDA approval pending

In addition, the existing exclusionary parenthetical note following code 77012 has been revised to restrict use of this code in conjunction with codes for thoracocentesis procedures (32554 and 32555) and pleural fluid drainage (32556 and 32557). For more information regarding the intended use for these codes, see the Rationale following these codes.

## Magnetic Resonance Guidance

**77021** Magnetic resonance guidance for needle placement (eg, for biopsy, needle aspiration, injection, or placement of localization device) radiological supervision and interpretation

(For procedure, see appropriate organ or site)

▶(Do not report 77021 in conjunction with 32554, 32555, 32556, 32557, 0232T)◀

 **Rationale**

The exclusionary parenthetical note following code 77021 has been revised to restrict use of this code in conjunction with codes for thoracocentesis procedures (32554 and 32555) and pleural fluid drainage (32556 and 32557). For more information regarding the intended use for these codes, see the Rationale following these codes.

# Radiation Oncology

## Radiation Treatment Management

**77435** Stereotactic body radiation therapy, treatment management, per treatment course, to 1 or more lesions, including image guidance, entire course not to exceed 5 fractions

(Do not report 77435 in conjunction with 77427-77432)

▶(The same physician should not report both stereotactic radiosurgery services [32701, 63620, 63621] and radiation treatment management [77435])◀

 **Rationale**

In support of the addition of new code 32701 for the reporting of thoracic target delineation for stereotactic body radiation therapy (SRS/SBRT), the instructional note following radiation treatment management code 77435 has been revised and updated to include code 32701. The revised cross-reference instructs that the same physician should not report both stereotactic radiosurgery services 32701, 63620, and 63621 and radiation treatment management code 77435. In addition, the phrase, "for extracranial lesions" has been deleted from the note to be consistent with current clinical practice for SRS/SBRT.

# Hyperthermia

⊙**77600**    Hyperthermia, externally generated; superficial (ie, heating to a depth of 4 cm or less)

⊙**77605**    deep (ie, heating to depths greater than 4 cm)

▶(For focused microwave thermotherapy of the breast, use 0301T)◀

 **Rationale**

In support of the establishment of Category III code 0301T to describe a new technology that includes interstitial placement of a catheter under ultrasound guidance and adaptive phased array wide-field focused microwave thermotherapy heat treatment for destruction/reduction of a malignant tumor (early and advanced stage breast cancer), a cross-reference note has been added following the hyperthermia codes 77600-77605 to direct users to report code 0301T for focused microwave thermotherapy of the breast.

## Nuclear Medicine

### Diagnostic

#### ENDOCRINE SYSTEM

▶(78000-78011 have been deleted. To report, see 78012-78014)◀

●**78012**    Thyroid uptake, single or multiple quantitative measurement(s) (including stimulation, suppression, or discharge, when performed)

●**78013**    Thyroid imaging (including vascular flow, when performed);

●**78014**    with single or multiple uptake(s) quantitative measurement(s) (including stimulation, suppression, or discharge, when performed)

 **Rationale**

Because code 78007, *thyroid imaging, with uptake; multiple determination,* was identified by the AMA/Specialty Society RVS Update Committee (RUC) as potentially misvalued, and to be surveyed as part of the Harvard-valued codes with volume greater than 30,000 screen, it was determined that the thyroid family in the Nuclear Medicine/Diagnostic Endocrine System subsection in the CPT code set would greatly benefit from revisions to modernize and consolidate the codes prior to performing RUC surveys.

Changes to this section include deletion of codes 78000-78011, addition of three new codes (78012-78014) describing thyroid uptake and imaging procedures, and revision of the parenthetical notes following codes 76376 and 76377 to include reference to new codes 78012-78014 and 78015.

⊘=Modifier 51 Exempt   ⊙=Moderate Sedation   ✚=Add-on Code   𝑁=FDA approval pending

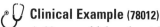 **Clinical Example (78012)**

A 32-year-old female with clinical symptoms of hyperthyroidism, blood thyroid function tests indicative of hyperthyroidism, and a diffusely enlarged non-nodular thyroid gland on physical examination.

**Description of Procedure (78012)**

The physician directs the technologist to adjust the acquisition protocol, as necessary, for the individual patient. The physician is available to answer questions for the technologist, review components of the study, and provide regulatory oversight throughout the procedure. The study typically consists of a single 24-hour uptake, and at times, multiple measurements every 4 to 6 hours plus the typical 24 hours are collected. A second standard capsule is maintained for comparison measurements. The patient should sit or lie with neck extended, and an open-faced collimated detector probe should be directed at the neck. Counts of the patient's neck and mid-thigh are obtained and repeated at varying time intervals as necessary. The physician verifies the adequacy of the data before completion of the study, and directs the technologist to obtain counts or reprocess the data, when necessary. The measurements are compared to relevant prior studies and formally interpreted (ie, a report is dictated for the medical record).

 **Clinical Example (78013)**

A 45-year-old female with two thyroid nodules on physical examination, without clinical symptoms of hyperthyroidism and with blood thyroid function tests indicative of euthyroidism.

**Description of Procedure (78013)**

The physician directs the technologist to adjust the acquisition protocol, as necessary, for the individual patient. The physician is available to answer questions for the technologist, review components of the study, and provide regulatory oversight throughout the procedure. Thyroid scintigraphy facilitates the detection of focal and/or global abnormalities of thyroid anatomy, correlation of anatomy with function, and detection of aberrant or residual normal tissue after therapy. Under the supervision of the physician, the technologist administers the radiopharmaceutical following the protocol determined. The complete study consists of administering the radiopharmaceutical by oral or typically by intravenous injection, acquiring multiple images in a variety of projections, and documenting the patient's position. Radioactive sources or lead markers may be used to identify anatomic landmarks such as the sternal notch and thyroid cartilage. When appropriate, the location of palpable nodules should be confirmed with the radioactive point source or lead marker image for anatomic correlation. The physician palpates and localizes any palpable nodules. The physician verifies the adequacy of the imaging data before completion of the study, and directs the technologist to obtain additional views or reprocess the data, when necessary. The data are formatted for film and/or digital display and analysis. The physician reviews the study for artifacts and abnormal distribution. The raw images (eg, upright or supine, anterior, obliques, etc) of the imaging are compared to any additional relevant prior studies and formally interpreted (ie, a report is dictated for the medical record). The data are formatted for film and/or digital display and analysis.

## Clinical Example (78014)

A 42-year-old female with clinical symptoms of hyperthyroidism, blood thyroid function tests indicative of hyperthyroidism, and a multi-nodular goiter on physical examination.

### Description of Procedure (78014)

Thyroid imaging with single or typically multiple uptakes is a combination of two radionuclide diagnostic imaging procedures that record the detection of focal and/or global abnormalities of thyroid anatomy, the correlation of anatomy with function, and the detection of aberrant or residual normal tissue after therapy. Under the supervision of the physician, the technologist administers the radiopharmaceutical(s) following the protocol determined. The complete study consists of administering the radiopharmaceutical(s) typically by oral or at times by intravenous injection, acquiring multiple images in a variety of projections, and documenting the patient's position. Radioactive sources or lead markers may be used to identify anatomic landmarks such as the sternal notch and thyroid cartilage. When appropriate, the location of palpable nodules should be confirmed with the radioactive point source or lead marker image for anatomic correlation. The physician palpates and localizes any palpable nodules. The physician verifies the adequacy of the imaging data before completion of the study, and directs the technologist to obtain additional views or reprocess the data, when necessary. The data are formatted for film and/or digital display and analysis. The physician reviews the study for artifacts and abnormal distribution. The raw images (eg, upright or supine, anterior, obliques, etc) of the imaging are compared to any additional relevant prior studies, as well as the single or multiple uptakes. The data are formatted for film and/or digital display and analysis. Additionally, single or typically multiple measurements at early 4 to 6 hours and/or 24 hours are collected.

The patient should sit or lie with neck extended, and an open-faced collimated detector probe should be directed at the neck. The study consists of single or typically multiple counts of the patient's neck and mid-thigh that are repeated at varying time intervals, as necessary. A second standard capsule is maintained for comparison measurements. The physician verifies the adequacy of the data before completion of the study, and directs the technologist to obtain additional views or reprocess the data, when necessary. The quantitative evaluations of measurements are compared to relevant prior and current studies and formally interpreted (ie, a report is dictated for the medical record).

The physician verifies the adequacy of the data before completion of the study, and directs the technologist to obtain counts or reprocess data, when necessary. The measurements are compared to relevant prior studies, and formally interpreted (ie, a report is dictated for the medical record).

▲**78070**  Parathyroid planar imaging (including subtraction, when performed);

●**78071**    with tomographic (SPECT)

●**78072**    with tomographic (SPECT), and concurrently acquired computed tomography (CT) for anatomical localization

---

⊘=Modifier 51 Exempt   ⊙=Moderate Sedation   ✚=Add-on Code   𝘕=FDA approval pending

# Rationale

Other changes to update and modernize the Nuclear Medicine/Diagnostic Endocrine System subsection in the CPT code set include revisions and additions to the current parathyroid code. A singular parathyroid code does not represent current clinical practice. SPECT and SPECT/CT parathyroid are frequently required in addition to planar imaging; there were no codes to report these clinically indicated procedures. To address these concerns and to clarify appropriate reporting, two new codes, SPECT (78071) and SPECT/CT (78072) have been established. To correlate with the new SPECT and SPECT/CT codes, the current code 78070 was revised by adding the word, "planar" and a parenthetical phrase, "(including subtraction, when performed)." This code is appropriate no matter what specific nuclear medicine technique (single or two injections) is used to acquire the planar data.

## Clinical Example (78070)

A 57-year-old female with elevated calcium levels and elevated PTH presents for evaluation of suspected hyperfunctioning parathyroid glands.

### Description of Procedure (78070)

The physician directs the technologist to adjust the acquisition protocol, as necessary, for the individual patient. The physician is available to answer questions for the technologist, review components of the study, and provide regulatory oversight throughout the procedure. The complete study consists of a minimum of two separate sets of planar imaging data encompassing the lower neck and the mediastinum, and techniques to differentiate radiopharmaceutical accumulation in anomalous or abnormal parathyroid glands from in the thyroid gland. The typical method involves the injection of a single radiopharmaceutical (99mTc-sestamibi) that is accumulated by both endocrine glands, but washes out of the thyroid gland faster than from parathyroid hyperplastic and adenomatous tissue. Anterior and bilateral anterior oblique images of the neck and anterior mediastinal images are acquired 10 to 30 minutes and again at 90 to 240 minutes after injection. A dual radiopharmaceutical technique, which is less commonly done, acquires similar but pre-timed sequential images for 5 minutes each, over a 30-minute period without moving the patient.

Whichever technique is used, thyroid and parathyroid imaging data are qualitatively compared to detect tissue uptake that is seen on the latter but is not present on the former to reveal discordant parathyroid uptake and its relative location. The physician verifies the adequacy of the imaging data before completion of the study, and directs the technologist to obtain additional views or reprocess the data, when necessary. The data are formatted for film and/or digital display and analysis. The physician reviews the study for artifacts and abnormal distribution. The imaging data are compared to relevant prior studies and formally interpreted (ie, a report is dictated for the medical record).

**Clinical Example (78071)**

A 47-year-old male with chronic renal failure and clinical evidence for hyperparathyroidism. Ultrasound shows suspicious nodule posterior to the right lobe of the thyroid.

**Description of Procedure (78071)**

The physician directs the technologist in the timing of the single photon emission computed tomography (SPECT) study and adjusts the acquisition protocol, as necessary, for the individual patient. The physician is available to answer questions from the technologist, review components of the study, and provide regulatory oversight throughout the procedure. The complete study consists of the following: (1) a minimum of two separate sets of planar imaging data encompassing the lower neck and the mediastinum; (2) techniques to differentiate radiopharmaceutical accumulation in anomalous or abnormal parathyroid glands from in the thyroid gland; and (3) a SPECT study of the same regions. The most commonly employed method is injection of a single radiopharmaceutical (99mTc-sestamibi) that is accumulated by both endocrine glands, but washes out of the thyroid gland faster than from parathyroid hyperplastic and adenomatous tissue. Anterior and bilateral anterior oblique planar images of the neck and anterior mediastinal images are acquired after 10 to 30 minutes and again at 90 to 240 minutes after injection. A SPECT study of the neck and mediastinum is acquired. A dual radiopharmaceutical technique, which is less commonly done, acquires similar but pre-timed sequential images for 5 minutes each, over a 30-minute period without moving the patient, followed by a SPECT study of the neck and mediastinum.

Whichever technique is used (single or dual radiopharmaceutical), thyroid and parathyroid imaging data are qualitatively compared to detect tissue uptake that is seen on the latter but is not present on the former to reveal discordant parathyroid uptake and its relative location for possible excision. The SPECT data are reconstructed in transaxial, sagittal, and coronal planes to facilitate the localization of abnormal parathyroid radiopharmaceutical accumulation. The physician verifies the adequacy of the imaging data before completion of the study, and directs the technologist to obtain additional views or reprocess the data when necessary. The data are formatted for film and/or digital display and analysis. The physician reviews the study for artifacts and abnormal distribution. The imaging data are compared to relevant prior studies and formally interpreted (ie, a report is dictated for the medical record).

 **Clinical Example (78072)**

A 68-year-old female with past history of neck exploration and resection of hyperplastic parathyroid glands now presents with evidence of recurrent hyperparathyroidism. Thyroid ultrasound is negative.

**Description of Procedure (78072)**

The physician directs the technologist in the timing of the single photon emission computed tomography/computed tomography (SPECT/CT) study and adjusts the acquisition protocol, as necessary, for the individual patient. The physician is available to answer questions from the technologist, review components of the study, and provide regulatory oversight throughout the procedure.

The complete study consists of a minimum of two separate sets of planar imaging data encompassing the lower neck and the mediastinum, and techniques to differentiate radiopharmaceutical accumulation in anomalous or abnormal parathyroid glands from in the thyroid gland, plus a SPECT/CT study of the same regions. The typical protocol is injection of a single radiopharmaceutical (99mTc-sestamibi) that is accumulated by both endocrine glands, but washes out of the thyroid gland faster than from parathyroid hyperplastic and adenomatous tissue. Anterior and bilateral anterior oblique planar images of the neck and anterior mediastinal images are acquired 10 to 30 minutes and again at 90 to 240 minutes after injection. A limited CT study of the neck and mediastinum is acquired, and without moving the patient, a SPECT study of the same regions is acquired. A dual radiopharmaceutical technique, which is less commonly done, acquires similar but pre-timed sequential images for 5 minutes each, over a 30-minute period without moving the patient, followed by a limited CT study of the neck and mediastinum, and again without moving the patient, acquisition of a SPECT study of the same regions.

Whichever technique is used (single or dual radiopharmaceutical), thyroid and parathyroid imaging data are qualitatively compared to detect tissue uptake that is seen on the latter but is not present on the former to reveal discordant parathyroid uptake and its relative location for possible excision. The SPECT and CT data are reconstructed in transaxial, sagittal, and coronal planes to facilitate the localization of abnormal parathyroid radiopharmaceutical accumulation. CT data are also used to generate attenuation corrected images in all three planes. Additional fused images from the SPECT and CT images are constructed to correlate the anatomic position of radiopharmaceutical accumulation with the current patient anatomy.

The physician verifies the adequacy of the imaging data before completion of the study, and directs the technologist to obtain additional views or reprocess the data, when necessary. The data are formatted for film and/or digital display and analysis. The physician reviews the study for artifacts and abnormal distribution. The imaging data are compared to relevant prior studies and formally interpreted (ie, a report is dictated for the medical record).

# Pathology and Laboratory

There have been numerous changes made to the Pathology and Laboratory section in the CPT code set. A major change to this section is the deletion of a set of procedures that are currently reported using the stacking codes 83890-83914 and array-based evaluation codes 88384-88386. In support of these deletions, a new multianalyte assays with algorithmic analyses (MAAAs), also known as IVDMIAs, subsection was added. The new subsection includes a new heading (Multianalyte Assays with Algorithmic Analyses), Category I introductory guidelines, an unlisted multianalyte assay with algorithmic analysis code, and eight new Category I multianalyte assay with algorithmic analyses codes. In concert with the addition of this new subsection, the CPT code set also contains a new Administrative Code List (Appendix O), which contains three new administrative and eight new Category I MAAA codes.

New definitions for inversion, loss of heterozygosity, and uniparental disomy have been added to the introduction of the Molecular Pathology section. Thirteen new codes have been added to Tier 1 codes, which are related to molecular pathology procedures in the CPT 2013 code set. The base descriptor of the 81400-81408 code series has been revised to include several new analytes.

Furthermore, 10 codes have been revised and 18 additional codes have been added throughout this section.

# Pathology and Laboratory

## Evocative/Suppression Testing

▶The following test panels involve the administration of evocative or suppressive agents, and the baseline and subsequent measurement of their effects on chemical constituents. These codes are to be used for the reporting of the laboratory component of the overall testing protocol. For the administration of the evocative or suppressive agents, see Hydration, Therapeutic, Prophylactic, Diagnostic Injections and Infusions, and Chemotherapy and Other Highly Complex Drug or Highly Complex Biologic Agent Administration (eg, 96365, 96366, 96367, 96368, 96372, 96374, 96375, 96376). In the code descriptors where reference is made to a particular analyte (eg, Cortisol: 82533 x 2) the "x 2" refers to the number of times the test for that particular analyte is performed.◀

### ✍ Rationale

The Evocative/Suppression Testing guidelines have been editorially revised to accurately reflect the entire family of therapeutic infusion codes. Also, the prolonged services code references have been deleted because it is not appropriate to report prolonged service codes for the time interval associated with therapeutic infusions. Omission of these references is consistent with the Prolonged Services guidelines in the Evaluation and Management Services section of the CPT code set.

## Molecular Pathology

Molecular pathology procedures are medical laboratory procedures involving the analyses of nucleic acid to detect variants in genes that may be indicative of germline (eg, constitutional disorders) or somatic (eg, neoplasia) conditions, or to test for histocompatibility antigens (eg, HLA). Code selection is typically based on the specific gene(s) that is being analyzed. Genes are described using Human Genome Organization (HUGO) approved gene names and are italicized in the code descriptors. Gene names were taken from tables of the HUGO Gene Nomenclature Commmittee (HGNC) at the time the CPT codes were developed. For the most part, Human Genome Variation Society (HGVS) recommendations were followed for the names of specific molecular variants. The familiar name is used for some variants because defined criteria were not in place when the variant was first described or because HGVS recommendations were changed over time (eg, intronic variants, processed proteins). When the gene name is represented by an abbreviation, the abbreviation is listed first, followed by the full gene name italicized in parentheses (eg, "F5 *[coagulation Factor V]*"), except for the HLA series of codes. Proteins or diseases commonly associated with the genes are listed as examples in the code descriptors. The examples do not represent all conditions in which testing of the gene may be indicated.

Codes that describe tests to assess for the presence of gene variants (see definitions) use common gene variant names. Typically, all of the listed variants would be tested. However, these lists are not exclusive. If other variants are also tested in the analysis, they would be included in the procedure and not reported separately. Full gene sequencing should not be reported using codes that assess for the presence of gene variants unless specifically stated in the code descriptor.

The molecular pathology codes include all analytical services performed in the test (eg, cell lysis, nucleic acid stabilization, extraction, digestion, amplification, and detection). Any procedures required prior to cell lysis (eg, microdissection, codes 88380 and 88381) should be reported separately.

The results of the procedure may require interpretation by a physician or other qualified health care professional. When only the interpretation and report are performed, modifier 26 may be appended to the specific molecular pathology code.

All analyses are qualitative unless otherwise noted.

For microbial identification, see 87149-87153 and 87470-87801, and 87900-87904. For in situ hybridization analyses, see 88271-88275 and 88365-88368.

▶Molecular pathology procedures that are not specified in 81200-81383 should be reported using either the appropriate Tier 2 code (81400-81408) or the unlisted molecular pathology procedure code, 81479.◀

### Rationale

The Molecular Pathology guidelines were revised to instruct and clarify that molecular pathology procedures not specified in 81200-81383 should be reported using the appropriate Tier 2 code (81400-81408) or the unlisted molecular pathology procedure code, 81479.

#### Definitions

For purposes of CPT reporting, the following definitions apply:

***Abnormal allele:*** an alternative form of a gene that contains a disease-related variation from the normal sequence.

***Intron:*** a nucleic acid sequence found between exons in human genes. An intron contains essential sequences for its proper removal (by a process known as *splicing*) to join exons together and thus facilitate production of a functional protein from a gene. An intron is sometimes referred to as an intervening sequence (IVS).

▶***Inversion:*** A defect in a chromosome in which a segment breaks and reinserts in the same place but in the opposite orientation.◀

▶***Loss of heterozygosity (LOH, allelic imbalance):*** An event that can occur in dividing cells that are heterozygous for one or more alleles, in which a daughter cell becomes hemizygous or homozygous for the allele(s) through mitotic recombination, deletion or other chromosomal event.◀

***Microarray:*** surface(s) on which multiple specific nucleic acid sequences are attached in a known arrangement. Sometimes referred to as a 'gene chip'. Examples of uses of microarrays include evaluation of a patient specimen for gains or losses of DNA sequences (copy number variants, CNVs), identification of the presence of specific nucleotide sequence variants (also known as single nucleotide polymorphisms, SNPs), mRNA expression levels, or DNA sequence analysis.

***Translocation:*** an abnormality resulting from the breakage of a chromosome and the relocation of a portion of that chromosome's DNA sequence to the same or another chromosome. Most common translocations involve a reciprocal exchange of DNA sequences between two differently numbered (ie, non-homologous) chromosomes, with or without a clinically significant loss of DNA.

⊘=Modifier 51 Exempt ⊙=Moderate Sedation ✚=Add-on Code ✗=FDA approval pending

▶ **Uniparental disomy (UPD):** Abnormal inheritance of both members of a chromosome pair from one parent, with absence of the other parent's chromosome for the pair. ◀

**Variant:** a nucleotide sequence difference from the "normal" (predominant) sequence for a given region. Variants are typically of two types: substitutions of one nucleotide for another, and deletions or insertions of nucleotides. Occasionally, variants reflect several nucleotide sequence changes in reasonably close proximity on the same chromosomal strand of DNA (a haplotype). These nucleotide sequence variants often result in amino acid changes in the protein made by the gene. The term *variant* does not itself carry a functional implication for those protein changes.

### 🔊 Rationale

New definitions for inversion, loss of heterozygosity, and uniparental disomy have been added to the introduction of the Molecular Pathology section. *Inversion* is defined as a defect in a chromosome in which a segment breaks and reinserts in the same place, but in the opposite orientation. *Loss of heterozygosity* is an event that can occur in dividing cells that are heterozygous for one or more alleles, in which a daughter cell becomes hemizygous or homozygous for the allele(s) through mitotic recombination, deletion or other chromosomal event. *Uniparental disomy* is an abnormal inheritance of both members of a chromosome pair from one parent, with absence of the other parent's chromosome for the pair.

## Tier 1 Molecular Pathology Procedures

81200    *ASPA (aspartoacylase)* (eg, Canavan disease) gene analysis, common variants (eg, E285A, Y231X)

●81201    APC (adenomatous polyposis coli) (eg, familial adenomatosis polyposis [FAP], attenuated FAP) gene analysis; full gene sequence

●81202       known familial variants

●81203       duplication/deletion variants

81228    Cytogenomic constitutional (genome-wide) microarray analysis; interrogation of genomic regions for copy number variants (eg, Bacterial Artificial Chromosome [BAC] or oligo-based comparative genomic hybridization [CGH] microarray analysis)

81229       interrogation of genomic regions for copy number and single nucleotide polymorphism (SNP) variants for chromosomal abnormalities

      (Do not report 81228 in conjunction with 81229)

●81235    *EGFR (epidermal growth factor receptor)* (eg, non-small cell lung cancer) gene analysis, common variants (eg, exon 19 LREA deletion, L858R, T790M, G719A, G719S, L861Q)

81251    *GBA (glucosidase, beta, acid)* (eg, Gaucher disease) gene analysis, common variants (eg, N370S, 84GG, L444P, IVS2+1G>A)

●81252    *GJB2 (gap junction protein, beta 2, 26kDa; connexin 26)* (eg, nonsyndromic hearing loss) gene analysis; full gene sequence

●81253       known familial variants

●81254    *GJB6 (gap junction protein, beta 6, 30kDa, connexin 30)* (eg, nonsyndromic hearing loss) gene analysis, common variants (eg, 309kb [del(GJB6-D13S1830)] and 232kb [del(GJB6-D13S1854)])

81264    *IGK@ (Immunoglobulin kappa light chain locus)* (eg, leukemia and lymphoma, B-cell), gene rearrangement analysis, evaluation to detect abnormal clonal population(s)

     ▶(For immunoglobulin lambda gene *[IGL@]* rearrangement or immunoglobulin kappa deleting element, *[IGKDEL]* analysis, use 81479)◀

81317    *PMS2 (postmeiotic segregation increased 2 [S. cerevisiae])* (eg, hereditary non-polyposis colorectal cancer, Lynch syndrome) gene analysis; full sequence analysis

81318      known familial variants

81319      duplication/deletion variants

●81321    *PTEN (phosphatase and tensin homolog)* (eg, Cowden syndrome, *PTEN* hamartoma tumor syndrome) gene analysis; full sequence analysis

●81322      known familial variant

●81323      duplication/deletion variant

●81324    *PMP22 (peripheral myelin protein 22)* (eg, Charcot-Marie-Tooth, hereditary neuropathy with liability to pressure palsies) gene analysis; duplication/deletion analysis

●81325      full sequence analysis

●81326      known familial variant

81342    *TRG@ (T cell antigen receptor, gamma)* (eg, leukemia and lymphoma), gene rearrangement analysis, evaluation to detect abnormal clonal population(s)

     ▶(For T cell antigen alpha [*TRA@*] gene rearrangement analysis, use 81479)◀

### Rationale

Thirteen new codes have been added to Tier 1 relating to molecular pathology procedures. Refer to the Molecular Pathology introductory guidelines in the CPT 2013 code set for more detailed information, instructions, and definitions for purposes of accurate CPT reporting.

To gain a thorough understanding of how these codes are reported, including how they are structured, use of abbreviations, and meaning of parenthetical content, see the special resource on Molecular Pathology included in the front matter of the *CPT Professional 2013* codebook. In addition, the May 2012 edition of the *CPT Assistant* newsletter also has a similar article on Molecular Pathology coding.

Codes 81201-81203 are used for tests that assess for the presence of adenomatous polyposis coli (APC), which may be indicative of familial adenomatosis polyposis (FAP) or attenuated FAP.

Code 81235 is used for a test that assesses for the presence of epidermal growth factor receptor (EGFR), which may be indicative of non-small cell lung cancer.

    ⊘=Modifier 51 Exempt   ⊙=Moderate Sedation   ✚=Add-on Code   ✗=FDA approval pending

Codes 81252 and 81253 are used for tests that assess for the presence of gap junction protein, beta 2, 26kDa, connexin 26 (GJB2), which may be indicative of nonsyndromic hearing loss.

Code 81254 is used for a test that assesses for the presence of gap junction protein, beta 6, 30kDa, connexin 30 (GJB6), which may be indicative of nonsyndromic hearing loss.

Code series 81321-81323 is used for tests that assess for the presence of phosphatase and tensin homolog (PTEN), which may be indicative of Cowden syndrome or PTEN hamartoma tumor syndrome.

Code series 81324-81326 is used for tests that assess for the presence of peripheral myelin protein 22 (PMP22), which may be indicative of Charcot-Marie-Tooth, hereditary neuropathy with liability to pressure palsies disorders.

The parenthetical note following code 81264 and the first parenthetical note following code 81342 have been revised, ie, by replacing the deleted stacking codes 83890-83914 with the new molecular pathology unlisted code 81479.

##  Clinical Example (81201)

A 40-year-old male patient presents to his physician with episodic hematochezia. The patient undergoes colonoscopy. A very large number of adenomatous polyps and a left-sided mass consistent with adenocarcinoma of the colon are identified. The patient's family history is positive for colon cancer in several relatives. Familial adenomatous polyposis (FAP) is suspected, and an anticoagulated peripheral blood sample is submitted for APC gene sequencing.

### Description of Procedure (81201)

High quality, genomic DNA is isolated from whole blood and subjected to 15 individual polymerase chain reaction (PCR) amplification reactions, whose products encompass the entire coding sequence, intron/exon boundaries, and portions of the 5' and 3' untranslated regions of the adenomatous polyposis coli (APC) gene. The PCR products from each reaction undergo bidirectional dideoxynucleotide chain termination sequencing using a capillary electrophoresis instrument. The pathologist or other qualified health care professional evaluates the sequencing electropherograms for potential nucleotide sequence variants, insertions, deletions, or other changes. The pathologist or other qualified health care professional compares this evaluation with possible variants suggested by computer software to ensure that all abnormalities are identified. The pathologist or other health care professional composes a report that specifies the patient's mutation status to include information from a database and literature search regarding the significance of the variants identified. The report is edited and signed, and the results are communicated to the appropriate caregivers.

## Clinical Example (81202)

A 10-year-old asymptomatic boy whose 40-year-old father was recently diagnosed with colon cancer and familial adenomatous polyposis (FAP) presents to his physician for genetic testing. The father has a disease-associated mutation in the APC gene. An anticoagulated peripheral blood sample from the asymptomatic boy is submitted for testing for this known familial mutation.

### Description of Procedure (81202)

High quality, genomic DNA is isolated from whole blood and subjected to polymerase chain reaction (PCR) amplification for the respective adenomatous polyposis coli (APC) exon that contains the known familial mutation. The PCR products undergo bidirectional dideoxynucleotide chain termination sequencing using a capillary electrophoresis instrument. The pathologist or other qualified health care professional evaluates the sequencing electropherograms for the known familial mutation and any other variants that may be present. The pathologist or other qualified health care professional composes a report that specifies the patient's mutation status. The report is edited and signed, and the results are communicated to the appropriate caregivers.

## Clinical Example (81203)

A 40-year-old male patient presents with episodic hematochezia. The patient undergoes colonoscopy. A very large number of adenomatous polyps and a left-sided mass consistent with adenocarcinoma of the colon are identified. Germline sequencing for the presence of an APC mutation does not reveal a mutation. Duplication/deletion analysis is performed.

### Description of Procedure (81203)

High quality, genomic DNA that was previously isolated from whole blood is subjected to multiplex ligation-dependent amplification (MLPA), which involves hybridization and ligation of multiple pairs of oligonucleotide probes specific for the 15 exons of the adenomatous polyposis coli (APC) gene to assess the dosage of each exon. The pathologist or other qualified health care professional examines the peak heights and calculated ratios of the individual exons to the control gene sequences to determine the dosage status for all of the exons tested in the APC gene. The pathologist or other qualified health care professional composes a report that specifies the patient's mutation status. The report is edited and signed, and the results are communicated to the appropriate caregivers.

## Clinical Example (81235)

A 50-year-old female with no history of tobacco use presents to her physician complaining of a chronic cough. A chest X-ray reveals a right-sided peripheral lung mass, which is determined by biopsy to be adenocarcinoma of the lung. An abdominal CT scan demonstrates liver opacities, which are confirmed to be metastatic lung cancer. A tissue block is submitted for EGFR mutation testing.

### Description of Procedure (81235)

Paraffin is removed and DNA is isolated from the patient's tumor tissue. DNA is subjected to four polymerase chain reaction (PCR) amplification reactions for exons 18-21 of the epidermal growth factor receptor (EGFR) gene. The PCR products from each exon undergo bidirectional dideoxynucleotide chain termination sequencing on a capillary electrophoresis instrument. The pathologist evaluates the electropherograms to identify any nucleotide sequence variants. The pathologist composes a report that specifies the patient's EGFR mutation status and includes a comment on the implications of the lower limit of detection of the test relative to the tumor content of the sample. The report is edited and signed, and the results are communicated to the appropriate caregivers.

### Clinical Example (81252)

An otherwise healthy 2-month-old boy was found to have moderate hearing loss on newborn hearing screening. He has normal vestibular function, does not display radiographic abnormalities of the inner ear, and does not have a family history of congenital deafness or hearing loss. His physical examination is otherwise unremarkable. His physician suspects a GJB2 mutation as a possible genetic cause for his hearing loss. An anticoagulated peripheral blood sample is submitted for GJB2 sequencing to assess for the presence of DFNB1 nonsyndromic hearing loss-related mutations.

### Description of Procedure (81252)

High quality, genomic DNA is isolated from whole blood and subjected to individual polymerase chain reaction (PCR) amplification reactions. The PCR products from each reaction undergo bidirectional dideoxynucleotide chain termination sequencing using a capillary electrophoresis instrument. The pathologist evaluates the sequencing electropherogram for potential nucleotide sequence variants, insertions, deletions, or other changes. The pathologist compares this evaluation with possible variations suggested by computer software to ensure that all abnormalities are identified. The pathologist composes a report that specifies the patient's GJB2 mutation status to include information from a database and literature search regarding the significance of the variants identified. The report is edited and signed, and the results are communicated to the appropriate caregivers.

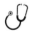
### Clinical Example (81253)

An otherwise healthy 1-month-old girl was found to have moderate hearing loss on newborn screening. Her older brother was found to have DFNB1 nonsyndromic hearing loss caused by two mutations in exon 2 of the GJB2 gene. Her physician suspects she has the same congenital hearing disorder as her brother. An anticoagulated peripheral blood sample is submitted for GJB2 exon 2 sequencing to assess for the presence of the known familial GJB2 mutations.

### Description of Procedure (81253)

High quality, genomic DNA is isolated from whole blood and subjected to polymerase chain reaction (PCR) amplification. The PCR products undergo bidirectional dideoxynucleotide chain termination sequencing using a capillary electrophoresis instrument. The pathologist evaluates the sequencing electropherogram for the known familial variants, as well as for other potential nucleotide sequence variants that may be present. The pathologist compares this evaluation with possible variations suggested by computer software to ensure that all abnormalities are identified. The pathologist composes a report that specifies the patient's GJB2 mutation status. The report is edited and signed, and the results are communicated to the appropriate caregivers.

## Clinical Example (81254)

An otherwise healthy 2-month-old boy was found to have moderate hearing loss on newborn hearing screening. He has normal vestibular function, does not display radiographic abnormalities of the inner ear, and does not have a family history of congenital deafness or hearing loss. His physical examination is otherwise unremarkable. His physician suspects a GJB2 mutation as a possible genetic cause for his hearing loss. An anticoagulated peripheral blood sample was previously submitted for GJB2 sequencing to assess for the presence of DFNB1 nonsyndromic hearing loss-related mutations, and only a single GJB2 mutation was identified. Targeted mutation testing for common GJB6 deletion mutations is performed.

**Description of Procedure (81254)**

High quality, genomic DNA that was previously isolated from whole blood is subjected to multiplex polymerase chain reaction (PCR) amplification with two primer sets that encompass the regions of the GJB6 common variants. The fluorescently-labeled PCR products are separated by capillary electrophoresis. The pathologist evaluates the electropherogram, comparing the relative sizes of the PCR product(s) to the control peaks to determine the GJB6 mutation status. The pathologist composes a report that specifies the GJB6 mutation status. The report is edited and signed, and the results are communicated to the appropriate caregivers.

## Clinical Example (81321)

A 30-year-old female presents to her physician complaining of facial growths. On physical examination she is found to have multiple papular lesions in her perioral and perinasal areas, as well as on her oral mucosa. She is also noted to have macrocephaly and bilateral breast nodules. She reports having a sister with similar facial lesions. Her physician suspects she may have Cowden Syndrome. An anticoagulated peripheral blood sample is submitted for PTEN gene sequencing to assess for the presence of a Cowden Syndrome-related mutation.

**Description of Procedure (81321)**

High quality, genomic DNA is isolated from whole blood and subjected to nine individual polymerase chain reaction (PCR) amplification reactions. The PCR products from each reaction undergo bidirectional dideoxynucleotide chain termination sequencing using a capillary electrophoresis instrument. The pathologist evaluates the sequencing electropherogram for potential nucleotide sequence variants, insertions, deletions, or other changes. The pathologist compares this evaluation with possible variations suggested by computer software to ensure that all abnormalities are identified. The pathologist composes a report that specifies the patient's phosphatase and tensin homolog (PTEN) mutation status to include information from a database and literature search regarding the significance of the variants identified. The report is edited and signed, and the results are communicated to the appropriate caregivers.

⊘=Modifier 51 Exempt   ⊙=Moderate Sedation   ✚=Add-on Code   ⁄V=FDA approval pending

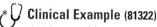

## Clinical Example (81322)

A 16-year-old asymptomatic male patient presents to his physician for genetic testing after his mother was diagnosed with breast cancer and PTEN Hamartoma Tumor Syndrome caused by a disease-associated PTEN gene mutation. An anticoagulated peripheral blood sample from the asymptomatic male patient is submitted for testing for the known familial mutation.

### Description of Procedure (81322)

High quality, genomic DNA is isolated from whole blood and subjected to polymerase chain reaction (PCR) amplification for the respective phosphatase and tensin homolog (PTEN) exon that contains the known familial mutation. The PCR products undergo bidirectional dideoxynucleotide chain termination sequencing using a capillary electrophoresis instrument. The pathologist evaluates the sequencing electropherograms for the known familial mutation and any other variants that may be present. The pathologist composes a report that specifies the patient's mutation status. The report is edited and signed, and the results are communicated to the appropriate caregivers.

## Clinical Example (81323)

A 40-year-old male presents to his physician with multiple papular facial and oral lesions, macrocephaly, palmar and plantar keratosis, and colorectal polyposis. He reports having a sister with similar facial lesions who developed breast cancer at age 38. His physician suspects he may have PTEN Hamartoma Tumor Syndrome. PTEN gene sequencing performed to assess the patient for the presence of a PTEN Hamartoma Tumor Syndrome-related mutation did not identify a mutation. Deletion/duplication analysis of the PTEN gene is requested.

### Description of Procedure (81323)

High quality, genomic DNA that was previously isolated from whole blood is subjected to multiplex ligation-dependent amplification (MLPA), which involves hybridization and ligation of multiple pairs of oligonucleotide probes specific for the nine exons of the phosphatase and tensin homolog (PTEN) gene to assess the dosage of each exon. The pathologist examines the peak heights and calculated ratios of the individual exons to the control gene sequences to determine the dosage status for all of the exons tested in the PTEN gene. The pathologist composes a report that specifies the patient's mutation status. The report is edited and signed, and the results are communicated to the appropriate caregivers.

## Clinical Example (81324)

A 12-year-old male is brought to his pediatrician for evaluation of foot and ankle weakness. He was delayed in walking and has difficulty running. His physical examination shows symmetrical atrophy of muscles below the knee (stork leg appearance), pes cavus deformity, absent deep tendon reflexes, and weakness with foot dorsiflexion. Nerve conduction studies demonstrate slowed velocity. The pediatrician suspects Charcot-Marie-Tooth neuropathy. A sample of anticoagulated peripheral blood is submitted for peripheral myelin protein 22 (PMP22) gene duplication/deletion analysis.

**Description of Procedure (81324)**

High-quality DNA is isolated from whole blood and subjected to multiplex liga-tion-dependent probe amplification (MLPA), which involves hybridization and ligation of multiple pairs of oligonucleotide probes specific to the five exons of the PMP22 gene to assess the dosage of each exon. The pathologist or other qualified health care professional examines the peak heights and calculated ratios of indi-vidual exons to the control gene sequences to determine the dosage status for all of the exons tested in the PMP22 gene. The pathologist or other qualified health care professional composes a report specifying the patient's mutation status. The report is edited, signed, and the results are communicated to the appropriate caregivers.

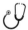 **Clinical Example (81325)**

A 20-year-old male presents to his physician complaining of progressive weakness of his feet and ankles. The physician notices that the patient has an abnormal gait with bilateral foot drop and bilateral pes cavus foot deformity. Electromyogram (EMG) studies demonstrate decreased nerve conduction velocities in the lower extremities. The patient reports that his father has had similar symptoms for many years. The patient's physician suspects Charcot-Marie-Tooth neuropathy. Peripheral myelin protein 22 (PMP22) gene testing performed to assess for the common duplication mutation of the PMP22 gene did not identify a mutation. Full gene sequencing of the PMP22 gene is requested to evaluate for a possible point mutation.

**Description of Procedure (81325)**

High-quality genomic DNA previously isolated from whole blood is subjected to four individual polymerase chain reaction (PCR) amplification reactions. The PCR products from each reaction undergo bidirectional dideoxynucleotide chain termination sequencing using a capillary electrophoresis instrument. The pathologist or other qualified health care professional evaluates the sequenc-ing electropherogram for potential point mutations or other possible nucleotide sequence variants such as insertions or deletions. The pathologist or other quali-fied health care professional compares this evaluation with possible variations suggested by computer software to ensure that all abnormalities are identified. The pathologist or other qualified health care professional composes a report that specifies the patient's PMP22 mutation status to include information from a data-base and literature search regarding the significance of the variants identified. The report is edited, signed, and the results are communicated to the appropriate caregivers.

**Clinical Example (81326)**

A 20-year-old male with a family history of Charcot-Marie-Tooth disease caused by a previously identified nucleotide point mutation in the Peripheral myelin protein 22 (PMP22) gene presents to his physician complaining of progressive weakness of his feet and ankles. The physician notices that the patient has an abnormal gait

⊘=Modifier 51 Exempt   ⊙=Moderate Sedation   ✚=Add-on Code   ✗=FDA approval pending

with bilateral foot drop and bilateral pes cavus foot deformity. An anticoagulated peripheral blood sample from the patient is submitted for assessment of the known familial PMP22 gene mutation.

**Description of Procedure (81326)**

High-quality genomic DNA is isolated from whole blood and subjected to polymerase chain reaction (PCR) amplification for the respective PMP22 exon that contains the known familial mutation. The PCR products undergo bidirectional dideoxynucleotide chain termination sequencing using a capillary electrophoresis instrument. The pathologist or other qualified health care professional evaluates the sequencing electropherogram for the known familial mutation and any other variants that may be present. The pathologist or other health care professional composes a report that specifies the patient's mutation status. The report is edited, signed, and the results are communicated to the appropriate caregivers.

# Tier 2 Molecular Pathology Procedures

The following molecular pathology procedure (Tier 2) codes are used to report procedures not listed in the Tier 1 molecular pathology codes (81200-81383). They represent medically useful procedures that are generally performed in lower volumes than Tier 1 procedures (eg, the incidence of the disease being tested is rare). They are arranged by level of technical resources and interpretive work by the physician or other qualified health care professional. The individual analyses listed under each code (ie, level of procedure) utilize the definitions and coding principles as described in the introduction preceding the Tier 1 molecular pathology codes. The parenthetical examples of methodologies presented near the beginning of each code provide general guidelines used to group procedures for a given level and are not all-inclusive.

▶Use the appropriate molecular pathology procedure level code that includes the specific analyte listed after the code descriptor. If the analyte tested is not listed under one of the Tier 2 codes or is not represented by a Tier 1 code, use the unlisted molecular pathology procedure code, 81479.◀

▲81400 Molecular pathology procedure, Level 1 *(eg, identification of single germline variant [eg, SNP] by techniques such as restriction enzyme digestion or melt curve analysis)*

▶*ABCC8 (ATP-binding cassette, sub-family C [CFTR/MRP], member 8) (eg, familial hyperinsulinism), F1388del variant*◀

▶*CLRN1 (clarin 1) (eg, Usher syndrome, type 3), N48K variant*◀

▶*FGFR3 (fibroblast growth factor receptor 3) (eg, Muenke syndrome), P250R variant*◀

▶*IVD (isovaleryl-CoA dehydrogenase) (eg, isovaleric acidemia), A282V variant*

*SERPINE1 (serpine peptidase inhibitor clade E, member 1, plasminogen activator inhibitor -1, PAI-1) (eg, thrombophilia), 4G variant*

*SHOC2 (soc-2 suppressor of clear homolog) (eg, Noonan-like syndrome with loose anagen hair), S2G variant*

*SMN1 (survival of motor neuron 1, telomeric) (eg, spinal muscular atrophy), exon 7 deletion*

*SRY (sex determining region Y) (eg, 46,XX testicular disorder of sex development, gonadal dysgenesis), gene analysis*

*TOR1A (torsin family 1, member A [torsin A])(eg, early-onset primary dystonia [DYT1]), 907_909delGAG (904_906delGAG) variant*◀

▲**81401**  Molecular pathology procedure, Level 2 (eg, 2-10 SNPs, 1 methylated variant, or 1 somatic variant [typically using nonsequencing target variant analysis], or detection of a dynamic mutation disorder/ triplet repeat)

APOB (apolipoprotein B) (eg, familial hypercholesterolemia type B), common variants (eg, R3500Q, R3500W)

*AR (androgen receptor)* (eg, spinal and bulbar muscular atrophy, Kennedy disease, X chromosome inactivation), characterization of alleles (eg, expanded size or methylation status)

*CBS (cystathionine-beta-synthase)* (eg, homocystinuria, cystathionine beta-synthase deficiency), common variants (eg, I278T, G307S)

*E2A/PBX1 (t(1;19))* (eg, acute lymphocytic leukemia), translocation analysis, qualitative, and quantitative, if performed

*EML4/ALK (inv(2))* (eg, non-small cell lung cancer), translocation or inversion analysis

*ETV6/RUNX1 (t(12;21))* (eg, acute lymphocytic leukemia), translocation analysis, qualitative, and quantitative, if performed

*EWSR1/ERG (t(21;22))* (eg, Ewing sarcoma/peripheral neuroectodermal tumor), translocation analysis, qualitative, and quantitative, if performed

*EWSR1/FLI1 (t(11;22))* (eg, Ewing sarcoma/peripheral neuroectodermal tumor), translocation analysis, qualitative, and quantitative, if performed

*FGFR3 (fibroblast growth factor receptor 3)* (eg, achondroplasia, hypochondroplasia), common variants (eg, 1138G>A, 1138G>C, 1620C>A, 1620C>G)

*FOXO1/PAX3 (t(1;13))* (eg, Ewing sarcoma/peripheral neuroectodermal tumor), translocation analysis, qualitative, and quantitative, if performed

*FOXO1/PAX7 (t(2;13))* (eg, Ewing sarcoma/peripheral neuroectodermal tumor), translocation analysis, qualitative, and quantitative, if performed

*FXN (frataxin)* (eg, Friedreich ataxia), evaluation to detect abnormal (expanded) alleles

*H19 (imprinted maternally expressed transcript [non-protein coding])* (eg, Beckwith-Wiedemann syndrome), methylation analysis

*KCNQ1OT1 (KCNQ1 overlapping transcript 1 [non-protein coding])* (eg, Beckwith-Wiedemann syndrome), methylation analysis

*MEG3/DLK1 (maternally expressed 3 [non-protein coding]/delta-like 1 homolog [Drosophila])* (eg, intrauterine growth retardation), methylation analysis

⊘=Modifier 51 Exempt   ⊙=Moderate Sedation   ✚=Add-on Code   𝒩=FDA approval pending

*MLL/AFF1 (t(4;11))* (eg, acute lymphoblastic leukemia), translocation analysis, qualitative, and quantitative, if performed

*MLL/MLLT3 (t(9;11))* (eg, acute myeloid leukemia), translocation analysis, qualitative, and quantitative, if performed

*MT-RNR1 (mitochondrially encoded 12S RNA)* (eg, nonsyndromic hearing loss), common variants (eg, m.1555A>G, m.1494C>T)

*MUTYH (mutY homolog [E. coli])* (eg, MYH-associated polyposis), common variants (eg, Y165C, G382D)

*MT-ATP6 (mitochondrially encoded ATP synthase 6)* (eg, neuropathy with ataxia and retinitis pigmentosa [NARP], Leigh syndrome), common variants (eg, m.8993T>G, m.8993T>C)

*MT-ND4, MT-ND6 (mitochondrially encoded NADH dehydrogenase 4, mitochondrially encoded NADH dehydrogenase 6)* (eg, Leber hereditary optic neuropathy [LHON]), common variants (eg, m.11778G>A, m.3460G>A, m.14484T>C)

*MT-TK (mitochondrially encoded tRNA lysine)* (eg, myoclonic epilepsy with ragged-red fibers [MERRF]), common variants (eg, m.8344A>G, m.8356T>C)

*MT-TL1 (mitochondrially encoded tRNA leucine 1 [UUA/G])* (eg, diabetes and hearing loss), common variants (eg, m.3243A>G, m.14709 T>C) MT-TL1

*MT-ND5 (mitochondrially encoded tRNA leucine 1 [UUA/G], mitochondrially encoded NADH dehydrogenase 5)* (eg, mitochondrial encephalopathy with lactic acidosis and stroke-like episodes [MELAS]), common variants (eg, m.3243A>G, m.3271T>C, m.3252A>G, m.13513G>A)

*MT-TS1, MT-RNR1 (mitochondrially encoded tRNA serine 1 [UCN], mitochondrially encoded 12S RNA)* (eg, nonsyndromic sensorineural deafness [including aminoglycoside-induced nonsyndromic deafness]), common variants (eg, m.7445A>G, m.1555A>G)

*NPM1/ALK (t(2;5))* (eg, anaplastic large cell lymphoma), translocation analysis PAX8/PPARG (t(2;3) (q13;p25)) (eg, follicular thyroid carcinoma), translocation analysis PRSS1 (protease, serine, 1 [trypsin 1]) (eg, hereditary pancreatitis), common variants (eg, N29I, A16V, R122H)

*PYGM (phosphorylase, glycogen, muscle)* (eg, glycogen storage disease type V, McArdle disease), common variants (eg, R50X, G205S)

*SMN1/SMN2 (survival of motor neuron 1, telomeric/survival of motor neuron 2, centromeric)* (eg, spinal muscular atrophy), dosage analysis (eg, carrier testing)

▲81402    Molecular pathology procedure, Level 3 (eg, >10 SNPs, 2-10 methylated variants, or 2-10 somatic variants [typically using non-sequencing target variant analysis], immunoglobulin and T-cell receptor gene rearrangements, duplication/deletion variants of 1 exon, loss of heterozygosity [LOH], uniparental disomy [UPD])

   ▶Chromosome 18q- (eg, D18S55, D18S58, D18S61, D18S64, and D18S69) (eg, colon cancer), allelic imbalance assessment (ie, loss of heterozygosity)◀

   ▶Uniparental disomy (UPD) (eg, Russell-Silver syndrome, Prader-Willi/Angelman syndrome), short tandem repeat (STR) analysis◀

▲**81403**    Molecular pathology procedure, Level 4 (eg, analysis of single exon by DNA sequence analysis, analysis of >10 amplicons using multiplex PCR in 2 or more independent reactions, mutation scanning or duplication/deletion variants of 2-5 exons)

▶*ANG (angiogenin, ribonuclease, RNase A family, 5)* (eg, amyotrophic lateral sclerosis), full gene sequence

*CEBPA (CCAAT/enhancer binding protein [C/EBP], alpha)* (eg, acute myeloid leukemia), full gene sequence

*CEL (carboxyl ester lipase [bile salt-stimulated lipase])* (eg, maturity-onset diabetes of the young [MODY]), targeted sequence analysis of exon 11 (eg, c.1785delC, c.1686delT)◀

▶*F8 (coagulation factor VIII)* (eg, hemophilia A), inversion analysis, intron 1 and intron 22A

*FGFR3 (fibroblast growth factor receptor 3)* (eg, isolated craniosynostosis), targeted sequence analysis (eg, exon 7)

(For targeted sequence analysis of multiple FGFR3 exons, use 81404)◀

▶*HBB (hemoglobin, beta, beta-globin)* (eg, beta thalassemia), duplication/deletion analysis

*HRAS (v-Ha-ras Harvey rat sarcoma viral oncogene homolog)* (eg, Costello syndrome), exon 2 sequence

*IDH1 (isocitrate dehydrogenase 1 [NADP+], soluble)* (eg, glioma), common exon 4 variants (eg, R132H, R132C)

*IDH2 (isocitrate dehydrogenase 2 [NADP+], mitochondrial)* (eg, glioma), common exon 4 variants (eg, R140W, R172M)◀

▶Known familial variant not otherwise specified, for gene listed in Tier 1 or Tier 2, DNA sequence analysis, each variant exon

(For a known familial variant that is considered a common variant, use specific common variant Tier 1 or Tier 2 code)

*KRAS (v-Ki-ras2 Kirsten rat sarcoma viral oncogene)* (eg, carcinoma), gene analysis, variant(s) in exon 3 (eg, codon 61)◀

▶*MT-RNR1 (mitochondrially encoded 12S RNA)* (eg, nonsyndromic hearing loss), full gene sequence

*MT-TS1 (mitochondrially encoded tRNA serine 1)* (eg, nonsyndromic hearing loss), full gene sequence

*SMN1 (survival of motor neuron 1, telomeric)* (eg, spinal muscular atrophy), known familial sequence variant(s)◀

▲**81404**    Molecular pathology procedure, Level 5 (eg, analysis of 2-5 exons by DNA sequence analysis, mutation scanning or duplication/deletion variants of 6-10 exons, or characterization of a dynamic mutation disorder/triplet repeat by Southern blot analysis)

▶*ACADS (acyl-CoA dehydrogenase, C-2 to C-3 short chain)* (eg, short chain acyl-CoA dehydrogenase deficiency), targeted sequence analysis (eg, exons 5 and 6)◀

*AQP2 (aquaporin 2 [collecting duct])* (eg, nephrogenic diabetes insipidus), full gene sequence

*ARX (aristaless related homeobox)* (eg, X-linked lissencephaly with ambiguous genitalia, X-linked mental retardation), full gene sequence◀

⊘=Modifier 51 Exempt   ⊙=Moderate Sedation   ✚=Add-on Code   ✗=FDA approval pending

▶ *CAV3 (caveolin 3)* (eg, CAV3-related distal myopathy, limb-girdle muscular dystrophy type 1C), full gene sequence

*CDKN2A (cyclin-dependent kinase inhibitor 2A)* (eg, CDKN2A-related cutaneous malignant melanoma, familial atypical mole-malignant melanoma syndrome), full gene sequence

*CLRN1 (clarin 1)* (eg, Usher syndrome, type 3), full gene sequence

*CPT2 (carnitine palmitoyltransferase 2)* (eg, carnitine palmitoyltransferase II deficiency), full gene sequence ◀

▶ *FGFR2 (fibroblast growth factor receptor 2)* (eg, craniosynostosis, Apert syndrome, Crouzon syndrome), targeted sequence analysis (eg, exons 8, 10)

*FGFR3 (fibroblast growth factor receptor 3)* (eg, achondroplasia, hypochondroplasia), targeted sequence analysis (eg, exons 8, 11, 12, 13) ◀

▶ *FXN (frataxin)* (eg, Friedreich ataxia), full gene sequence ◀

▶ *HNF1B (HNF1 homeobox B)* (eg, maturity-onset diabetes of the young [MODY]), duplication/deletion analysis

*HRAS (v-Ha-ras Harvey rat sarcoma viral oncogene homolog)* (eg, Costello syndrome), full gene sequence ◀

▶ *MEN1 (multiple endocrine neoplasia I)* (eg, multiple endocrine neoplasia type 1, Wermer syndrome), duplication/deletion analysis ◀

▶ *PDX1 (pancreatic and duodenal homeobox 1)* (eg, maturity-onset diabetes of the young [MODY]), full gene sequence

*PRNP (prion protein)* (eg, genetic prion disease), full gene sequence

*PRSS1 (protease, serine, 1 [trypsin 1])* (eg, hereditary pancreatitis), full gene sequence

*RAF1 (v-raf-1 murine leukemia viral oncogene homolog 1)* (eg, LEOPARD syndrome), targeted sequence analysis (eg, exons 7, 12, 14, 17) ◀

▶ *SLC25A4 (solute carrier family 25 [mitochondrial carrier; adenine nucleotide translocator], member 4)* (eg, progressive external ophthalmoplegia), full gene sequence

*TP53 (tumor protein 53)* (eg, tumor samples), targeted sequence analysis of 2-5 exons

*TTR (transthyretin)* (eg, familial transthyretin amyloidosis), full gene sequence

*TYR (tyrosinase [oculocutaneous albinism IA])* (eg, oculocutaneous albinism IA), full gene sequence

*USH1G (Usher syndrome 1G [autosomal recessive])* (eg, Usher syndrome, type 1), full gene sequence ◀

▲ **81405** Molecular pathology procedure, Level 6 (eg, analysis of 6-10 exons by DNA sequence analysis, mutation scanning or duplication/deletion variants of 11-25 exons)

▶ *ABCD1 (ATP-binding cassette, sub-family D [ALD], member 1)* (eg, adrenoleukodystrophy), full gene sequence

*ACADS (acyl-CoA dehydrogenase, C-2 to C-3 short chain)* (eg, short chain acyl-CoA dehydrogenase deficiency), full gene sequence

---

*ACTC1 (actin, alpha, cardiac muscle 1)* (eg, familial hypertrophic cardiomyopathy), full gene sequence

*APTX (aprataxin)* (eg, ataxia with oculomotor apraxia 1), full gene sequence

*AR (androgen receptor)* (eg, androgen insensitivity syndrome), full gene sequence

*CHRNA4 (cholinergic receptor, nicotinic, alpha 4)* (eg, nocturnal frontal lobe epilepsy), full gene sequence

*CHRNB2 (cholinergic receptor, nicotinic, beta 2 [neuronal])* (eg, nocturnal frontal lobe epilepsy), full gene sequence◄

►*DFNB59 (deafness, autosomal recessive 59)* (eg, autosomal recessive nonsyndromic hearing impairment), full gene sequence

*DHCR7 (7-dehydrocholesterol reductase)* (eg, Smith-Lemli-Opitz syndrome), full gene sequence

*EYA1 (eyes absent homolog 1 [Drosophila])* (eg, branchio-oto-renal [BOR] spectrum disorders), duplication/deletion analysis

*F9 (coagulation factor IX)* (eg, hemophilia B), full gene sequence

*FH (fumarate hydratase)* (eg, fumarate hydratase deficiency, hereditary leiomyomatosis with renal cell cancer), full gene sequence◄

►*GFAP (glial fibrillary acidic protein)* (eg, Alexander disease), full gene sequence

*GLA (galactosidase, alpha)* (eg, Fabry disease), full gene sequence

*HBA1/HBA2 (alpha globin 1 and alpha globin 2)* (eg, thalassemia), full gene sequence

*HNF1A (HNF1 homeobox A)* (eg, maturity-onset diabetes of the young [MODY]), full gene sequence

*HNF1B (HNF1 homeobox B)* (eg, maturity-onset diabetes of the young [MODY]), full gene sequence

*KRAS (v-Ki-ras2 Kirsten rat sarcoma viral oncogene homolog)* (eg, Noonan syndrome), full gene sequence

*LAMP2 (lysosomal-associated membrane protein 2)* (eg, Danon disease), full gene sequence

*MEN1 (multiple endocrine neoplasia I)* (eg, multiple endocrine neoplasia type 1, Wermer syndrome), full gene sequence

*MPZ (myelin protein zero)* (eg, Charcot-Marie-Tooth), full gene sequence

*MYL2 (myosin, light chain 2, regulatory, cardiac, slow)* (eg, familial hypertrophic cardiomyopathy), full gene sequence

*MYL3 (myosin, light chain 3, alkali, ventricular, skeletal, slow)* (eg, familial hypertrophic cardiomyopathy), full gene sequence

*MYOT (myotilin)* (eg, limb-girdle muscular dystrophy), full gene sequence

*NEFL (neurofilament, light polypeptide)* (eg, Charcot-Marie-Tooth), full gene sequence

*NF2 (neurofibromin 2 [merlin])* (eg, neurofibromatosis, type 2), duplication/deletion analysis

*NSD1 (nuclear receptor binding SET domain protein 1)* (eg, Sotos syndrome), duplication/deletion analysis

*OTC (ornithine carbamoyltransferase)* (eg, ornithine transcarbamylase deficiency), full gene sequence◄

►*RET (ret proto-oncogene)* (eg, multiple endocrine neoplasia, type 2A and familial medullary thyroid carcinoma), targeted sequence analysis (eg, exons 10, 11, 13-16)◄

►*SDHC (succinate dehydrogenase complex, subunit C, integral membrane protein, 15kDa)* (eg, hereditary paraganglioma-pheochromocytoma syndrome), full gene sequence

*SGCA (sarcoglycan, alpha [50kDa dystrophin-associated glycoprotein])* (eg, limb-girdle muscular dystrophy), full gene sequence

*SGCB (sarcoglycan, beta [43kDa dystrophin-associated glycoprotein])* (eg, limb-girdle muscular dystrophy), full gene sequence

*SGCD (sarcoglycan, delta [35kDa dystrophin-associated glycoprotein])* (eg, limb-girdle muscular dystrophy), full gene sequence

*SGCG (sarcoglycan, gamma [35kDa dystrophin-associated glycoprotein])* (eg, limb-girdle muscular dystrophy), full gene sequence

*SHOC2 (soc-2 suppressor of clear homolog)* (eg, Noonan-like syndrome with loose anagen hair), full gene sequence

*SMN1 (survival of motor neuron 1, telomeric)* (eg, spinal muscular atrophy), full gene sequence

*SPRED1 (sprouty-related, EVH-1 domain containing 1)* (eg, Legius syndrome), full gene sequence ◄

►*TNNI3 (troponin I, type 3 [cardiac])* (eg, familial hypertrophic cardiomyopathy), full gene sequence

*TP53 (tumor protein 53)* (eg, Li-Fraumeni syndrome, tumor samples), full gene sequence or targeted sequence analysis of >5 exons

*TPM1 (tropomyosin 1 [alpha])* (eg, familial hypertrophic cardiomyopathy), full gene sequence

*TSC1 (tuberous sclerosis 1)* (eg, tuberous sclerosis), duplication/deletion analysis◄

▲81406    Molecular pathology procedure, Level 7 (eg, analysis of 11-25 exons by DNA sequence analysis, mutation scanning or duplication/deletion variants of 26-50 exons, cytogenomic array analysis for neoplasia)

►*ACADVL (acyl-CoA dehydrogenase, very long chain)* (eg, very long chain acyl-coenzyme A dehydrogenase deficiency), full gene sequence

*ACTN4 (actinin, alpha 4)* (eg, focal segmental glomerulosclerosis), full gene sequence

*ANO5 (anoctamin 5)* (eg, limb-girdle muscular dystrophy), full gene sequence

*APP (amyloid beta [A4] precursor protein)* (eg, Alzheimer disease), full gene sequence

*ATP7B (ATPase, Cu++ transporting, beta polypeptide)* (eg, Wilson disease), full gene sequence

*BRAF (v-raf murine sarcoma viral oncogene homolog B1)* (eg, Noonan syndrome), full gene sequence◄

►*CBS (cystathionine-beta-synthase)* (eg, homocystinuria, cystathionine beta-synthase deficiency), full gene sequence

*CDH1 (cadherin 1, type 1, E-cadherin [epithelial])* (eg, hereditary diffuse gastric cancer), full gene sequence

*CDKL5 (cyclin-dependent kinase-like 5)* (eg, early infantile epileptic encephalopathy), full gene sequence◄

►*DLAT (dihydrolipoamide S-acetyltransferase)* (eg, pyruvate dehydrogenase E2 deficiency), full gene sequence

*DLD (dihydrolipoamide dehydrogenase)* (eg, maple syrup urine disease, type III), full gene sequence

*EYA1 (eyes absent homolog 1 [Drosophila])* (eg, branchio-oto-renal [BOR] spectrum disorders), full gene sequence

*F8 (coagulation factor VIII)* (eg, hemophilia A), duplication/deletion analysis

*GAA (glucosidase, alpha; acid)* (eg, glycogen storage disease type II [Pompe disease]), full gene sequence◄

►*GCDH (glutaryl-CoA dehydrogenase)* (eg, glutaricacidemia type 1), full gene sequence

*GCK (glucokinase [hexokinase 4])* (eg, maturity-onset diabetes of the young [MODY]), full gene sequence

*HADHA (hydroxyacyl-CoA dehydrogenase/3-ketoacyl-CoA thiolase/enoyl-CoA hydratase [trifunctional protein] alpha subunit)* (eg, long chain acyl-coenzyme A dehydrogenase deficiency), full gene sequence◄

►*HNF4A (hepatocyte nuclear factor 4, alpha)* (eg, maturity-onset diabetes of the young [MODY]), full gene sequence

*IVD (isovaleryl-CoA dehydrogenase)* (eg, isovaleric acidemia), full gene sequence

*JAG1 (jagged 1)* (eg, Alagille syndrome), duplication/deletion analysis

*LDB3 (LIM domain binding 3)* (eg, familial dilated cardiomyopathy, myofibrillar myopathy), full gene sequence◄

►*MAP2K1 (mitogen-activated protein kinase 1)* (eg, cardiofaciocutaneous syndrome), full gene sequence

*MAP2K2 (mitogen-activated protein kinase 2)* (eg, cardiofaciocutaneous syndrome), full gene sequence

*MCCC2 (methylcrotonoyl-CoA carboxylase 2 [beta])* (eg, 3-methylcrotonyl carboxylase deficiency), full gene sequence

*MUTYH (mutY homolog [E. coli])* (eg, MYH-associated polyposis), full gene sequence

*NF2 (neurofibromin 2 [merlin])* (eg, neurofibromatosis, type 2), full gene sequence

*NOTCH3 (notch 3)* (eg, cerebral autosomal dominant arteriopathy with subcortical infarcts and leukoencephalopathy [CADASIL]), targeted sequence analysis (eg, exons 1-23)

*NSD1 (nuclear receptor binding SET domain protein 1)* (eg, Sotos syndrome), full gene sequence

*OPA1 (optic atrophy 1)* (eg, optic atrophy), duplication/deletion analysis

*PAH (phenylalanine hydroxylase)* (eg, phenylketonuria), full gene sequence

*PALB2 (partner and localizer of BRCA2)* (eg, breast and pancreatic cancer), full gene sequence

*PAX2 (paired box 2)* (eg, renal coloboma syndrome), full gene sequence

⃠=Modifier 51 Exempt  ⊙=Moderate Sedation  ✚=Add-on Code  𝒩=FDA approval pending

*PC (pyruvate carboxylase)* (eg, pyruvate carboxylase deficiency), full gene sequence

*PCCB (propionyl CoA carboxylase, beta polypeptide)* (eg, propionic acidemia), full gene sequence

*PDHA1 (pyruvate dehydrogenase [lipoamide] alpha 1)* (eg, lactic acidosis), full gene sequence

*PDHX (pyruvate dehydrogenase complex, component X)* (eg, lactic acidosis), full gene sequence◄

▶*PRKAG2 (protein kinase, AMP-activated, gamma 2 non-catalytic subunit)* (eg, familial hypertrophic cardiomyopathy with Wolff-Parkinson-White syndrome, lethal congenital glycogen storage disease of heart), full gene sequence

*PSEN2 (presenilin 2 [Alzheimer disease 4])* (eg, Alzheimer disease), full gene sequence

*PTPN11 (protein tyrosine phosphatase, non-receptor type 11)* (eg, Noonan syndrome, LEOPARD syndrome), full gene sequence

*PYGM (phosphorylase, glycogen, muscle)* (eg, glycogen storage disease type V, McArdle disease), full gene sequence

*RAF1 (v-raf-1 murine leukemia viral oncogene homolog 1)* (eg, LEOPARD syndrome), full gene sequence

*RET (ret proto-oncogene)* (eg, Hirschsprung disease), full gene sequence◄

▶*SLC9A6 (solute carrier family 9 [sodium/hydrogen exchanger], member 6)* (eg, Christianson syndrome), full gene sequence

*SLC26A4 (solute carrier family 26, member 4)* (eg, Pendred syndrome), full gene sequence

*SOS1 (son of sevenless homolog 1)* (eg, Noonan syndrome, gingival fibromatosis), full gene sequence

*TAZ (tafazzin)* (eg, methylglutaconic aciduria type 2, Barth syndrome), full gene sequence

*TNNT2 (troponin T, type 2 [cardiac])* (eg, familial hypertrophic cardiomyopathy), full gene sequence

*TSC1 (tuberous sclerosis 1)* (eg, tuberous sclerosis), full gene sequence

*TSC2 (tuberous sclerosis 2)* (eg, tuberous sclerosis), duplication/deletion analysis

*UBE3A (ubiquitin protein ligase E3A)* (eg, Angelman syndrome), full gene sequence◄

▲**81407**  Molecular pathology procedure, Level 8 (eg, analysis of 26-50 exons by DNA sequence analysis, mutation scanning or duplication/deletion variants of >50 exons, sequence analysis of multiple genes on one platform)

▶*ABCC8 (ATP-binding cassette, sub-family C [CFTR/MRP], member 8)* (eg, familial hyperinsulinism), full gene sequence

*CHD7 (chromodomain helicase DNA binding protein 7)* (eg, CHARGE syndrome), full gene sequence

*F8 (coagulation factor VIII)* (eg, hemophilia A), full gene sequence

*JAG1 (jagged 1)* (eg, Alagille syndrome), full gene sequence

*MYBPC3 (myosin binding protein C, cardiac)* (eg, familial hypertrophic cardiomyopathy), full gene sequence

*MYH6 (myosin, heavy chain 6, cardiac muscle, alpha)* (eg, familial dilated cardiomyopathy), full gene sequence

*MYH7 (myosin, heavy chain 7, cardiac muscle, beta)* (eg, familial hypertrophic cardiomyopathy, Liang distal myopathy), full gene sequence

*MYO7A (myosin VIIA)* (eg, Usher syndrome, type 1), full gene sequence

*NOTCH1 (notch 1)* (eg, aortic valve disease), full gene sequence

*OPA1 (optic atrophy 1)* (eg, optic atrophy), full gene sequence

*PCDH15 (protocadherin-related 15)* (eg, Usher syndrome, type 1), full gene sequence

*SCN1A (sodium channel, voltage-gated, type 1, alpha subunit)* (eg, generalized epilepsy with febrile seizures), full gene sequence

*SCN5A (sodium channel, voltage-gated, type V, alpha subunit)* (eg, familial dilated cardiomyopathy), full gene sequence

*TSC2 (tuberous sclerosis 2)* (eg, tuberous sclerosis), full gene sequence◄

▲**81408**   Molecular pathology procedure, Level 9 (eg, analysis of >50 exons in a single gene by DNA sequence analysis)

►*ATM (ataxia telangiectasia mutated)* (eg, ataxia telangiectasia), full gene sequence

*CDH23 (cadherin-related 23)* (eg, Usher syndrome, type 1), full gene sequence

*COL1A1 (collagen, type I, alpha 1)* (eg, osteogenesis imperfecta, type I), full gene sequence

*COL1A2 (collagen, type I, alpha 2)* (eg, osteogenesis imperfecta, type I), full gene sequence

*DYSF (dysferlin, limb girdle muscular dystrophy 2B [autosomal recessive])* (eg, limb-girdle muscular dystrophy), full gene sequence◄

►*USH2A (Usher syndrome 2A [autosomal recessive, mild])* (eg, Usher syndrome, type 2), full gene sequence◄

●**81479**   Unlisted molecular pathology procedure

### ✍ Rationale

The Tier 2 molecular pathology codes have been editorially revised with the inclusion of additional tests that have been determined to fall under the level of Tier 2 reporting.

The base descriptor of code 81402 has been revised to specify loss of heterozygosity (LOH), uniparental disomy [UPD]). Several new analytes have been added to codes 81400 through 81408. These revisions are editorial.

Also in code 81402, the analyte *TRD@* was listed as *TCD@* in error. This correction will be included in the 2013 CPT errata document and posted to the AMA CPT Web site at www.ama-assn.org/ama/pub/physician-resources/solutions-managing-your-practice/coding-billing-insurance/cpt/about-cpt/errata.page.

In code 81401, the analyte FGFR3 was revised to include common variants 1620C>A and 1620C>G to the examples in parentheses. In code 81403, an instructional parenthetical note was added instructing users to report the specific common variant Tier 1 or Tier 2 code for a known familial variant that is

⊘=Modifier 51 Exempt   ⊙=Moderate Sedation   ✚=Add-on Code   ⁄ =FDA approval pending considered a common variant. Also, the new analyte that has been added to code 81401, APOB (apolipoprotein B) *(eg, familial hypercholesterolemia type B), common variants (eg, R3500Q, R3500W),* was inadvertently listed at the end of the descriptor for *ADRB2.* This correction will be included in the 2013 CPT errata document and posted to the AMA CPT Web site at www.ama-assn.org/ama/pub/physician-resources/solutions-managing-your-practice/coding-billing-insurance/cpt/about-cpt/errata.page.

In code 81401, the analyte EWSR1/WT1 (t(11;22)) *(eg, Ewing sarcoma/peripheral neuroectodermal tumor), translocation analysis, qualitative, and quantitative, if performed,* was inadvertently omitted from the listing of analytes included in code 81401. This correction will be included in the 2013 CPT errata document and posted to the AMA CPT Web site at www.ama-assn.org/ama/pub/physician-resources/solutions-managing-your-practice/coding-billing-insurance/cpt/about-cpt/errata.page.

The analyte description for KRAS in code 81403 has been editorially revised by changing the number of exons in the KRAS test from 2 to 3 and providing an example in parentheses. The analyte descriptor for NOTCH3 in code 81406 has been editorially revised to describe autosomal dominant.

Code 81479 was developed to allow reporting of services formerly identified by deleted codes 83890-83914 and 88384-88386.

# ►Multianalyte Assays with Algorithmic Analyses◄

►Multianalyte Assays with Algorithmic Analyses (MAAAs) are procedures that utilize multiple results derived from assays of various types, including molecular pathology assays, fluorescent in situ hybridization assays and non-nucleic acid based assays (eg, proteins, polypeptides, lipids, carbohydrates). Algorithmic analysis using the results of these assays as well as other patient information (if used) is then performed, and reported typically as a numeric score(s) or as a probability. MAAAs are typically unique to a single clinical laboratory or manufacturer. The results of individual component procedure(s) that are inputs to the MAAAs may be provided on the associated laboratory report, however these assays are not reported separately using additional codes.

The format for the code descriptors of MAAAs usually include (in order):

- Disease type (eg, oncology, autoimmune, tissue rejection),

- Material(s) analyzed (eg, DNA, RNA, protein, antibody),

- Number of markers (eg, number of genes, number of proteins),

- Methodology(ies) (eg, microarray, real-time [RT]-PCR, in situ hybridization [ISH], enzyme linked immunosorbent assays [ELISA]),

- Number of functional domains (if indicated),

- Specimen type (eg, blood, fresh tissue, formalin-fixed paraffin embedded),

- Algorithm result type (eg, prognostic, diagnostic),

- Report (eg, probability index, risk score)

MAAAs, including those that do not have a Category I code, may be found in Appendix O. MAAAs that do not have a Category I code are identified in Appendix O by a four-digit number followed by the letter "M." The Category I MAAA codes that are included in this subsection are also included in Appendix O. All MAAA codes are listed in Appendix O along with the procedure's proprietary name.

When a specific MAAA procedure is not listed below or in Appendix O, the procedure must be reported using the Category I MAAA unlisted code (81599).

These codes encompass all analytical services required (eg, cell lysis, nucleic acid stabilization, extraction, digestion, amplification, hybridization, and detection) in addition to the algorithmic analysis itself. Procedures that are required prior to cell lysis (eg, microdissection, codes 88380 and 88381) should be reported separately.◄

●**81500**　Oncology (ovarian), biochemical assays of two proteins (CA-125 and HE4), utilizing serum, with menopausal status, algorithm reported as a risk score

▶(Do not report 81500 in conjunction with 86304, 86305)◄

●**81503**　Oncology (ovarian), biochemical assays of five proteins (CA-125, apoliproprotein A1, beta-2 microglobulin, transferrin, and pre-albumin), utilizing serum, algorithm reported as a risk score

▶(Do not report 81503 in conjunction with 82172, 82232, 83695, 83700, 84134, 84466, 86304)◄

●**81506**　Endocrinology (type 2 diabetes), biochemical assays of seven analytes (glucose, HbA1c, insulin, hs-CRP, adoponectin, ferritin, interleukin 2-receptor alpha), utilizing serum or plasma, algorithm reporting a risk score

▶(Do not report 81506 in conjunction with constituent components [ie, 82728, 82947, 83036, 83525, 86141], 84999 [for adopectin], and 83520 [for interleukin 2-receptor alpha])◄

●**81508**　Fetal congenital abnormalities, biochemical assays of two proteins (PAPP-A, hCG [any form]), utilizing maternal serum, algorithm reported as a risk score

▶(Do not report 81508 in conjunction with 84163, 84702)◄

●**81509**　Fetal congenital abnormalities, biochemical assays of three proteins (PAPP-A, hCG [any form], DIA), utilizing maternal serum, algorithm reported as a risk score

▶(Do not report 81509 in conjunction with 84163, 84702, 86336)◄

●**81510**　Fetal congenital abnormalities, biochemical assays of three analytes (AFP, uE3, hCG [any form]), utilizing maternal serum, algorithm reported as a risk score

▶(Do not report 81510 in conjunction with 82105, 82677, 84702)◄

●**81511**　Fetal congenital abnormalities, biochemical assays of four analytes (AFP, uE3, hCG [any form], DIA) utilizing maternal serum, algorithm reported as a risk score (may include additional results from previous biochemical testing)

▶(Do not report 81511 in conjunction with 82105, 82677, 84702, 86336)◄

●**81512**　Fetal congenital abnormalities, biochemical assays of five analytes (AFP, uE3, total hCG, hyperglycosylated hCG, DIA) utilizing maternal serum, algorithm reported as a risk score

▶(Do not report 81512 in conjunction with 82105, 82677, 84702, 86336◄

　⊘=Modifier 51 Exempt　⊙=Moderate Sedation　+=Add-on Code　𝘕=FDA approval pending

●**81599**    Unlisted multianalyte assay with algorithmic analysis

▶(Do not use 81599 for multianalyte assays with algorithmic analyses listed in Appendix O)◄

 **Rationale**

Having completed the large project to construct a new subsection of the CPT Pathology and Laboratory section, including guidelines, definitions, and new codes to report the molecular pathology services that are a cornerstone of testing for personalized medicine, the next step was to address the addition of the last major set of procedures that are currently reported using the stacking codes 83890-83914 and array-based evaluation codes 88384-88386.

These tests are the multianalyte assays with algorithmic analyses (MAAAs), also known as in vitro diagnostic multivariate index assays (IVDMIAs). MAAAs utilize multiple results derived from molecular pathology assays, as well as fluorescent in situ hybridization and other non-nucleic acid-based assays, which are then used as inputs into algorithmic analyses to derive a single result, reported typically as a numeric score, index, or probability. These services are typically performed by and generally available from only a single laboratory or vendor.

To facilitate accurate reporting of MAAA services, a new subsection was added to the Pathology and Laboratory section, which includes a new heading (Multianalyte Assays with Algorithmic Analyses), Category I introductory guidelines, an unlisted multianalyte assay with algorithmic analysis code (81599), and eight new Category I multianalyte assay with algorithmic analyses codes (81500, 81503, 81506, 81508, 81509, 81510, 81511, and 81512). The CPT code set also contains a new administrative code list (Appendix O). Appendix O contains three new administrative and eight new multianalyte assays with algorithmic analyses (MAAA) codes. Also included are introductory guidelines that provide specific guidance on how to accurately report or assign codes and the specific requirements for inclusion in the administrative code list or as a Category I code.

To assist users in reporting the most recently approved administrative codes, the AMA's CPT Web site features updates of the CPT Editorial Panel actions and early publication of the administrative codes in March, June, and November in a given CPT cycle. These dates for early release correspond with the completion of the actions following each of the three annual CPT Editorial Panel meetings in each CPT cycle (May, October, and February).

Code 81500 is used for a qualitative serum test that combines the results of two analytes and menopausal status into a numeric score using an algorithm.

Code 81503 is used for a multianalyte assay that provides a risk index for malignancy of an ovarian mass.

Code 81506 is used for a multianalyte assay that develops a single risk score correlated with the probability of developing a disease.

Codes 81508, 81509, 81510, 81511, and 81512 are used for multianalyte assays that provide maternal serum screening results.

Finally, code 81559 was established to indentify unlisted MAAA procedures.

### Clinical Example (81500)

The patient is a 64-year-old female who presents with complaints of pelvic pressure and pain. The pelvic examination finds an 8-cm firm, fixed, right adnexal mass. The patient is sent for a pelvic ultrasound, which shows a complex cystic and solid adnexal mass. The physician and the patient agree to surgery. Prior to scheduling the surgery, the physician requests a risk of ovarian malignancy algorithm (ROMA) test so as to determine whether the case should be triaged to a physician with special expertise in gynecologic malignancy management.

### Description of Procedure (81500)

The patient's serum is analyzed for CA125 using chemiluminescent microparticle immunoassay (CMIA) methodology and for HE4 using an enzyme immunometric assay (EIA) methodology. The results of the CA125 and HE4 assays along with the patient's menopausal status are entered into computer software that uses an algorithm.

### Clinical Example (81503)

A 43-year-old female presents with pelvic discomfort. On examination, an ovarian mass is identified. A transvaginal ultrasound reveals an indeterminate, complex-appearing solid mass in the right adnexae, and surgical removal is planned. The OVA1 test is ordered to help distinguish between malignant and benign conditions and determine whether referral to a gynecologic oncologist is appropriate.

### Description of Procedure (81503)

A routine blood draw is taken. The specimen is sent to a clinical laboratory at which the five analytes are measured using conventional immunoassay technology. The values of the analytes are input into the OvaCalc® software and the index score is automatically generated, which is reported to the physician.

### Clinical Example (81506)

A 44-year-old female sees her primary care physician for her annual physical examination. She has had impaired fasting glucose during the past two annual check-ups (values 103 mg/dL and 105 mg/dL, respectively). Her physician has recommended she lose 5% to 7% of her body weight, but at each consecutive visit she has increased her weight by 5 lbs. At this examination, her physician orders a Type 2 diabetes five-year Diabetes Risk Score to determine whether the patient should be put into an aggressive diabetes prevention program.

### Description of Procedure (81506)

A fasting venipuncture blood sample is taken by a phlebotomist, processed (serum and whole blood), and shipped refrigerated to the testing laboratory. The samples are processed using quantitative chemistry and immunoassay platforms to generate concentrations for each of the seven biomarkers required. The seven results are analyzed with a multivariate algorithm to generate a Diabetes Risk Score between 1 and 10 that can be correlated to the absolute risk of the patient developing Type 2 diabetes within five years. The numeric score and the concentrations of the individual biomarkers are delivered to the ordering physician.

## Clinical Example (81508)

A patient of advanced maternal age discussed the risk, benefits, and utility of maternal marker screening for neural tube defects and chromosomal abnormalities. She elects to undergo maternal serum screening. A 35-year-old patient presents to the obstetrics office at 11 weeks' gestation. She is leery of diagnostic testing but fears maternal serum screening due to high false positive rates. She wants screening but wants to minimize the false positive rate. She states she would pursue early diagnostic testing, if found to be at very high risk for Down syndrome. The physician reviews the maternal serum screening options with the patient. Sequential 1 screening, which tests for levels of pregnancy-associated plasma protein A (PAPP-A) and human chorionic gonadotropin (hCG), has a less than 1% false positive rate and a 70% Down syndrome detection rate in the first trimester when combined with fetal nuchal translucency measurements and maternal demographic data. The patient notes that she will proceed with chorionic villus sampling (CVS) if she is found to be "screen positive." If she is not screen positive, she will proceed with Sequential 2 testing in the second trimester. She is informed that Sequential 2 testing has an overall detection rate for Down syndrome of 92% and a 3% false positive rate. She opts to proceed with Sequential 1 screening due to the availability of first trimester diagnostic testing if screen positive, and the overall lower false positive rate and higher detection rate than other maternal serum screening tests.

### Description of Procedure (81508)

Laboratory procedures to test the patient's PAPP-A and hCG levels are performed. The patient's risk score is determined by applying the algorithm to the two lab results along with fetal nuchal translucency (NT) measurements and maternal patient demographic data. Note: Performing the NT procedure is not included in code 81503.

## Clinical Example (81509)

A 40-year-old female presents to the obstetrics office. The patient states that she wants to have the option of chorionic villus sampling (CVS), if she is found to be "screen positive" for Down syndrome. She states that she would discontinue an affected pregnancy, but second trimester termination is not an option for her. She states she would like to proceed with the first trimester screening test, which provides the highest detection rate. The physician reviews with her the options for first trimester screening and the results of both the First and Second Trimester Evaluation of Risk (FASTER) study and the Serum, Urine, and Ultrasound Screening Study (SURUSS), which found the high detection rates when combining pregnancy-associated plasma protein A (PAPP-A), human chorionic gonadotropin (hCG), and dimeric inhibin A (DIA) levels with fetal ultrasound markers and maternal demographic data.

### Description of Procedure (81509)

Laboratory procedures PAPP-A, hCG, and DIA levels are performed. The patient's risk score is determined by applying the algorithm to the three lab results along with fetal nuchal translucency (NT) measurements and maternal patient demographic data. Note: Performing the NT procedure is not included in code 81509.

### ⚕ Clinical Example (81510)

A 25-year-old female presents for obstetrics care at 15 weeks' gestation. Laboratory procedures to test the patient's alpha-fetoprotein (AFP), unconjugated estriol (uE3), and human chorionic gonadotropin (hCG) levels are performed. The patient's risk score is determined by applying the algorithm to the three lab results and maternal patient demographic data. The option of maternal serum screening for Down syndrome versus diagnostic testing is reviewed. At her current gestational age, Triple/X-tra or Quad/Tetra screening are the available maternal serum screening options. The patient opts to proceed with Triple/X-tra screening, which when combined with maternal age, weight, race, and diabetic status, has a 60% detection rate with a 5% false positive rate.

### Description of Procedure (81510)

Laboratory procedures to test the patient's alpha-fetoprotein (AFP), unconjugated estriol (uE3), and human chorionic gonadotropin (hCG) levels are performed. The patient's risk score is determined by applying the algorithm to the three lab results and maternal patient demographic data. Note: Performing the NT procedure is not included in code 81510.

### ⚕ Clinical Example (81511)

A 35-year-old patient returns to the obstetrics office at 15 weeks' gestation. She has previously obtained the first part of a sequential screen in the first trimester of her pregnancy. The patient discusses with her physician the results of the first trimester portion of the test, which were not positive. The patient is interested in reassurance that her fetus's risk of Down syndrome is low and would like screening for open spina bifida, which is not available in the first trimester. She opts to complete the second trimester portion of the sequential panel, which includes testing for levels of alpha-fetoprotein (AFP), unconjugated estriol (uE3), human chorionic gonadotropin (hCG), and dimeric inhibin A (DIA) (AFP, uE3, hCG (any form), DIA in order to get the Down syndrome detection rate of 92% and false positive rate of ~3% associated with the completion of both halves of sequential testing as well as screening for open spina bifida.

### Description of Procedure (81511)

Laboratory procedures to test the patient's AFP, uE3, hCG, and DIA levels are performed. The patient's risk score is determined by applying the algorithm to the four lab results along with fetal nuchal translucency (NT) measurements and maternal patient demographic data. Note: Performing the NT procedure is not included in code 81511.

### ⚕ Clinical Example (81512)

A 34-year-old pregnant female presents to her physician at 16 weeks' gestation for a routine visit. The physician recommends that the patient has blood drawn for a maternal serum screening test, which screens for the risk of neural tube defects, Down syndrome, and trisomy 18. The physician recommends the five-analyte panel, including alpha-fetoprotein (AFP), unconjugated estriol (uE3), human chorionic gonadotropin (hCG), hyperglycosylated hCG, and dimeric inhibin A (DIA).

⊘=Modifier 51 Exempt   ⊙=Moderate Sedation   ✚=Add-on Code   𝒩=FDA approval pending

## Description of Procedure (81512)

Laboratory procedures to test the patient's AFP, uE3, total hCG, hyperglycosyl-ated hCG, and DIA levels are performed. The patient's risk score is determined by applying the algorithm to the five lab results along with the fetal nuchal translucency (NT) measurements and maternal patient demographic data. Note: Performing the NT procedure is not included in code 81512.

## Chemistry

The material for examination may be from any source unless otherwise specified in the code descriptor. When an analyte is measured in multiple specimens from different sources, or in specimens that are obtained at different times, the analyte is reported separately for each source and for each specimen. The examination is quantitative unless specified. To report an organ or disease oriented panel, see codes 80048-80076.

When a code describes a method where measurement of multiple analytes may require one or several procedures, each procedure is coded separately (eg, 82491-82492, 82541-82544). For example, if two analytes are measured using column chromatography using a single stationary or mobile phase, use 82492. If the same two analytes are measured using different stationary or mobile phase conditions, 82491 would be used twice. If a total of four analytes are measured where two analytes are measured with a single stationary and mobile phase, and the other two analytes are measured using a different stationary and mobile phase, use 82492 twice. If a total of three analytes are measured where two analytes are measured using a single stationary or mobile phase condition, and the third analyte is measured separately using a different stationary or mobile phase procedure, use 82492 once for the two analytes measured under the same condition, and use 82491 once for the third analyte measured separately.

▶Clinical information or mathematically calculated values, which are not specifically requested by the ordering physician and are derived from the results of other ordered or performed laboratory tests, are considered part of the ordered test procedure(s) and therefore are not separately reportable service(s).◀

▶When the requested analyte result is derived using a calculation that requires values from non-requested laboratory analyses, only the requested analyte code should be reported.◀

▶When the calculated analyte determination requires values derived from other requested and nonrequested laboratory analyses, the requested analyte codes (including those calculated) should be reported.◀

▶An exception to the above is when an analyte (eg, urinary creatinine) is performed to compensate for variations in urine concentration (eg, microalbumin, thromboxane metabolites) in random urine samples; the appropriate CPT code is reported for both the ordered analyte and the additional required analyte. When the calculated result(s) represent an algorithmically derived numeric score or probability, see the appropriate multianalyte assay with algorithmic analyses (MAAA) code or the MAAA unlisted code (81599).◀

## Rationale

The Chemistry guidelines were editorially revised to provide more detailed coding instruction regarding reporting calculated analyte determinations using values derived from other analyses. In addition, in support of the establishment of codes, descriptors, and guidelines to describe multanalyte assays with algorithmic analyses (MAAA) codes, the Chemistry guidelines have been updated to facilitate accurate reporting of these services.

| | |
|---|---|
| **82000** | Acetaldehyde, blood |
| ▲**82009** | Ketone body(s) (eg, acetone, acetoacetic acid, beta-hydroxybutyrate); qualitative |
| ▲**82010** | quantitative |

## Rationale

Codes 82009 and 82010 have been revised to reflect current clinical practice. The specimen source has been removed, and a parenthetical list of examples (eg, acetone, acetoacetic acid and beta-hydroxybutyrate) describing ketone bodies were added to the descriptor of codes 82009 and 82010. These codes are intended to describe qualitative and quantitative tests for ketone bodies such as acetone, acetoacetic acid, or beta-hydroxybutyrate present in blood. These procedures are primarily used to screen for, detect, and monitor diabetic ketoacidosis (DKA) in people with Type 1, and sometimes, Type 2 diabetes.

| | |
|---|---|
| **82775** | Galactose-1-phosphate uridyl transferase; quantitative |
| **82776** | screen |
| ●**82777** | Galectin-3 |

## Rationale

Code 82777 was added to report the Galectin-3 assay, which is an enzyme immunoassay that uses two highly specific monoclonal antibodies for the direct measurement of Galectin-3 in human plasma and serum. This code has been developed to measure Galectin-3, related Galectins or the progressive cardiac fibrogenesis associated with Galectin-3 elevation.

## Clinical Example (82777)

A 68-year-old male visits the emergency room with shortness of breath attributed to heart failure. The patient has a history of chronic, mildly symptomatic heart failure with recent gradual decline despite guideline-indicated therapy. Upon further examination, the patient is classified as New York Heart Association (NYHA) Class III with left ventricular ejection fraction (LVEF) of 34%. An ethylenediaminetetraacetic acid (EDTA) sample was obtained and spun. After separation, plasma was frozen at −20°C for analysis the next day at the hospital's laboratory facility. The assay reported a high plasma Galectin-3 level of 42 ng/mL suggestive of cardiac remodeling resulting in poor prognosis. Based on the results of the Galectin-3 assay and clinical (eg, furosemide dose now 80 mg/day; systolic BP, 110 mmHg; QRS duration, 140 msec; echo left ventricular ejection fraction [LVEF], 34%) and other laboratory (eg, serum creatinine upper limit of normal)

⊘=Modifier 51 Exempt  ⊙=Moderate Sedation  ✚=Add-on Code  ✚=FDA approval pending

features, the cardiologist decided to recommend a bi-ventricular pacemaker (CRT) treatment in addition to medical therapy despite the fact that the patient rapidly improved to NYHA Class II with intensified diuretic therapy.

### Description of Procedure (82777)

A female with metastatic breast cancer presents to her physician for a follow-up examination. An anticoagulated blood sample is submitted to the laboratory for cell enumeration using immunologic selection and identification in fluid specimen (eg, circulating tumor cells in blood).

**83887**   Nicotine

▶(83890-83914 have been deleted. To report, see 81200-81479)◄

### ✎ Rationale

In support of the establishment of Tier 1 and Tier 2 Molecular Pathology Procedures codes (81200-81383, 81400-81408), the current stacking-code method of reporting molecular pathology services (83890-83914) and the array-based evaluation codes (88384-88386) code set have been deleted.

To gain a thorough understanding of how to appropriately report Tier 1 and Tier 2 codes, several resources have been created, including introductory guidelines and definitions included in the Molecular Pathology subsection of the CPT 2013 code set. Another resource developed to help code molecular pathology procedures is a special CPT insert in the front matter of the *CPT 2013 Professional Edition codebook*. The special insert offers additional information to help users understand the Tier 1 and Tier 2 code structure, use of abbreviation within code descriptors, and the meaning of the parenthetical content included in the code descriptors. In addition, the May 2012 edition of *CPT Assistant* also contains an article that includes an overview of the CPT Editorial Panel Molecular Pathology Coding Workgroup's charge and its current and future activities.

## Immunology

**#●86152**   Cell enumeration using immunologic selection and identification in fluid specimen (eg, circulating tumor cells in blood);

▶(For physician interpretation and report, use 86153. For cell enumeration with interpretation and report, use 86152 and 86153)◄

**#●86153**      physician interpretation and report, when required

▶(For cell enumeration, use 86152. For cell enumeration with interpretation and report, use 86152 and 86153)◄

▶(For flow cytometric immunophenotyping, see 88184-88189)◄

▶(For flow cytometric quantitation, see 86355, 86356, 86357, 86359, 86360, 86361, 86367)◄

**Rationale**

Two codes (86152, 86153) have been established to report cell enumeration using immunologic selection and identification. This test is also referred to as *circulating tumor cells (CTC) enumeration*. The purpose of this test is to determine disease prognosis in cancer patients and for use in deciding the course of treatment.

In support of the establishment of codes 86152 and 86153, Category III codes 0279T and 0280T have been deleted from the CPT code set. A parenthetical note has been added following code 86152 to indicate that code 86153 should be reported for physician interpretation and report, when required. The note also indicates that codes 86152 and 86153 should be reported for cell enumeration with interpretation and report. A similar note has been added following code 86153 indicating that code 86152 should be reported for cell enumeration and that codes 86152 and 86153 should be reported for cell enumeration with interpretation and report. A second parenthetical note has been added following code 86153 directing users to the appropriate codes to report for flow cytometric immunophenotyping or flow cytometric quantitation services.

 **Clinical Example (86152)**

A female with metastatic breast cancer presents to her physician for a follow-up examination. An anticoagulated blood sample is submitted to the laboratory for cell enumeration using immunologic selection and identification in fluid specimen (eg, circulating tumor cells in blood).

**Description of Procedure (86152)**

Following centrifugation of 10 mL of blood received in an ethylenediaminetetraacetic acid (EDTA) tube with special preservative, the buffy coat and plasma are separated from the red blood cells and placed in a buffer. A semi-automated system is used to separate, stain, and fluorescently label cells from the buffy coat and packed red cells. The resulting mixture of fluorescently labeled cells is disbursed onto a flat plane for image analysis. A series of fluorescent images are recorded at high magnification by a photographic scanning device in each of four channels for cytokeratin, DAPI, white cell markers, and controls. The resulting images are compiled by a computer and presented as an image gallery. Cells conforming to the characteristic immunofluorescent pattern are scored. A final circulating epithelial cell count is enumerated and the results are entered into the laboratory information system (LIS).

**Clinical Example (86153)**

A female with metastatic breast cancer presents to her physician for follow-up. Results of the cell enumeration using immunologic selection and identification in fluid specimen (eg, circulating tumor cells in blood) require interpretation by physician.

**Description of Procedure (86153)**

The physician examines the entire image file and classifies the circulating cells as epithelial tumor cells, white blood cells, or other, based on strict cytomorphological criteria and experience in fluorescent microscopy. The physician reviews the

⊘=Modifier 51 Exempt ⊙=Moderate Sedation ✚=Add-on Code 𝒩=FDA approval pending

relevant findings in the patient's case history. The physician prepares and signs an interpretive written report.

**86148**     Anti-phosphatidylserine (phospholipid) antibody

►(To report antiprothrombin [phospholipid cofactor] antibody, use 86849)◄

 **Rationale**

In support of the deletion of code 0030T, a parenthetical note has been added following code 86148 to direct users to use of 86849 to report antiprothrombin phospholipid cofactor antibody.

**86152**     ►Code is out of numerical sequence. See 86000-86804◄

**86153**     ►Code is out of numerical sequence. See 86000-86804◄

**86485**     Skin test; candida

**86580**          tuberculosis, intradermal

(For tuberculosis test, cell mediated immunity measurement of gamma interferon antigen response, use 86480)

►(For skin tests for allergy, see 95012-95199)◄

 **Rationale**

In response to the deletion of code 95010 from the CPT code set, the second parenthetical note following 86580 has been revised with the removal of code 95010, in order to reflect the appropriate range of codes to report allergy testing.

**86710**     Antibody; influenza virus

●**86711**          JC (John Cunningham) virus

 **Rationale**

A new laboratory code, 86711, has been established to report detection of John Cunningham (JC) virus. The purpose of this test is to determine disease prognosis in patients with progressive multifocal leukoencephalopathy (PML) and for use in determining the course of treatment.

**Clinical Example (86711)**

A 55-year-old female patient presents with relapsing-remitting multiple sclerosis (MS). The patient is being treated with disease modifying agents, and the physician is considering a change in treatment regimen. The physician orders the JC virus antibody enzyme-linked immunosorbent assay (ELISA) to detect the presence of antibodies so that the patient's antibody status can be used in conjunction with other clinical data as an aid in risk stratification for progressive multifocal leukoencephalopathy (PML), and in assessing a potential change in treatment regimen.

# Tissue Typing

● **86828**     Antibody to human leukocyte antigens (HLA), solid phase assays (eg, microspheres or beads, ELISA, flow cytometry); qualitative assessment of the presence or absence of antibody(ies) to HLA Class I and Class II HLA antigens

● **86829**     qualitative assessment of the presence or absence of antibody(ies) to HLA Class I or Class II HLA antigens

    ▶(If solid phase testing is performed to assess presence or absence of antibody to both HLA classes, use 86828)◀

● **86830**     antibody identification by qualitative panel using complete HLA phenotypes, HLA Class I

● **86831**     antibody identification by qualitative panel using complete HLA phenotypes, HLA Class II

● **86832**     high definition qualitative panel for identification of antibody specificities (eg, individual antigen per bead methodology), HLA Class I

● **86833**     high definition qualitative panel for identification of antibody specificities (eg, individual antigen per bead methodology), HLA Class II

    ▶(If solid phase testing is performed to test for HLA Class I or II antibody after treatment [eg, to remove IgM antibodies or other interfering substances], report 86828-86833 once for each panel with the untreated serum and once for each panel with the treated serum)◀

● **86834**     semi-quantitative panel (eg, titer), HLA Class I

● **86835**     semi-quantitative panel (eg, titer), HLA Class II

### ✐ Rationale

New test platforms have been developed for antibody to human leukocyte antigen (HLA) solid phase assays. These platforms use solid phase assays covering the most common HLA Class I and Class II antigens. The technology uses microspheres, chips, or ELISA trays coated with purified or recombinant HLA molecules. Eight new codes have been established for reporting antibody to human leukocyte antigen (HLA) solid phase assays. Code 86828 describes qualitative assessment of the presence or absence of antibody(ies) to HLA Class I and Class II HLA antigens. Code 86829 describes qualitative assessment of the presence or absence of antibody(ies) to HLA Class I or Class II HLA antigens. A parenthetical note following code 86829 directs users to code 86828, if solid phase testing is performed to assess presence or absence of antibody to both HLA classes. Code 86830 describes antibody identification by qualitative panel using complete HLA phenotypes, HLA Class I. Code 86831 describes antibody identification by qualitative panel using complete HLA phenotypes, HLA Class II. Code 86832 describes high definition qualitative panel for identification of antibody specificities (eg, individual antigen per bead methodology), HLA Class I. Code 86833 describes high definition qualitative panel for identification of antibody specificities (eg, individual antigen per bead methodology), HLA Class II.

An instructional parenthetical note following code 86833 instructs users to report 86828-86833 once for each panel with the untreated serum and once for each panel with the treated serum if solid phase testing is performed to test for HLA Class I or II antibody after treatment, for example, to remove IgM antibodies or other interfering substances.

 ### Clinical Example (86828)

A patient with end-stage renal disease (ESRD) is being considered for a kidney transplant and is listed on the United Network for Organ Sharing (UNOS) waiting list. Testing to determine the presence or absence of antibody to human leukocyte antigen (HLA) Class I and Class II HLA antigens is requested. A blood sample is submitted.

### Description of Procedure (86828)

Serum is prepared from a blood sample and tested for antibodies by mixing the serum with beads coated with Class I HLA antigens and beads coated with Class II HLA antigens. The beads are analyzed on an instrument designed to detect binding of antibody using fluorescent anti-IgG. If antibody is bound to the beads with Class I HLA, it indicates that the patient is sensitized to Class I HLA antigens. If antibody is bound to the beads with Class II HLA, it indicates that the patient is sensitized to Class II HLA antigens.

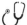 ### Clinical Example (86829)

A patient presents with a low platelet count, and platelet transfusions do not produce a lasting increment. An immunologic mechanism is suspected. Testing to determine the presence or absence of antibody to human leukocyte antigen (HLA) Class I HLA antigens is requested. A blood sample is submitted.

### Description of Procedure (86829)

Serum is prepared from a blood sample and tested for antibodies by mixing the serum with beads coated with Class I HLA antigens. The beads are analyzed on an instrument designed to detect binding of antibody to the HLA antigen coated beads binding using fluorescent anti-IgG. If antibody is bound to the beads, it indicates that the patient has antibody to Class I HLA antigens.

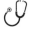 ### Clinical Example (86830)

A patient with end-stage renal disease (ESRD) is being considered for a kidney transplant and is listed on the United Network for Organ Sharing (UNOS) waiting list. The patient has been found to have antibody to Class I human leukocyte antigen (HLA) antigens by qualitative testing of previous samples, followed by testing to define the specificity of these antibodies using high-definition bead panels. A blood sample is submitted to monitor the patient for changes in the antibody profile.

### Description of Procedure (86830)

Serum is prepared from a blood sample and tested for antibodies by mixing the serum with a panel of up to 100 identifiable beads that are each coated with a different complete set of Class I HLA antigens from a single individual. The beads are analyzed for binding of antibody to the HLA antigens using an instrument designed to detect antibody binding using fluorescent anti-IgG. If antibody is present, the reactivity is compared to the patient's antibody profile for changes.

Changes in the profile may indicate new specificities that should be confirmed by high-definition testing.

###  Clinical Example (86831)

A patient with end-stage renal disease (ESRD) is being considered for a kidney transplant and is listed on the United Network for Organ Sharing (UNOS) waiting list. The patient has been found to have antibody to Class II human leukocyte antigen (HLA) antigens by qualitative testing of previous samples, followed by testing to define the specificity of these antibodies using high-definition bead panels. A blood sample is submitted to monitor the patient for changes in the antibody profile.

### Description of Procedure (86831)

Serum is prepared from a blood sample and tested for antibodies by mixing the serum with a panel of up to 100 identifiable beads that are each coated with a different complete set of Class II HLA antigens from a single individual. The beads are analyzed for binding of antibody to these antigens using an instrument designed to detect antibody binding using fluorescent anti-IgG. If antibody is present, the reactivity is compared to the patient's antibody profile for changes. Changes in the profile may indicate new specificities that should be confirmed by high-definition testing.

###  Clinical Example (86832)

A patient with kidney failure due to end-stage renal disease (ESRD) is being considered for a kidney transplant and is listed on the United Network for Organ Sharing (UNOS) waiting list. The patient was found to be sensitized to Class I human leukocyte antigen (HLA) antigens based on qualitative testing for anti-HLA antibody. Testing is requested to identify the specificity(ies) of the antibody to HLA Class I antigens in order to assign unacceptable HLA antigens for transplant. A blood sample is submitted for testing.

### Description of Procedure (86832)

Serum is prepared from a blood sample and tested for antibodies by mixing it with a panel of beads coated with specific (recombinant) HLA class I antigens. The beads are analyzed on an instrument designed to detect antibody binding to the beads using fluorescent anti-IgG. HLA specificities are determined by analyzing the bead reactivity. These specificities are compared with the patient typing, and unacceptable antigens are determined for entry into the UNOS computer to be used in donor selection.

###  Clinical Example (86833)

A patient with kidney failure due to end-stage renal disease (ESRD) is being considered for a kidney transplant and is listed on the United Network for Organ Sharing (UNOS) waiting list. The patient was found to be sensitized to Class II human leukocyte antigen (HLA) antigens based on qualitative testing for anti-HLA antibody. Testing is requested to identify the specificity(ies) of the antibody to HLA Class II antigens, in order to assign unacceptable HLA antigens for transplant. A blood sample is submitted for testing.

**Description of Procedure (86833)**

Serum is prepared from a blood sample and tested for antibodies by mixing it with a panel of beads coated with specific (recombinant) HLA class II antigens. The beads are analyzed on an instrument designed to detect antibody binding to the beads using fluorescent anti-IgG. HLA specificities are determined by analyzing the bead reactivity. These specificities are compared with the patient typing, and unacceptable antigens are determined for entry into the UNOS computer to be used in donor selection.

 **Clinical Example (86834)**

A patient with kidney failure due to end-stage renal disease (ESRD) is being considered for a kidney transplant and is listed on the United Network for Organ Sharing (UNOS) waiting list. The patient has been found to be sensitized to Class I human leukocyte antigen (HLA) antigens. A potential living donor has been identified, but the patient's antibodies are directed to a donor Class I HLA antigen, resulting in a positive crossmatch. A desensitization protocol is initiated. As part of a desensitization protocol, a titration of the patient's antibody is requested to determine whether the donor-specific antibody level has decreased after desensitization. A blood sample is submitted for testing.

**Description of Procedure (86834)**

Serum is prepared from a blood sample and tested in dilutions by mixing it with a panel of beads coated with individual (recombinant) HLA Class I (A, B, C) antigens. The beads are analyzed on an instrument designed to detect antibody binding using fluorescent anti-IgG. At each dilution, the antibody binding is compared to the binding prior to desensitization.

 **Clinical Example (86835)**

A patient with kidney failure due to end-stage renal disease (ESRD) is being considered for a kidney transplant and is listed on the United Network for Organ Sharing (UNOS) waiting list. The patient has been found to be sensitized to Class II human leukocyte antigen (HLA) antigens. A potential living donor has been identified, but the patient's antibodies are directed to a donor Class II HLA antigen, resulting in a positive crossmatch. A desensitization protocol is initiated. As part of a desensitization protocol, a titration of the patient's antibody is requested to determine whether the donor-specific antibody level has decreased after desensitization. A blood sample is submitted for testing.

**Description of Procedure (86835)**

Serum is prepared from a blood sample and tested in dilutions by mixing it with a panel of beads coated with individual (recombinant) Class II (DR, DQ, or DP) HLA antigens. The beads are analyzed on an instrument designed to detect antibody binding using fluorescent anti-IgG. At each dilution, the antibody binding is compared to the binding prior to desensitization.

# Transfusion Medicine

**86890**   Autologous blood or component, collection processing and storage; predeposited

**86891**      intra- or postoperative salvage

(For physician services to autologous donors, see 99201-99204)

**86950**   Leukocyte transfusion

▶(For allogeneic lymphocyte infusion, use 38242)◀

(For leukapheresis, use 36511)

### ✍ Rationale

The parenthetical note following collection processing and storage codes 86890 and 86891 was deleted for the CPT 2013 code set. However, the note was retained in error. This correction will be included in the 2013 CPT errata document and posted to the AMA CPT Web site at www.ama-assn.org/ama/pub/physician-resources/solutions-managing-your-practice/coding-billing-insurance/cpt/about-cpt/errata.page. In concert with the revisions to the family of codes 38240-38242, a cross-reference has been added following code 86950 directing users to the appropriate code for reporting allogeneic lymphocyte infusion (38242).

# Microbiology

▶Presumptive identification of microorganisms is defined as identification by colony morphology, growth on selective media, Gram stains, or up to three tests (eg, catalase, oxidase, indole, urease). Definitive identification of microorganisms is defined as an identification to the genus or species level that requires additional tests (eg, biochemical panels, slide cultures). If additional studies involve molecular probes, nucleic acid sequencing, chromatography, or immunologic techniques, these should be separately coded using 87140-87158, in addition to definitive identification codes. The molecular diagnostic codes (eg, 81200-81408) are not to be used in combination with or instead of the procedures represented by 87140-87158. For multiple specimens/sites use modifier 59. For repeat laboratory tests performed on the same day, use modifier 91.◀

**87140**   Culture, typing; immunofluorescent method, each antiserum

**87149**      identification by nucleic acid (DNA or RNA) probe, direct probe technique, per culture or isolate, each organism probed

▶(Do not report 87149 in conjunction with 81200-81408)◀

**87150**      identification by nucleic acid (DNA or RNA) probe, amplified probe technique, per culture or isolate, each organism probed

▶(Do not report 87150 in conjunction with 81200-81408)◀

**87152**      identification by pulse field gel typing

▶(Do not report 87152 in conjunction with 81200-81408)◀

►These codes are intended for primary source only. For similar studies on culture material, refer to codes 87140-87158. Infectious agents by antigen detection, immunofluorescence microscopy, or nucleic acid probe techniques should be reported as precisely as possible. The molecular pathology procedures codes (81200-81408) are not to be used in combination with or instead of the procedures represented by 87470-87801. The most specific code possible should be reported. If there is no specific agent code, the general methodology code (eg, 87299, 87449, 87450, 87797, 87798, 87799, 87899) should be used. For identification of antibodies to many of the listed infectious agents, see 86602-86804. When separate results are reported for different species or strain of organisms, each result should be coded separately. Use modifier 59 when separate results are reported for different species or strains that are described by the same code.◄

## 🖎 Rationale

To accommodate the deletion of stacking codes 83890-83914 and their replacement with Molecular Pathology codes 81200-81479, the Microbiology guidelines and the instructional parenthetical notes following codes 87149, 87150, and 87152 have been revised to reflect this change.

| | |
|---|---|
| **87470** | Infectious agent detection by nucleic acid (DNA or RNA); Bartonella henselae and Bartonella quintana, direct probe technique |
| ▲**87498** | enterovirus, reverse transcription and amplified probe technique |
| ▲**87521** | hepatitis C, reverse transcription and amplified probe technique |
| ▲**87522** | hepatitis C, reverse transcription and quantification |
| ▲**87535** | HIV-1, reverse transcription and amplified probe technique |
| ▲**87536** | HIV-1, reverse transcription and quantification |
| ▲**87538** | HIV-2, reverse transcription and amplified probe technique |
| ▲**87539** | HIV-2, reverse transcription and quantification |

## 🖎 Rationale

Prior to 2013, infectious agent detection by nucleic acid (DNA or RNA) codes 87498, 87521, 87522, 87535, 87536, 87538, and 87539 did not reflect that reverse transcriptase is used in these assays. RNA is fragile and must be treated with chemicals to avoid degradation. RNA is then reverse transcribed to cDNA before amplification can occur. To accurately reflect the performance of these tests, codes 87498, 87521, 87522, 87535, 87536, 87538, and 87539 for enterovirus, hepatitis C, HIV-1, and HIV-2 have been editorially revised to include reverse transcription.

| | |
|---|---|
| **87622** | papillomavirus, human, quantification |
| ●**87631** | respiratory virus (eg, adenovirus, influenza virus, coronavirus, metapneumovirus, parainfluenza virus, respiratory syncytial virus, rhinovirus), multiplex reverse transcription and amplified probe technique, multiple types or subtypes, 3-5 targets |
| ●**87632** | respiratory virus (eg, adenovirus, influenza virus, coronavirus, metapneumovirus, parainfluenza virus, respiratory syncytial virus, rhinovirus), multiplex reverse transcription and amplified probe technique, multiple types or subtypes, 6-11 targets |

●**87633**        respiratory virus (eg, adenovirus, influenza virus, coronavirus, metapneumovirus, parainfluenza virus, respiratory syncytial virus, rhinovirus), multiplex reverse transcription and amplified probe technique, multiple types or subtypes, 12-25 targets

▶(Use 87631-87633 for nucleic acid assays which detect multiple respiratory viruses in a multiplex reaction [ie, single procedure with multiple results])◀

▶(For assays that are used to type or subtype influenza viruses only, see 87501-87503)◀

▶(For assays that include influenza viruses with additional respiratory viruses, see 87631-87633)◀

▶(For detection of multiple infectious agents not otherwise specified which report a single result, see 87800, 87801)◀

**87800**     Infectious agent detection by nucleic acid (DNA or RNA), multiple organisms; direct probe(s) technique

**87801**        amplified probe(s) technique

(For each specific organism nucleic acid detection from a primary source, see 87470-87660. For detection of specific infectious agents not otherwise specified, see 87797, 87798, or 87799 1 time for each agent)

▶(For detection of multiple infectious agents not otherwise specified which report a single result, see 87800, 87801)◀

▶(Do not use 87801 for nucleic acid assays that detect multiple respiratory viruses in a multiplex reaction [ie, single procedure with multiple results], see 87631-87633)◀

### ✍️ Rationale

Three codes have been established to report infectious agent detection of respiratory viruses by nucleic acid (87631-87633). These codes more accurately define the number and potential types of respiratory viral targets simultaneously assessed. Instructional parenthetical notes have been added and existing notes have been revised to provide further clarification on the appropriate use of these codes.

### 🩺 Clinical Example (87631)

A pediatric patient presents to his or her physician with a cough, fever, and respiratory distress compatible with an influenza-like illness. The physician obtains a nasopharyngeal swab specimen, places it in a transport medium, and sends it to the laboratory for testing. The physician orders a multiplex reverse transcription polymerase chain reaction (RT-PCR) based assay for influenza A, influenza B, and respiratory syncytial virus (RSV).

**Description of Procedure (87631)**

Upon receipt of the nasopharyngeal swab specimen, high quality total nucleic acid is isolated and stored under RNase-free conditions. Reverse transcription is used to convert RNA to cDNA followed by real-time PCR amplification using primers for influenza A, influenza B, and RSV, along with a control gene.

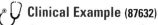 **Clinical Example** (87632)

A patient presents to his or her physician with a cough, fever, and respiratory distress compatible with an influenza-like illness. The physician suspects the patient may be infected with the H1N1 virus. The physician obtains a nasopharyngeal swab specimen, places it in a transport medium, and sends it to the laboratory for reverse transcription polymerase chain reaction (RT-PCR) testing for influenza A, influenza B, influenza A H1, novel H1N1, and H3 subtyping, and RSV.

**Description of Procedure** (87632)

Upon receipt of the nasopharyngeal swab specimen, high quality total nucleic acid is isolated and stored under RNase-free conditions. Reverse transcription is used to convert RNA to cDNA followed by real-time PCR amplification using primers for five influenza types and subtypes, RSV, and a control gene.

 **Clinical Example** (87633)

A patient presents to his or her physician with a cough, fever, and respiratory distress. The physician suspects the patient may be infected with the H1N1 virus. The physician obtains a nasopharyngeal swab specimen, places it in a transport medium, and sends it to the laboratory for multiplex reverse transcription polymerase chain reaction (RT-PCR) testing for twelve viruses.

**Description of Procedure** (87633)

Upon receipt of the nasopharyngeal swab specimen, high quality total nucleic acid is isolated and stored under RNase-free conditions. Multiplexed reverse transcription is used to convert RNA to cDNA followed by PCR-based amplification using primers for multiple virus types and a control gene. The amplification products are hybridized to fluorescently color-coded microspheres for simultaneous detection and identification of twelve respiratory viruses and subtypes.

| | |
|---|---|
| 87900 | Infectious agent drug susceptibility phenotype prediction using regularly updated genotypic bioinformatics |
| #●87910 | Infectious agent genotype analysis by nucleic acid (DNA or RNA); cytomegalovirus |
| ▲87901 | HIV-1, reverse transcriptase and protease regions |
| #87906 | HIV-1, other region (eg, integrase, fusion) |
| #●87912 | Hepatitis B virus |
| 87902 | Hepatitis C virus |

**Rationale**

Codes for two new Category I infectious agent genotype analysis by nucleic acid (DNA or RNA) procedures were added to the CPT code set. These procedures help to determine drug resistance and treatment options for viral diseases. Specifically, code 87910 is used for nucleic acid probe techniques for the detection of cytomegalovirus, and 87912 is used for nucleic acid probe techniques for the detection of Hepatitis B virus. To maintain consistency and uniformity, code 87901 was also revised from a parent code to a child code under new code 87910. Codes 87910 and 87912 appear with a hash (#) symbol to indicate that these codes are out of numerical sequence.

## Clinical Example (87910)

A 45-year-old male presents to the emergency room with symptoms of pneumonia. This patient had received a lung transplant four months earlier from an organ donor, who was sero-positive for cytomegalovirus (CMV). The patient was sero-negative for CMV at the time of the transplant, and was therefore, prescribed gancyclovir prophylactically for 3 months. Suspecting CMV infection, the physician initiates therapy with gancyclovir. In addition, the physician orders diagnostic testing and a CMV genotype test. The diagnostic tests confirm a diagnosis of CMV pneumonia. The results of the genotype test report a mutation in UL97. This mutation is associated with gancyclovir resistance, and therefore, the patient is placed on foscarnet therapy because a mutation in UL97 does not confer resistance to this drug.

### Description of Procedure (87910)

This test uses the viral DNA sequence and associates it to known drug resistance mutations in the UL97 and UL54 regions of CMV. The assay consists of automated viral DNA extraction, DNA amplification by polymerase chain reaction (PCR) with specific primers, cycle sequencing of PCR products, and association of mutations at selected codons in the UL97 and UL54 genes with resistance to ganciclovir, foscarnet, and cidofovir.

## Clinical Example (87912)

The patient is a 30-year-old male who is hepatitis B surface antigen (HBsAg) and hepatitis B e antigen (HBeAg)–positive. The patient has been on a nucleoside/nucleotide treatment (lamivudine) for six months. His hepatitis B plasma viral load is 1,500 IU/mL, his alanine transaminase (ALT) level is slightly elevated, and his liver biopsy shows minimal inflammation. A DNA-sequencing test for the hepatitis B virus (HBV) genotype is requested to interrogate potential resistance mutations specific for lamivudine and other nucleoside/nucleotide analogues. Based on the findings, therapy may be adjusted to a new nucleoside/nucleotide agent to provide the greatest benefit for the patient, with subsequent evaluation and management based on response to that therapy.

### Description of Procedure (87912)

Polymerase chain reaction (PCR) with HBV-specific primers is used to amplify two regions of the HBV genome containing relevant portions of the DNA polymerase S, BCP, and precore genes. Resulting PCR products are sequenced and sequence data are analyzed for mutations at codons rt169, 173, 180, 181, 184, 194, 202, 204, 207, 236, and 250 of the polymerase gene; at nucleotides 1762 and 1764 of the BCP region; and at nucleotide 1896 of the precore region. The HBV genotype is determined by computer-aided alignment and phylogenetic analysis of the amplified portion of the S gene.

⊘=Modifier 51 Exempt   ⊙=Moderate Sedation   ✛=Add-on Code   𝑁=FDA approval pending

# Cytopathology

**88184** Flow cytometry, cell surface, cytoplasmic, or nuclear marker, technical component only; first marker

**✛88185** each additional marker (List separately in addition to code for first marker)

(Report 88185 in conjunction with 88184)

**88187** Flow cytometry, interpretation; 2 to 8 markers

**88188** 9 to 15 markers

**88189** 16 or more markers

(Do not report 88187-88189 for interpretation of 86355, 86356, 86357, 86359, 86360, 86361, 86367)

►(For assessment of circulating antibodies by flow cytometric techniques, see analyte and method-specific codes in the Chemistry section [83516-83520] or Immunology section [86000-86849])◄

## 🔏 Rationale

Before 2013, there had been confusion regarding the appropriate use of flow cytometry codes 88184, 88185, 88187, 88188, and 88189. The codes have been mistakenly interpreted as general-method codes for technologies utilizing flow cytometry as the means of reaction detection or measurement regardless of the specimen type and analyte being detected. These codes were being reported for procedures to detect patients' antibodies in serum, which is not the intent of these codes.

Codes 88184, 88185, and 88187-88189 describe testing performed on patient's cells to detect markers, such as antigens on the surface of cells for the assessment of potential hematologic conditions.

# Cytogenetic Studies

►Molecular pathology procedures should be reported using either the appropriate Tier 1 (81200-81383), Tier 2 (81400-81408) or the unlisted molecular pathology procedure code 81479.◄

## 🔏 Rationale

In accordance with the deletion of Appendix I, **Genetic Testing Code Modifiers**, the Cytogenetic Studies guideline, which indicated that an Appendix I modifier should be used when molecular diagnostic procedures are performed to test for oncologic or inherited disorders, has been deleted. A new guideline has been added directing users to the Tier 1 or Tier 2 codes or the unlisted molecular pathology code to report molecular pathology procedures.

●88375  Optical endomicroscopic image(s), interpretation and report, real-time or referred, each endoscopic session

▶(Do not report 88375 in conjunction with 43206 or 43252)◀

### ✍ Rationale

Code 88375 has been established to identify the interpretation and report of the optical endomicroscopic image(s) provided (whether done real-time or referred) and includes review of all images provided during the endoscopic session. This code is intended to identify provision of the interpretation and report service for optical endomicroscopy when provided by a separate practitioner such as a pathologist. Codes 43206 and 43252 are used to identify provision of both the optical endomicroscopic procedure and the interpretation and report for the specimens obtained by the same practitioner. Because interpretation is inherently included as part of the optical endomicroscopy procedure, an exclusionary parenthetical note has been listed following code 88375 to restrict use of this code in conjunction with the aforementioned "surgical" codes. For more information regarding the intended use for codes 43206 and 43252, see the Rationale for these codes.

### 🩺 Clinical Example (88375)

A 57-year-old female with reflux symptoms unresponsive to pharmacologic therapy undergoes esophagogastroduodenoscopy (EGD). A suspicious 3-cm segment in the distal esophagus is identified, and endoscopic biopsies are taken with real-time interpretive assessment of the optical endomicroscopy images by a pathologist, to identify the areas of highest yield for biopsy for subsequent anatomic pathology examination.

**Description of Procedure (88375)**

The pathologist reviews the clinical history and referred information, reviews the optical endomicroscopy images in real time, and informs and guides the endoscopist through concurrent electronic or telephone communication regarding the need for specimens and the topography from which to obtain them. The pathologist issues a report of the interpretation of the image(s) and any recommendations made.

88380  Microdissection (ie, sample preparation of microscopically identified target); laser capture

88381      manual

(Do not report 88380 in conjunction with 88381)

▶(88384-88386 have been deleted. To report, see 81200-81479)◀

### ✍ Rationale

In support of the establishment of Tier 1 and Tier 2 Molecular Pathology Procedures (81200-81383, 81400-81408), the current stacking-code method of reporting molecular pathology services codes (83890-83914) and array-based evaluation codes (88384-88386) have been deleted.

---

⊘=Modifier 51 Exempt  ⊙=Moderate Sedation  ✚=Add-on Code  ✗=FDA approval pending

# Reproductive Medicine Procedures

**89300**   Semen analysis; presence and/or motility of sperm including Huhner test (post coital)

**89310**       motility and count (not including Huhner test)

**89320**       volume, count, motility, and differential

▶(Skin tests, see 86485-86580 and 95012-95199)◀

## ✎ Rationale

In response to the deletion of code 95010 from the CPT code set, the cross-reference note following code 89320 has been revised with the removal of code 95010, in order to reflect the appropriate range of codes to report skin testing.

# Medicine

The Medicine section includes a total of 51 new codes and 47 deletions. Several codes have also been revised including revisions related to nomenclature reporting neutrality, which is discussed in the CPT Nomenclature Reporting Neutrality section beginning on page 1 of this book.

Many guidelines throughout the Medicine section have also been revised with the addition of explicit code-range listings. These changes are discussed in the Explicit Code Ranges section beginning on page 45 of this book.

Among the various changes in the Vaccines, Toxoids subsection are four influenza vaccine codes that have been editorially revised to state "trivalent" to differentiate them from new code 90672 to describe a quadrivalent influenza virus vaccine.

The Psychiatry subsection has undergone significant changes with a new coding structure and coding concepts to facilitate an accurate reflection of the work performed by physicians and other qualified health care professionals. Among the numerous changes is the deletion of a total of 24 individual psychotherapy codes, which have been replaced with a new series of six psychotherapy codes.

The Cardiovascular subsection has many changes, including a new coding structure for percutaneous coronary interventions with 13 new codes and guidelines. Other changes include the deletion of intracardiac ablation codes and the addition of three new codes, which combine comprehensive electrophysiologic evaluation with intracardiac ablation of arrhythmogenic focus services.

Other changes to the Medicine section include the revision of the allergy testing codes and many changes to the Neurology and Neuromuscular subsection. Sleep testing, nerve conduction tests, intraoperative neurophysiology, and autonomic function tests are all areas with new and revised codes.

# Medicine

## Immunization Administration for Vaccines/Toxoids

**90460** Immunization administration through 18 years of age via any route of administration, with counseling by physician or other qualified health care professional; first or only component of each vaccine or toxoid administered

**90471** Immunization administration (includes percutaneous, intradermal, subcutaneous, or intramuscular injections); 1 vaccine (single or combination vaccine/toxoid)

**+90472** each additional vaccine (single or combination vaccine/toxoid) (List separately in addition to code for primary procedure)

▶(Use 90472 in conjunction with 90460, 90471, 90473)◀

**90473** Immunization administration by intranasal or oral route; 1 vaccine (single or combination vaccine/toxoid)

**+90474** each additional vaccine (single or combination vaccine/toxoid) (List separately in addition to code for primary procedure)

▶(Use 90474 in conjunction with 90460, 90471, 90473)◀

### Rationale

The parenthetical note following the non-counseling immunization administration add-on codes 90472 and 90474 was revised to allow reporting of these services, in addition to the primary counseling immunization administration code 90460 to report circumstances when counseling is provided before immunization administration for one vaccine, and when counseling for the additional vaccine is not required.

## ▶Vaccines, Toxoids◀

**●90653** Influenza vaccine, inactivated, subunit, adjuvanted, for intramuscular use

### Rationale

A vaccine product code, 90653, was established for an adjuvanted influenza vaccine. Adjuvants are included in vaccines to increase the immune response, and in some instances reduce the number of doses required to achieve adequate immunogenicity. Code 90653 appears in the CPT codebook with the US Food and Drug Administration (FDA) approval pending symbol ( ⋉ ). Updates on the FDA status of this code will be available on the AMA CPT Web site under Category I Vaccine Codes (www.ama-assn.org/ama/pub/physician-resources/solutions-managing-your-practice/coding-billing-insurance/cpt/about-cpt/category-i-vaccine-codes.shtml), and in subsequent publications of the CPT codebook. The service associated with the administration of the vaccine is separately reported using Immunization Administration for Vaccines/Toxoids codes (90460-90474).

 **Clinical Example (90653)**

A 77-year-old male with congestive heart failure and chronic obstructive pulmonary disease presents to his primary care physician for a routine visit immediately before the influenza season. He is a candidate for immunization, and the physician chooses the adjuvanted influenza preparation due to impaired immunogenicity because of his age and because of his use of inhaled steroids.

**Description of Procedure (90653)**

A new vaccine product is described to the patient. The service associated with the administration of the vaccine is separately reported using the Immunization Administration for Vaccines/Toxoids codes (90460-90474).

90654   Influenza virus vaccine, split virus, preservative-free, for intradermal use

▲90655   Influenza virus vaccine, trivalent, split virus, preservative free, when administered to children 6-35 months of age, for intramuscular use

▲90656   Influenza virus vaccine, trivalent, split virus, preservative free, when administered to individuals 3 years and older, for intramuscular use

▲90657   Influenza virus vaccine, trivalent, split virus, when administered to children 6-35 months of age, for intramuscular use

▲90658   Influenza virus vaccine, trivalent, split virus, when administered to individuals 3 years of age and older, for intramuscular use

 **Rationale**

Influenza virus vaccine product codes 90655, 90656, 90657, and 90658 were editorially revised to specify "trivalent" to prepare for the new quadrivalent influenza vaccines, which is expected to be available for use in 2013 and assigned to four new codes that will be available on the CPT Web site with the US Food and Drug Administration (FDA) approval pending symbol ( ✔ ). The current trivalent influenza vaccines include coverage for three (trivalent) strains, 2 A strains and 1 B strain. The quadrivalent vaccine includes an additional B strain, thereby covering both of the B lineages for a total of four (quadrivalent) strains, two type A strains and two type B strains. To obtain the quadrivalent influenza vaccines and to get future updates on the FDA status of the quadrivalent codes, please visit the CPT Web site under Category I Vaccine Codes (www.ama-assn.org/ama/pub/physician-resources/solutions-managing-your-practice/coding-billing-insurance/cpt/about-cpt/category-i-vaccine-codes.shtml). Use of the trivalent and quadrivalent influenza vaccines will co-exist for now, and will be selected based on specific patient populations. The service associated with the administration of these vaccine products is separately reported using Immunization Administration for Vaccines/Toxoids codes (90460-90474).

Ⓢ=Modifier 51 Exempt   ⊙=Moderate Sedation   ✚=Add-on Code   ✔=FDA approval pending

| ▲90660 | Influenza virus vaccine, trivalent, live, for intranasal use |
| #●90672 | Influenza virus vaccine, quadrivalent, live, for intranasal use |
| 90670 | Pneumococcal conjugate vaccine, 13 valent, for intramuscular use |
| 90672 | ▶Code is out of numerical sequence. See 90476-90749◀ |

##  Rationale

A new vaccine product code 90672 was established for a quadrivalent intranasal live influenza virus vaccine receiving FDA approval in February 2012. The quadrivalent product offers coverage for four virus strains (two type A and two type B). Code 90672 appears with a hash symbol (#) to indicate that it is out of numerical sequence. A reference note was added (where this code would have been found numerically) to direct users to the appropriate code range 90476-90749. The intranasal live influenza vaccine code 90660 contains coverage for three virus strains (two type A and one type B) and was editorially revised to include the term, "trivalent." The service associated with the administration of these intranasal vaccines is separately reported using Immunization Administration for Vaccines/Toxoids codes (90460-90474).

Code 90665 for reporting Lyme Disease vaccine product introduced to the market in 1998 and added to CPT 1999 code set was deleted, as it is no longer available.

## Clinical Example (90672)

A 10-year-old healthy male presents for an annual influenza vaccine in September. He has not received an influenza vaccine for the current season. A quadrivalent, live attenuated influenza vaccine is administered intranasally.

### Description of Procedure (90672)

The service associated with the administration of the vaccine is separately reported using the Immunization Administration for Vaccines/Toxoids codes (90460-90474).

▶(90701 has been deleted)◀

## Rationale

The vaccine product code 90701 for reporting the whole cell Pertussis vaccine composed of whole cells of killed Bordetella pertussis bacilli, combined with Diphtheria and tetanus toxoids (DTP) was deleted, as it is no longer used in the United States.

▶(90718 has been deleted)◀

### Rationale

Code 90718 to report preservative containing tetanus and diphtheria toxoid (Td) vaccine was deleted to eliminate confusion, because no Td product currently on the market is considered "preservative containing." Code 90714 is appropriate for reporting all available Td vaccines. The ingredients in the available products are not considered preservatives because they are byproducts of the manufacturing process and exist in trace amounts.

⁄ ●**90739**   Hepatitis B vaccine, adult dosage (2 dose schedule), for intramuscular use

▲**90746**   Hepatitis B vaccine, adult dosage (3 dose schedule), for intramuscular use

### Rationale

A vaccine product code 90739 was established for a 2-dose hepatitis B vaccine enhanced with an immunostimulatory adjuvant. The 3-dose hepatitis B vaccine code 90746 has been editorially revised to state "3 dose schedule" to differentiate it from new code 90739. Code 90739 appears in the CPT codebook with the US Food and Drug Administration (FDA) approval pending symbol ( ⁄ ). Updates on the FDA status of this code will be reflected on the AMA CPT Web site under Category I Vaccine Codes (www.ama-assn.org/ama/pub/physician-resources/solutions-managing-your-practice/coding-billing-insurance/cpt/about-cpt/category-i-vaccine-codes.shtml), and in subsequent publications of the CPT codebook. The service associated with the administration of the hepatitis B vaccine is separately reported using Immunization Administration for Vaccines/Toxoids codes (90460-90474).

### Clinical Example (90739)

A 50-year-old female presents to her primary care physician seeking a vaccination against hepatitis B, as next month she will be traveling to East Asia and is concerned about getting infected.

### Description of Procedure (90739)

A new vaccine product is described to the patient. The service associated with the administration of the vaccine is reported separately using the Immunization Administration for Vaccines/Toxoids codes (90460-90474).

## Psychiatry

▶Psychiatry services include diagnostic services, psychotherapy, and other services to an individual, family, or group. Patient condition, characteristics, or situational factors may require services described as being with interactive complexity. Services may be provided to a patient in crisis. Services are provided in all settings of care and psychiatry services codes are reported without regard to setting. Services may be provided by a physician or other qualified health care professional. Some psychiatry services may be reported with **Evaluation and Management Services** (99201-99255, 99281-99285, 99304-99337, 99341-99350) or other services when performed. **Evaluation and Management Services** (99201-99285, 99304-99337, 99341-99350) may be reported for treatment of psychiatric conditions, rather than using **Psychiatry Services** codes, when appropriate.

⊘=Modifier 51 Exempt  ⊙=Moderate Sedation  ✚=Add-on Code  ⁄=FDA approval pending

Hospital care in treating a psychiatric inpatient or partial hospitalization may be initial or subsequent in nature (see 99221-99233).

Some patients receive hospital evaluation and management services only and others receive hospital evaluation and management services and other procedures. If other procedures such as electroconvulsive therapy or psychotherapy are rendered in addition to hospital evaluation and management services, these may be listed separately (eg, hospital care services [99221-99223, 99231-99233] plus electroconvulsive therapy [90870]), or when psychotherapy is done, with appropriate code(s) defining psychotherapy services.

Consultation for psychiatric evaluation of a patient includes examination of a patient and exchange of information with the primary physician and other informants such as nurses or family members, and preparation of a report. These services may be reported using consultation codes (see **Consultations**).◄

### ✏️ Rationale

A new coding structure in the Psychiatry section was established to incorporate new coding concepts to facilitate an accurate reflection of the different work performed by physicians and other qualified health care professionals. The new series of codes added to the Psychiatry section captures the dramatic changes in the way psychotherapy services are provided since the inception of these codes into the CPT code set in 1998. Examples of these changes include the shift from the treatment of single disorders to the management of multiple medical co-morbidities and the shift of site of service from the hospital to the office setting.

As part of this restructuring, the introductory guidelines in the Psychiatry section were revised to provide appropriate instruction on the reporting of E/M services for treatment of psychiatric conditions.

## ►Interactive Complexity◄

►Code 90785 is an add-on code for interactive complexity to be reported in conjunction with codes for diagnostic psychiatric evaluation (90791, 90792), psychotherapy (90832, 90834, 90837), psychotherapy when performed with an evaluation and management service (90833, 90836, 90838, 99201-99255, 99304-99337, 99341-99350), and group psychotherapy (90853).

Interactive complexity refers to specific communication factors that complicate the delivery of a psychiatric procedure. Common factors include more difficult communication with discordant or emotional family members and engagement of young and verbally undeveloped or impaired patients. Typical patients are those who have third parties, such as parents, guardians, other family members, interpreters, language translators, agencies, court officers, or schools involved in their psychiatric care.

These factors are typically present with patients who:

■ Have other individuals legally responsible for their care, such as minors or adults with guardians, or

■ Request others to be involved in their care during the visit, such as adults accompanied by one or more participating family members or interpreter or language translator, or

- Require the involvement of other third parties, such as child welfare agencies, parole or probation officers, or schools.

Psychiatric procedures may be reported "with interactive complexity" when at least one of the following is present:

1. The need to manage maladaptive communication (related to, eg, high anxiety, high reactivity, repeated questions, or disagreement) among participants that complicates delivery of care.

2. Caregiver emotions or behavior that interferes with the caregiver's understanding and ability to assist in the implementation of the treatment plan.

3. Evidence or disclosure of a sentinel event and mandated report to third party (eg, abuse or neglect with report to state agency) with initiation of discussion of the sentinel event and/or report with patient and other visit participants.

4. Use of play equipment, other physical devices, interpreter, or translator to communicate with the patient to overcome barriers to therapeutic or diagnostic interaction between the physician or other qualified health care professional and a patient who:

- Is not fluent in the same language as the physician or other qualified health care professional, or

- Has not developed, or has lost, either the expressive language communication skills to explain his/her symptoms and response to treatment, or the receptive communication skills to understand the physician or other qualified health care professional if he/she were to use typical language for communication.◄

When provided in conjunction with the psychotherapy services (90832-90838), the amount of time spent by a physician or other qualified health care professional providing interactive complexity services should be reflected in the timed service code for psychotherapy (90832, 90834, 90837) or the psychotherapy add-on code performed with an evaluation and management service (90833, 90836, 90838) and must relate to the psychotherapy service only. Interactive complexity is not a factor for evaluation and management services selection (99201-99255, 99281-99285, 99304-99337, 99341-99350), except as it directly affects key components as defined in the Evaluation and Management Services Guidelines (ie, history, examination, and medical decision making).◄

+ ●90785    Interactive complexity (List separately in addition to the code for primary procedure)

▶(Use 90785 in conjunction with codes for diagnostic psychiatric evaluation [90791, 90792], psychotherapy [90832, 90834, 90837], psychotherapy when performed with an evaluation and management service [90833, 90836, 90838, 99201-99255, 99304-99337, 99341-99350], and group psychotherapy [90853])◄

▶(Do not report 90785 in conjunction with 90839, 90840, or in conjunction with E/M services when no psychotherapy service is also reported)◄

## ✍ Rationale

A new subsection was added to the Psychiatry section for reporting interactive complexity. Interactive complexity is specific and recognized communication difficulties for various types of patients and situations (eg, maladaptive communication among visit participants, interference from caregiver emotions or behavior, disclosure and discussion of a sentinel event, and language difficulties) that represent significant complicating factors that may increase the intensity of the primary psychiatric procedure.

Add-on code 90785 was established to report interactive complexity in conjunction with the following new psychiatric codes: Psychiatric Diagnostic Evaluation (90791, 90792); Psychotherapy (90832, 90834, 90837); Psychotherapy performed with an Evaluation and Management service (90833, 90836, 90838, 99201-99255, 99304-99337, 99341-99350); and Group Psychotherapy (90853). Code 90785 may not be reported with an evaluation and management service that is not provided in conjunction with a psychotherapy service.

New guidelines and parenthetical notes were added in the Interactive Complexity section to provide instruction on the appropriate reporting of code 90785. The guidelines include a list of requirements or factors to consider when determining appropriate use of the interactive complexity code 90785. Interactive complexity will be reported in addition to primary procedure codes when communication difficulties are present and it becomes necessary to involve other family members, translators, third-party payers, agencies and school representatives, including compliance with mandates for reporting abuse and or neglect. It may also involve addressing any language barriers that may exist between the patient and physician or other qualified health care professional.

### Clinical Example (90785)

Psychotherapy for an older elementary school-aged child accompanied by divorced parents, reporting declining grades, temper outbursts, and bedtime difficulties. Parents are extremely anxious and repeatedly ask questions about the treatment process. Each parent continually challenges the other's observations of the patient.

### Description of Procedure (90785)

Review chart from previous sessions. Therapeutic communication with child and parents to obtain interval history and examine mental status. A variety of psychotherapeutic approaches with the child is used to address patient's mood and behaviors. Meet with parents without the child to discuss patient's progress and parents' concerns. Manage parents' anxiety and conflict with redirection to their child's symptoms, strengths, deficits, and treatment needs. Discuss next steps to clarify diagnoses and treatment options. Document services and coordinate care with patient's other health care providers and school, paying particular attention to sorting through and attempting to validate parents' differing observations and concerns in communication with the child's teachers.

## ▶Psychiatric Diagnostic Procedures◀

▶Psychiatric diagnostic evaluation is an integrated biopsychosocial assessment, including history, mental status, and recommendations. The evaluation may include communication with family or other sources and review and ordering of diagnostic studies.

Psychiatric diagnostic evaluation with medical services is an integrated biopsychosocial and medical assessment, including history, mental status, other physical examination elements as indicated, and recommendations. The evaluation may include communication with family or other sources, prescription of medications, and review and ordering of laboratory or other diagnostic studies.

In certain circumstances one or more other informants (family members, guardians, or significant others) may be seen in lieu of the patient. Codes 90791, 90792 may be reported more than once for the patient when separate diagnostic evaluations are conducted with the patient and other informants. Report services as being provided to the patient and not the informant or other party in such circumstances. Codes 90791, 90792 may be reported once per day and not on the same day as an evaluation and management service performed by the same individual for the same patient.

The psychiatric diagnostic evaluation may include interactive complexity services when factors exist that complicate the delivery of the psychiatric procedure. These services should be reported with add-on code 90785 used in conjunction with the diagnostic psychiatric evaluation codes 90791, 90792.

Codes 90791, 90792 are used for the diagnostic assessment(s) or reassessment(s), if required, and do not include psychotherapeutic services. Psychotherapy services, including for crisis, may not be reported on the same day.◄

● **90791** Psychiatric diagnostic evaluation

● **90792** Psychiatric diagnostic evaluation with medical services

▶(Do not report 90791 or 90792 in conjunction with 99201-99337, 99341-99350, 99366-99368, 99401-99444)◄

▶(Use 90785 in conjunction with 90791, 90792 when the diagnostic evaluation includes interactive complexity services)◄

▶(90801 and 90802 have been deleted. To report diagnostic evaluations, see 90791, 90792)◄

## ✍ Rationale

The Psychiatric Diagnostic Procedures section was revised with new codes, deleted codes, and new guidelines to describe psychiatric diagnostic procedures. Prior to 2013, the section described psychiatric diagnostic or evaluative interview procedures. However, psychiatric diagnostic interview codes 90801 and 90802 were deleted. Two new codes for psychiatric diagnostic evaluation (90791, 90792) were established to replace codes 90801 and 90802. Codes 90791 and 90792 differentiate between diagnostic services done with medical services (90792) and without medical services (90791). The interactive component of the diagnostic evaluation, formerly included in code 90802, is now captured by the new interactive complexity add-on code 90785, which may be reported in conjunction with the new psychiatric diagnostic evaluation codes 90791 and 90792.
See the Rationale for code 90785.

## 🩺 Clinical Example (90791)

Diagnostic evaluation of an adult with co-morbid medical conditions who reports increasing anxiety, irritability, and trouble sleeping. Although on antidepressant medication, the patient has been feeling increasingly depressed and helpless, and is unable to go to work. The patient was referred by the primary care provider for psychotherapy services.

**Description of Procedure (90791)**

The procedure is explained and informed consent is obtained. A psychiatric history, including present illness, past history, family history, and complete mental status examination is obtained. Referrals for other tests and evaluations are obtained as needed. Diagnostic studies are ordered and reviewed, and a definitive diagnosis or at least a narrow enough differential to warrant a treatment plan is established. A decision is made concerning the need for degree of supervision (eg, hospitalization). Patient is counseled concerning the diagnosis and options for treatment and proposed options, including explaining the need for and process of psychotherapy. May also include communication with the patient's family or other informants in addition to or in lieu of the patient.

 **Clinical Example (90792)**

Diagnostic evaluation of an adult with co-morbid medical conditions who reports worsening depression and agitation. The patient has been feeling hopeless and sleeping poorly, and reports deteriorating work performance and marital problems. The patient was referred by the primary care provider after a six-week trial of an antidepressant medication with little improvement.

**Description of Procedure (90792)**

Introduce self to patient, obtain informed consent and discuss mandatory reporting. The purposes of the evaluation may include assessing competence, assessing safety, establishing a presumptive diagnosis(es), and formulating a treatment plan, including consideration of additional medical evaluation, medication, psychotherapy, or both, and the appropriate site of service based on acuity and level of risk for potentially harmful behaviors, among other criteria (eg, inpatient, day-treatment, or outpatient).

In order to accomplish the above, an extensive history is obtained, including present illness, past psychiatric history, chemical dependency history, family history, social history, and treatments, as well as a medical history, review of systems, and focused questions related to safety, lethality, aggression, and/or competence, as indicated. A specialty specific examination is completed as well. A working therapeutic relationship is established.

The findings are integrated into a diagnostic formulation, including specific medical psychiatric diagnoses, personality considerations, contributing general medical factors, psychosocial stressors, and current level of functioning.

Based on these multifaceted diagnoses, a treatment plan is formulated, which includes the consideration of medications, psychotherapy, general medical laboratory, or other tests, as well as the level of care needed (eg, inpatient, day-hospital, intensive outpatient, or outpatient). This plan is discussed with the patient (and other parties as indicated/appropriate), treatment options are reviewed, and informed consent is obtained. Prescriptions are provided for medication and additional medical diagnostic tests, when indicated.

▶(90804, 90805, 90806, 90807, 90808, 90809 have been deleted. To report, see psychotherapy codes 90832, 90834, 90837 or psychotherapy add-on codes when performed with an evaluation and management service [90833, 90836, 90838, 99201-99255, 99304-99337, 99341-99350])◀

▶(90810, 90811, 90812, 90813, 90814, 90815 have been deleted. To report interactive psychotherapy, report 90785 in conjunction with psychotherapy codes 90832, 90834, 90837 or psychotherapy add-on codes when performed with an evaluation and management service [90833, 90836, 90838, 99201-99255, 99304-99337, 99341-99350])◀

▶(90816, 90817, 90818, 90819, 90821, 90822 have been deleted. To report, see psychotherapy codes 90832, 90834, 90837 or psychotherapy add-on codes when performed with an evaluation and management service [90833, 90836, 90838, 99201-99255, 99304-99337, 99341-99350])◀

▶(90823, 90824, 90826, 90827, 90828, 90829 have been deleted. To report interactive psychotherapy, report 90785 in conjunction with psychotherapy codes 90832, 90834, 90837 or psychotherapy add-on codes when performed with an evaluation and management service [90833, 90836, 90838, 99201-99255, 99304-99337, 99341-99350])◀

## ✍ Rationale

As part of the new coding structure in the Psychiatry section, subsections Office or Other Outpatient Facility (90804-90809) and Inpatient Hospital, Partial Hospital or Residential Care Facility (90816-90829) were deleted. These services should now be reported using new psychotherapy code 90832, 90834, or 90837. When reporting these services with an evaluation and management (E/M) service, the appropriate E/M service code should be reported in conjunction with new psychotherapy add-on codes 90833, 90836, and 90838. Cross-reference parenthetical notes were added to direct users to the appropriate codes for these services.

### ▶PSYCHOTHERAPY◀

▶ Psychotherapy is the treatment of mental illness and behavioral disturbances in which the physician or other qualified health care professional, through definitive therapeutic communication, attempts to alleviate the emotional disturbances, reverse or change maladaptive patterns of behavior, and encourage personality growth and development.

The psychotherapy service codes 90832-90838 include ongoing assessment and adjustment of psychotherapeutic interventions, and may include involvement of family member(s) or others in the treatment process.

Psychotherapy times are for face-to-face services with patient and/or family member. The patient must be present for all or some of the service. For family psychotherapy without the patient present, use 90846. In reporting, choose the code closest to the actual time (ie, 16-37 minutes for 90832 and 90833, 38-52 minutes for 90834 and 90836, and 53 or more minutes for 90837 and 90838). Do not report psychotherapy of less than 16 minutes duration. (See instructions for the usage of Time in the Introduction of the CPT code set).

Psychotherapy provided to a patient in a crisis state is reported with codes 90839 and 90840 and cannot be reported in addition to the psychotherapy codes 90832-90838. For psychotherapy for crisis, see "Other Psychotherapy."

Code 90785 is an add-on code to report interactive complexity services when provided in conjunction with the psychotherapy codes 90832-90838. The amount of time spent by a physician or other qualified health care professional providing interactive complexity services should be reflected in the timed service code for psychotherapy (90832, 90834, 90837) or the psychotherapy add-on code performed with an evaluation and management service (90833, 90836, 90838).

Some psychiatric patients receive a medical evaluation and management (E/M) service on the same day as a psychotherapy service by the same physician or other qualified health care professional. To report both E/M and psychotherapy, the two services must be significant and separately identifiable. These services are reported by using codes specific for psychotherapy when performed with evaluation and management services (90833, 90836, 90838) as add-on codes to the evaluation and management service.

Medical symptoms and disorders inform treatment choices of psychotherapeutic interventions, and data from therapeutic communication are used to evaluate the presence, type, and severity of medical symptoms and disorders. For the purposes of reporting, the medical and psychotherapeutic components of the service may be separately identified as follows:

1. The type and level of E/M service is selected first based upon the key components of history, examination, and medical decision-making.

2. Time associated with activities used to meet criteria for the E/M service is not included in the time used for reporting the psychotherapy service (ie, time spent on history, examination and medical decision making **when used for the E/M service** is not psychotherapy time). Time may not be used as the basis of E/M code selection and Prolonged Services may not be reported when psychotherapy with E/M (90833, 90836, 90838) are reported.

3. A separate diagnosis is not required for the reporting of E/M and psychotherapy on the same date of service.◄

● **90832**    Psychotherapy, 30 minutes with patient and/or family member

✚ ● **90833**    Psychotherapy, 30 minutes with patient and/or family member when performed with an evaluation and management service (List separately in addition to the code for primary procedure)

    ►(Use 90833 in conjunction with 99201-99255, 99304-99337, 99341-99350)◄

● **90834**    Psychotherapy, 45 minutes with patient and/or family member

✚ ● **90836**    Psychotherapy, 45 minutes with patient and/or family member when performed with an evaluation and management service (List separately in addition to the code for primary procedure)

    ►(Use 90836 in conjunction with 99201-99255, 99304-99337, 99341-99350)◄

● **90837**    Psychotherapy, 60 minutes with patient and/or family member

✚ ● **90838**    Psychotherapy, 60 minutes with patient and/or family member when performed with an evaluation and management service (List separately in addition to the code for primary procedure)

    ►(Use 90838 in conjunction with 99201-99255, 99304-99337, 99341-99350)◄

    ►(Use the appropriate prolonged services code [99354-99357] for psychotherapy services 68 minutes or longer)◄

    ►(Use 90785 in conjunction with 90832, 90833, 90834, 90836, 90837, 90838 when psychotherapy includes interactive complexity services)◄

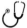 **Rationale**

A new series of psychotherapy codes (90832-90838) and guidelines were established to replace the individual psychotherapy codes 90804-90829. The differences between codes 90832-90838 and the former psychotherapy codes (90804-90829) are outlined below:

• Site of service is no longer a criterion for code selection.

• Time specifications were changed to be consistent with CPT convention.

• "Individual" is not in the code titles and psychotherapy time may include face-to-face time with family members, as long as the patient is present for part of the session.

• Interactive psychotherapy codes were replaced with reporting psychotherapy in conjunction with an interactive complexity add-on code 90785, expanding the types of communication difficulties that are recognized (see Rationale for code 90785).

• Codes for individual psychotherapy without medical evaluation and management services (90804, 90806, 90808, 90810, 90812, 90814, 90816, 90818, 90821, 90823, 90826, 90828) were replaced with psychotherapy codes 90832, 90834, 90837.

• Codes for psychotherapy with medical evaluation and management |services (90805, 90807, 90809, 90811, 90813, 90815, 90817, 90819, 90822, 90824, 90827, 90829) were replaced with psychotherapy add-on codes 90833, 90836, 90838, which are to be reported in conjunction with codes for Evaluation and Management (E/M) services.

**Note:** To report both an E/M code and a psychotherapy add-on code, the two services must be significant and separately identifiable, as follows: the type and level of E/M service is selected first, based on the key components of history, examination, and medical decision making. The psychotherapy must be 16 minutes or more, face-to-face with patient and/or family. Time associated with activities used to meet criteria for the E/M service is not included in the time used for reporting the psychotherapy service (ie, time spent on history, examination, and medical decision making **when used for the E/M service** is not psychotherapy time). Time may not be used as the basis of E/M code selection. The E/M service and the psychotherapy service may be for the same diagnosis.

Parenthetical notes were added to instruct users on the appropriate use of the new codes.

## Clinical Example (90832)

Psychotherapy for a young adult with the diagnoses of depression, anxiety, and attention deficit disorder, who has relationship problems and recently moved away from family. Patient is taking stimulant and antidepressant medications.

### Description of Procedure (90832)

Face-to-face therapeutic communication is conducted with the patient and/or the patient's family. Objective information and an interval history are obtained. The patient's mental state is examined, including an evaluation and exploration of the intensity and complexity of the patient's symptoms, feelings, thoughts, and behaviors in the context of the patient's psychosocial and health stressors and coping styles. A range of psychotherapy approaches are used to reduce the patient's distress and morbidity, and ongoing behavioral- and mental-status changes in the patient are addressed.

 ### Clinical Example (90833)

Psychotherapy for a young adult with the diagnoses of depression, anxiety, and attention deficit disorder, who has relationship problems and recently moved away from family. Patient is taking stimulant and antidepressant medications.

**Description of Procedure (90833)**

Data from various sources, including past interactions with the patient, current history and mental status findings, information that may have come to light from other historians or outside records, and the patient's behavior, descriptions, and responses to intrasession interventions, are all reviewed or considered, and a working therapeutic interpretation, behavioral treatment plan, or supportive intervention strategy is formulated and enacted. Examples of the focus of this intervention could include a current acute situation, suicidal thought/safety plan, or a pattern of dysfunctional behavior. Evidence of behavioral change, demonstration of insight, or reduction in symptoms (eg, anxiety, depression, irritability) is sought based on the psychotherapeutic interventions.

 ### Clinical Example (90834)

Psychotherapy for an adult suffering from co-morbid medical conditions, depression, and agitation of two-months duration, which resulted in loss of job after several emotional outbursts at work. Patient is anxious about loss of income and inability to find another job.

**Description of Procedure (90834)**

Face-to-face therapeutic communication is conducted with the patient and/or the patient's family. Objective information and an interval history are obtained. The patient's mental state is examined, including an evaluation and exploration of the intensity and complexity of the patient's symptoms, feelings, thoughts, and behaviors in the context of the patient's psychosocial and health stressors and coping styles. A range of psychotherapy approaches are used to reduce the patient's distress and morbidity, and ongoing behavioral- and mental-status changes in the patient are addressed.

 ### Clinical Example (90836)

Psychotherapy for an adult suffering from co-morbid medical conditions, depression, and agitation of two-months duration, which resulted in loss of job after several emotional outbursts at work. Patient is anxious about loss of income and inability to find another job.

**Description of Procedure (90836)**

Data from various sources, including past interactions with the patient, current history and mental status findings, information that may have come to light from other historians or outside records, and the patient's behavior, descriptions, and responses to intrasession interventions, are all reviewed or considered, and a working therapeutic interpretation, behavioral treatment plan, or supportive intervention strategy is formulated and enacted. Examples of the focus of this intervention could include a current acute situation, suicidal thought/safety plan, or a pattern of dysfunctional behavior. Evidence of behavioral change, demonstration of insight, or reduction in symptoms (eg, anxiety, depression, irritability) is sought based on the psychotherapeutic interventions.

###  Clinical Example (90837)

Psychotherapy for adult with anxiety and depressive symptoms, who is on several medications for two co-morbid medical conditions. Patient has returned to work after a recent psychiatric hospitalization for depression. Psychosocial stressors at work and home have increased anxiety and depression since discharge.

### Description of Procedure (90837)

Face-to-face therapeutic communication is conducted with the patient and/or the patient's family. Objective information and an interval history are obtained. The patient's mental state is examined, including an evaluation and exploration of the intensity and complexity of the patient's symptoms, feelings, thoughts, and behaviors in the context of the patient's psychosocial and health stressors and coping styles. A range of psychotherapy approaches are used to reduce the patient's distress and morbidity, and ongoing behavioral- and mental-status changes in the patient are addressed.

###  Clinical Example (90838)

Psychotherapy for adult with anxiety and depressive symptoms, who is on several medications for these conditions and two co-morbid medical conditions. Patient has returned to work after a recent psychiatric hospitalization for depression. Psychosocial stressors at work and home have increased anxiety and depression since discharge.

### Description of Procedure (90838)

Data from various sources, including past interactions with the patient, current history and mental status findings, information that may have come to light from other historians or outside records, and the patient's behavior, descriptions, and responses to intrasession interventions, are all reviewed or considered, and a working therapeutic interpretation, behavioral treatment plan, or supportive intervention strategy is formulated and enacted. Examples of the focus of this intervention could include a current acute situation, suicidal thought/safety plan, or a pattern of dysfunctional behavior. Evidence of behavioral change, demonstration of insight, or reduction in symptoms (eg, anxiety, depression, irritability) is sought based on the psychotherapeutic interventions.

## OTHER PSYCHOTHERAPY

### ►Psychotherapy for Crisis◄

►Psychotherapy for crisis is an urgent assessment and history of a crisis state, a mental status exam, and a disposition. The treatment includes psychotherapy, mobilization of resources to defuse the crisis and restore safety, and implementation of psychotherapeutic interventions to minimize the potential for psychological trauma. The presenting problem is typically life threatening or complex and requires immediate attention to a patient in high distress.

Codes 90839, 90840 are used to report the total duration of time face-to-face with the patient and/or family spent by the physician or other qualified health care professional providing psychotherapy for crisis, even if the time spent on that date is not continuous. For any given period of time spent providing psychotherapy for crisis state, the physician or other qualified health care professional must devote his or her full attention to the patient and, therefore, cannot provide services to any other patient during the same time period. The patient must be present for all or some of the service. Do not report with 90791 or 90792.

Code 90839 is used to report the first 30-74 minutes of psychotherapy for crisis on a given date. It should be used only once per date even if the time spent by the physician or other health care professional is not continuous on that date. Psychotherapy for crisis of less than 30 minutes total duration on a given date should be reported with 90832 or 90833 (when provided with evaluation and management services). Code 90840 is used to report additional block(s) of time, of up to 30 minutes each beyond the first 74 minutes.◄

●**90839**   Psychotherapy for crisis; first 60 minutes

+ ●**90840**      each additional 30 minutes (List separately in addition to code for primary service)

►(Use 90840 in conjunction with 90839)◄

►(Do not report 90839, 90840 in conjunction with 90791, 90792, psychotherapy codes 90832-90838 or other psychiatric services, or 90785-90899)◄

### ✎ Rationale

A major new concept and addition to the psychotherapy section is the addition of codes for Psychotherapy for Crisis when psychotherapy services are provided to a patient, who presents in high distress with complex or life threatening circumstances that require urgent and immediate attention. A new subsection, Psychotherapy for Crisis, new guidelines, and two new codes (90839 and 90840) were established to report services performed in these circumstances. Code 90839 is reported for the first 60 minutes of psychotherapy performed for crisis. Add-on code 90840 is reported for each additional 30 minutes. These codes may not be reported with the psychiatric diagnostic evaluation codes (90791, 90792), the psychotherapy codes (90832-90838), or 90785-90899. Parenthetical notes have been added to provide additional instruction on the appropriate use of these new codes.

---

**Clinical Example (90839)**

Psychotherapy for crisis with young adult who has been seen in psychotherapy for depression, and is now severely depressed and distraught. The patient expresses suicidal ideation with an imminent plan.

**Description of Procedure (90839)**

Depression and risk assessments are conducted and a family member is contacted. The patient is encouraged to reveal and discuss what has been going on with the family member and therapist. Options for protection and treatment are discussed and an extensive safety plan is designed and agreed upon, to the satisfaction of patient, family member, and therapist. Document services and coordinate care with patient's other health care providers.

 **Clinical Example (90840)**

Psychotherapy for crisis with young adult who has been seen in psychotherapy for depression, and is now severely depressed and distraught. The patient expresses suicidal ideation with an imminent plan. Late in the session, the patient disclosed a history of a recent sexual assault, and the therapy is continued beyond the time threshold of the primary service reported separately. This is an add-on time-based code.

**Description of Procedure (90840)**

Depression and risk assessments are conducted and a family member is contacted. The patient is encouraged to reveal and discuss what has been going on with the family member and therapist. Options for protection and treatment are discussed and an extensive safety plan is designed and agreed upon, to the satisfaction of patient, family member, and therapist. Document services and coordinate care with patient's other health care providers.

**90845**   Psychoanalysis

**90846**   Family psychotherapy (without the patient present)

**90847**   Family psychotherapy (conjoint psychotherapy) (with patient present)

**90849**   Multiple-family group psychotherapy

**90853**   Group psychotherapy (other than of a multiple-family group)
►(Use 90853 in conjunction with 90785 for the specified patient when group psychotherapy includes interactive complexity)◄
►(90857 has been deleted. To report, use 90785 in conjunction with 90853)◄

 **Rationale**

Code 90857 for interactive group therapy was deleted, and a parenthetical note to instruct the use of code 90853 for group therapy with code 90785 for interactive complexity for psychotherapy provided in a group setting requiring interactive complexity services was added. Please see Rationale for code 90785, which explains interactive complexity services.

⃠=Modifier 51 Exempt   ⦿=Moderate Sedation   ✚=Add-on Code   ⅄=FDA approval pending

## ▶OTHER PSYCHIATRIC SERVICES OR PROCEDURES◀

(For analysis/programming of neurostimulators used for vagus nerve stimulation therapy, see 95970, 95974, 95975)

▶(90862 has been deleted. To report, see 90863 or Evaluation and Management services codes 99201-99255, 99281-99285, 99304-99337, 99341-99350)◀

**+ ●90863**  Pharmacologic management, including prescription and review of medication, when performed with psychotherapy services (List separately in addition to the code for primary procedure)

▶(Use 90863 in conjunction with 90832, 90834, 90837)◀

▶(For pharmacologic management with psychotherapy services performed by a physician or other qualified health care professional who may report evaluation and management codes, use the appropriate evaluation and management codes 99201-99255, 99281-99285, 99304-99337, 99341-99350 and the appropriate psychotherapy with evaluation and management service 90833, 90836, 90838)◀

▶(Do not count time spent on providing pharmacologic management services in the time used for selection of the psychotherapy service)◀

###  Rationale

The final major change in the Psychiatry section includes the addition of a new code for pharmacologic management (90863) and the deletion of the former pharmacologic management code 90862. Several parenthetical notes were added to instruct users on the appropriate use of add-on code 90863, and the Evaluation and Management (E/M) services codes 99201-99255, 99281-99285, 99304-99337, 99341-99350. Qualified health care professionals who are not authorized to report E/M codes may report the new add-on pharmacologic management code 90863, in conjunction with psychotherapy codes 90832, 90834, and 90837. Physicians and other qualified health care professionals who may report E/M services may report pharmacologic management with psychotherapy services using E/M codes 99201-99255, 90836, 99281-99285, 99304-99337, 99341-99350, along with the psychotherapy codes 90833, 90836, 90838.

###  Clinical Example (90863)

A 66-year-old married female with Major Depressive Disorder diagnosis; established patient on antidepressant medication with psychotherapy. Patient is experiencing increased lability, depressed mood, and sleep disturbance following recent move from independent living in family home to senior citizen apartments.

**Description of Procedure (90863)**

Qualified health care professional provides 45 minutes of psychotherapy to address increased depressive symptomatology and relationship issues along with pharmacologic management to evaluate possible dosage adjustment and possible change in anti-depressant medication.

**90865** Narcosynthesis for psychiatric diagnostic and therapeutic purposes (eg, sodium amobarbital (Amytal) interview)

**90867** Therapeutic repetitive transcranial magnetic stimulation (TMS) treatment; initial, including cortical mapping, motor threshold determination, delivery and management

(Report only once per course of treatment)

▶(Do not report 90867 in conjunction with 90868, 90869, 95860, 95870, 95928, 95929, 95939)◀

**90868** subsequent delivery and management, per session

**90869** subsequent motor threshold re-determination with delivery and management

▶(Do not report 90869 in conjunction with 90867, 90868, 95860-95870, 95928, 95929, 95939)◀

▶(If a significant, separately identifiable evaluation and management, medication management, or psychotherapy service is performed, the appropriate E/M or psychotherapy code may be reported in addition to 90867-90869. Evaluation and management activities directly related to cortical mapping, motor threshold determination, delivery and management of TMS are not separately reported)◀

▶(For transcranial magnetic stimulation motor function mapping for therapeutic planning other than for repetitive transcranial magnetic stimulation, use 0310T)◀

▶(Do not count time spent on providing pharmacologic management services in the time used for selection of the psychotherapy service)◀

### ✍ Rationale

New and revised parentheticals were included following the transcranial magnetic stimulation (TMS) codes 90867-90869 to: (1) instruct users to not report code 90869 in conjunction with needle electromyography codes 95860-95870 and central motor evoked potential studies, 95928, 95929, 95939; (2) update the instructions pertaining to the psychotherapy codes to correspond to the changes in the Psychiatry section; (3) reference the use of code 0310T for navigated transcranial magnetic stimulation (nTMS); and (4) provide instructions that pharmacologic management should not be included in the time counted for psychotherapy.

**90870** Electroconvulsive therapy (includes necessary monitoring)

▲**90875** Individual psychophysiological therapy incorporating biofeedback training by any modality (face-to-face with the patient), with psychotherapy (eg, insight oriented, behavior modifying or supportive psychotherapy); 30 minutes

▲**90876** 45 minutes

### ✍ Rationale

Codes 90875 and 90876 were revised; time ranges were replaced by single-time designations of 30 minutes (90875) and 45 minutes (90876).

---

⊘=Modifier 51 Exempt   ⊙=Moderate Sedation   ✚=Add-on Code   𝑵=FDA approval pending

**91022**   Duodenal motility (manometric) study

(If gastrointestinal endoscopy is performed, use 43235)

(If fluoroscopy is performed, use 76000)

(If gastric motility study is performed, use 91020)

▶(Do not report 91020, 91022 in conjunction with 91112)◀

**▲91111**   Gastrointestinal tract imaging, intraluminal (eg, capsule endoscopy), esophagus with interpretation and report

(Do not report 91111 in conjunction with 91110)

▶(For measurement of gastrointestinal tract transit times or pressure using wireless capsule, use 91112)◀

**●91112**   Gastrointestinal transit and pressure measurement, stomach through colon, wireless capsule, with interpretation and report

▶(Do not report 91112 in conjunction with 83986, 91020, 91022, 91117)◀

**91117**   Colon motility (manometric) study, minimum 6 hours continuous recording (including provocation tests, eg, meal, intracolonic balloon distension, pharmacologic agents, if performed), with interpretation and report

▶(For wireless capsule pressure measurements, use 91112)◀

## 🖎 Rationale

New code 91112 is used to report gastrointestinal tract transit and pressure measurements taken from the stomach to the colon via wireless capsule. This code is intended to replace code 0242T. To accommodate this change, the parenthetical note's cross-references and exclusionary parenthetical notes were revised to reference the new code. This includes the parenthetical that follows code 91022 (which excludes the use of the new code in conjunction with codes 91020 and 91022), the note that follows code 91111 (which directs use of code 91112 for the measurement of gastrointestional tract transit time or pressure using wireless capsules), and the exclusionary note that follows code 91112 itself (which excludes the use of code 91112 in conjunction with the procedures identified by the use of codes 83986 [pH body fluid measurement], 91020 [Gastric motility {manometric} studies], 91022 [Duodenal motility {manometric} study], and 91117 for colonic motility study). In addition, a parenthetical cross-reference in place of deleted code 0242T alerts users to the appropriate code to report for this procedure. For more information regarding the deletion of code 0242T, see the Rationale for this code. See also discussion on CPT nomenclature reporting neutrality.

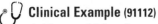 **Clinical Example (91112)**

A 35-year-old female is referred for evaluation of nausea, bloating, abdominal discomfort and constipation. Previous diagnostic studies were negative and confirmed absence of a luminal obstructing lesion. The patient has failed to respond to pharmacological therapy.

**Description of Procedure (91112)**

Physician observes the patient while the patient ingests the capsule. Patient wears a data receiver for 3 to 7 days while transit and pressure measurements are recorded. After the receiver has been returned to the physician's office, the data are downloaded to the computer. The physician reviews the data collected by the reviever.

# Ophthalmology

## Special Ophthalmological Services

**92015**    Determination of refractive state

▶(For instrument based ocular screening, use 99174)◀

###  Rationale

A parenthetical note was added following determination of refractive state code 92015 instructing users to use code 99174 for instrument-based ocular screening. See also the Rationale for the revision of code 99174.

**92132**    Scanning computerized ophthalmic diagnostic imaging, anterior segment, with interpretation and report, unilateral or bilateral

▶(For specular microscopy and endothelial cell analysis, use 92286)◀

▶OTHER SPECIALIZED SERVICES◀

▲**92286**    Anterior segment imaging with interpretation and report; with specular microscopy and endothelial cell analysis

▲**92287**        with fluorescein angiography

### Rationale

As part of the AMA RUC Relativity Assessment Workgroup (RAW) (formerly Five-Year Review Identification Workgroup) analysis of codes, it was determined that code 92286 was a high volume, frequently reported code, but it was never valued by the AMA/Specialty Society RVS Update Committee (RUC), as it was Harvard-valued. In preparation for review of code 92286 to undergo RUC valuation, the involved societies from ophthalmology requested a revision of code 92286 so it could be appropriately valued by the RUC, and to better reflect the technology that exists for this procedure. Originally, the use of code 92286 required the use of film to perform specular endothelial microscopy and cell count. As digital

⃠=Modifier 51 Exempt    ⊙=Moderate Sedation    ✚=Add-on Code    𝒩=FDA approval pending

photography matured in the clinical arena, film became rare and subsequently obsolete for this service; thus the word, "photography" has been replaced with the term "imaging" and the term "cell analysis" replaces the term "cell count," because the technology has progressed from the use of sound waves to topography, which enables not only a cell count but an assessment of the thickness of the cornea and angle of the iris to determine the presence or absence of glaucoma. A cross-reference following code 92132 was added to reference the anterior segment imaging procedure as now described.

 **Clinical Example (92286)**

A 72-year-old female with visually significant cataracts is noted to have slit-lamp evidence of endothelial dystrophy prior to planned cataract surgery.

**Description of Procedure (92286)**

Images are acquired and reviewed for adequate quality before analysis. Cells to be counted are outlined and marked. Software is used to calculate endothelial cell density. Images and cell density measurements are evaluated. A report is prepared and sent to the referring physician.

# Cardiovascular

## Therapeutic Services and Procedures

**92920**   ▶Code is out of numerical sequence. See 92998-93000◀

**92921**   ▶Code is out of numerical sequence. See 92998-93000◀

**92924**   ▶Code is out of numerical sequence. See 92998-93000◀

**92925**   ▶Code is out of numerical sequence. See 92998-93000◀

**92928**   ▶Code is out of numerical sequence. See 92998-93000◀

**92929**   ▶Code is out of numerical sequence. See 92998-93000◀

**92933**   ▶Code is out of numerical sequence. See 92998-93000◀

**92934**   ▶Code is out of numerical sequence. See 92998-93000◀

**92937**   ▶Code is out of numerical sequence. See 92998-93000◀

**92938**   ▶Code is out of numerical sequence. See 92998-93000◀

**92941**   ▶Code is out of numerical sequence. See 92998-93000◀

**92943**   ▶Code is out of numerical sequence. See 92998-93000◀

**92944**   ▶Code is out of numerical sequence. See 92998-93000◀

**✐ Rationale**

In support of the new percutaneous coronary intervention coding structure, codes 92920-92944 are out of numerical sequence and are now located in the new Coronary Therapeutic Services and Procedures subsection. See the Rationale regarding the percutaneous coronary intervention changes for further information.

### ▶OTHER THERAPEUTIC SERVICES AND PROCEDURES◀

⊙**92953**    Temporary transcutaneous pacing

⊙**92960**    Cardioversion, elective, electrical conversion of arrhythmia; external

⊙**92961**        internal (separate procedure)

▶(Do not report 92961 in conjunction with 93282-93284, 93287, 93289, 93295, 93296, 93618-93624, 93631, 93640-93642, 93650, 93653-93657, 93662)◀

**✐ Rationale**

In support of the changes to the Intracardiac Electrophysiological Procedures/ Studies section, the parenthetical note following codes 92960 and 92961 was revised. Deleted code 93652 was removed and codes 93653-93657 were added to the note to indicate that codes 92960 and 92961 should not be reported with these codes.

**92970**    Cardioassist-method of circulatory assist; internal

**92971**        external

(For balloon atrial-septostomy, use 92992)

(For placement of catheters for use in circulatory assist devices such as intra-aortic balloon pump, use 33970)

**92973**    ▶Code is out of numerical sequence. See 92998-93000◀

**92974**    ▶Code is out of numerical sequence. See 92998-93000◀

**92975**    ▶Code is out of numerical sequence. See 92998-93000◀

**92977**    ▶Code is out of numerical sequence. See 92998-93000◀

**92978**    ▶Code is out of numerical sequence. See 92998-93000◀

**92979**    ▶Code is out of numerical sequence. See 92998-93000◀

▶(92980, 92981, 92982, 92984 have been deleted. To report, see 92920-92944)◀

⊙**92986**    Percutaneous balloon valvuloplasty; aortic valve

⊙**92987**        mitral valve

**92990**        pulmonary valve

**92992**    Atrial septectomy or septostomy; transvenous method, balloon (eg, Rashkind type) (includes cardiac catheterization)

---

⊘=Modifier 51 Exempt   ⊙=Moderate Sedation   ✚=Add-on Code   =FDA approval pending

**92993**        blade method (Park septostomy) (includes cardiac catheterization)

►(92995, 92996 have been deleted. To report, see 92924, 92925, 92933-92944)◄

**92997**   Percutaneous transluminal pulmonary artery balloon angioplasty; single vessel

**+92998**        each additional vessel (List separately in addition to code for primary procedure)

(Use 92998 in conjunction with 92997)

## ►CORONARY THERAPEUTIC SERVICES AND PROCEDURES◄

►Codes 92920-92944 describe percutaneous revascularization services performed for occlusive disease of the coronary vessels (major coronary arteries, coronary artery branches, or coronary artery bypass grafts). These percutaneous coronary intervention (PCI) codes are built on progressive hierarchies with more intensive services inclusive of lesser intensive services. These PCI codes all include the work of accessing and selectively catheterizing the vessel, traversing the lesion, radiological supervision and interpretation directly related to the intervention(s) performed, closure of the arteriotomy when performed through the access sheath, and imaging performed to document completion of the intervention in addition to the intervention(s) performed. These codes include angioplasty (eg, balloon, cutting balloon, wired balloons, cryoplasty), atherectomy (eg, directional, rotational, laser), and stenting (eg, balloon expandable, self-expanding, bare metal, drug eluting, covered). Each code in this family includes balloon angioplasty, when performed. Diagnostic coronary angiography may be reported separately under specific circumstances.

Diagnostic coronary angiography codes (93454-93461) and injection procedure codes (93563-93564) should not be used with percutaneous coronary revascularization services (92920-92944) to report:

1. Contrast injections, angiography, roadmapping, and/or fluoroscopic guidance for the coronary intervention,

2. Vessel measurement for the coronary intervention, or

3. Post-coronary angioplasty/stent/atherectomy angiography, as this work is captured in the percutaneous coronary revascularization services codes (92920-92944).

Diagnostic angiography performed at the time of a coronary interventional procedure may be separately reportable if:

1. No prior catheter-based coronary angiography study is available, and a full diagnostic study is performed, and a decision to intervene is based on the diagnostic angiography, **or**

2. A prior study is available, but as documented in the medical record:

   a. The patient's condition with respect to the clinical indication has changed since the prior study, **or**

   b. There is inadequate visualization of the anatomy and/or pathology, **or**

   c. There is a clinical change during the procedure that requires new evaluation outside the target area of intervention.

Diagnostic coronary angiography performed at a separate session from an interventional procedure is separately reportable.

**Major coronary arteries:** The major coronary arteries are the left main, left anterior descending, left circumflex, right, and ramus intermedius arteries. All PCI procedures performed in all segments (proximal, mid, distal) of a single major coronary artery through the native coronary circulation are reported with one code. When one segment of a major coronary artery is treated through the native circulation and treatment of another segment of the same artery requires access through a coronary artery bypass graft, the intervention through the bypass graft is reported separately.

**Coronary artery branches:** Up to two coronary artery branches of the left anterior descending (diagonals), left circumflex (marginals), and right (posterior descending, posterolaterals) coronary arteries are recognized. The left main and ramus intermedius coronary arteries do not have recognized branches for reporting purposes. All PCI(s) performed in any segment (proximal, mid, distal) of a coronary artery branch is reported with one code. PCI is reported for up to two branches of a major coronary artery. Additional PCI in a third branch of the same major coronary artery is not separately reportable.

**Coronary artery bypass grafts:** ach coronary artery bypass graft represents a coronary vessel. A sequential bypass graft with more than one distal anastomosis represents only one graft. A branching bypass graft (eg, Y graft) represents a coronary vessel for the main graft, and each branch off the main graft constitutes an additional coronary vessel. PCI performed on major coronary arteries or coronary artery branches by access through a bypass graft is reported using the bypass graft PCI codes. All bypass graft PCI codes include the use of coronary artery embolic protection devices when performed.

Only one base code from this family may be reported for revascularization of a major coronary artery and its recognized branches. Only one base code should be reported for revascularization of a coronary artery bypass graft, its subtended coronary artery, and recognized branches of the subtended coronary artery. If one segment of a major coronary artery and its recognized branches is treated through the native circulation, and treatment of another segment of the same vessel requires access through a coronary artery bypass graft, an additional base code is reported to describe the intervention performed through the bypass graft. The PCI base codes are 92920, 92924, 92928, 92933, 92937, 92941, and 92943. The PCI base code that includes the most intensive service provided for the target vessel should be reported. The hierarchy of these services is built on an intensity of service ranked from highest to lowest as 92943 = 92941 = 92933 > 92924 > 92937 = 92928 > 92920.

PCI performed during the same session in additional recognized branches of the target vessel should be reported using the applicable add-on code(s). The add-on codes are 92921, 92925, 92929, 92934, 92938, and 92944 and follow the same principle in regard to reporting the most intensive service provided. The intensity of service is ranked from highest to lowest as 92944 = 92938 > 92934 > 92925 > 92929 > 92921.

PCI performed during the same session in additional major coronary or in additional coronary artery bypass grafts should be reported using the applicable additional base code(s). PCI performed during the same session in additional coronary artery branches should be reported using the applicable additional add-on code(s).

If a single lesion extends from one target vessel (major coronary artery, coronary artery bypass graft, or coronary artery branch) into another target vessel, but can be revascularized with a single intervention bridging the two vessels, this PCI should be reported with a single code despite treating more than one vessel. or example, if a left main coronary lesion extends into the proximal left circumflex coronary artery and a single stent is placed to treat the entire lesion, this PCI should be

⊘=Modifier 51 Exempt  ⊙=Moderate Sedation  ✚=Add-on Code  �=FDA approval pending

reported as a single vessel stent (92928). In this example, a code for additional vessel treatment (92929) would not be additionally reported.

When bifurcation lesions are treated, PCI is reported for both vessels treated. or example, when a bifurcation lesion involving the left anterior descending artery and the first diagonal artery is treated by stenting both vessels, 92928 and 92929 are both reported.

Target vessel PCI for acute myocardial infarction is inclusive of all balloon angioplasty, atherectomy, stenting, manual aspiration thrombectomy, distal protection, and intracoronary rheolytic agent administration performed. Mechanical thrombectomy is reported separately.

Chronic total occlusion of a coronary vessel is present when there is no antegrade flow through the true lumen, accompanied by suggestive angiographic and clinical criteria (eg, antegrade "bridging" collaterals present, calcification at the occlusion site, no current presentation with ST elevation or Q wave acute myocardial infarction attributable to the occluded target lesion). Current presentation with ST elevation or Q wave acute myocardial infarction attributable to the occluded target lesion, subtotal occlusion, and occlusion with dye staining at the site consistent with fresh thrombus are not considered chronic total occlusion.

Codes 92973 (percutaneous transluminal coronary thrombectomy, mechanical), 92974 (coronary brachytherapy), 92978 and 92979 (intravascular ultrasound), and 93571 and 93572 (intravascular Doppler velocity and/or pressure [fractional flow reserve (FFR) or coronary flow reserve (CR)]) are add-on codes for reporting procedures performed in addition to coronary and bypass graft diagnostic and interventional services, unless included in the base code. Non-mechanical, aspiration thrombectomy is not reported with 92973, and is included in the PCI code for acute myocardial infarction (92941), when performed.◄

►(To report transcatheter placement of radiation delivery device for coronary intravascular brachytherapy, use 92974)◄

►(For intravascular radioelement application, see 77785-77787)◄

(For nonsurgical septal reduction therapy [eg, alcohol ablation], use 93799)

#⊙●92920   Percutaneous transluminal coronary angioplasty; single major coronary artery or branch

#⊙✛●92921       each additional branch of a major coronary artery (List separately in addition to code for primary procedure)

►(Use 92921 in conjunction with 92920, 92924, 92928, 92933, 92937, 92941, 92943)◄

#⊙●92924   Percutaneous transluminal coronary atherectomy, with coronary angioplasty when performed; single major coronary artery or branch

#⊙✛●92925       each additional branch of a major coronary artery (List separately in addition to code for primary procedure)

►(Use 92925 in conjunction with 92924, 92928, 92933, 92937, 92941, 92943)◄

#⊙●92928   Percutaneous transcatheter placement of intracoronary stent(s), with coronary angioplasty when performed; single major coronary artery or branch

#⊙✛●92929       each additional branch of a major coronary artery (List separately in addition to code for primary procedure)

►(Use 92929 in conjunction with 92928, 92933, 92937, 92941, 92943)◄

**# ⊙ ● 92933** Percutaneous transluminal coronary atherectomy, with intracoronary stent, with coronary angioplasty when performed; single major coronary artery or branch

**# ⊙ ✚ ● 92934** each additional branch of a major coronary artery (List separately in addition to code for primary procedure)

►(Use 92934 in conjunction with 92933, 92937, 92941, 92943)◄

**# ⊙ ● 92937** Percutaneous transluminal revascularization of or through coronary artery bypass graft (internal mammary, free arterial, venous), any combination of intracoronary stent, atherectomy and angioplasty, including distal protection when performed; single vessel

**# ⊙ ✚ ● 92938** each additional branch subtended by the bypass graft (List separately in addition to code for primary procedure)

►(Use 92938 in conjunction with 92937)◄

**# ⊙ ● 92941** Percutaneous transluminal revascularization of acute total/subtotal occlusion during acute myocardial infarction, coronary artery or coronary artery bypass graft, any combination of intracoronary stent, atherectomy and angioplasty, including aspiration thrombectomy when performed, single vessel

►(For additional vessels treated, see 92920-92938, 92943, 92944)◄

**# ⊙ ● 92943** Percutaneous transluminal revascularization of chronic total occlusion, coronary artery, coronary artery branch, or coronary artery bypass graft, any combination of intracoronary stent, atherectomy and angioplasty; single vessel

**# ⊙ ✚ ● 92944** each additional coronary artery, coronary artery branch, or bypass graft (List separately in addition to code for primary procedure)

►(Use 92944 in conjunction with 92924, 92928, 92933, 92937, 92941, 92943)◄

►(To report transcatheter placement of radiation delivery device for coronary intravascular brachytherapy, use 92974)◄

►(For intravascular radioelement application, see 77785-77787)◄

**# ⊙ ✚ ▲ 92973** Percutaneous transluminal coronary thrombectomy mechanical (List separately in addition to code for primary procedure)

►(Use 92973 in conjunction with 92920, 92924, 92928, 92933, 92937, 92941, 92943, 92975, 93454-93461, 93563, 93564)◄

►(Do not report 92973 for aspiration thrombectomy)◄

**# ⊙ ✚ 92974** Transcatheter placement of radiation delivery device for subsequent coronary intravascular brachytherapy (List separately in addition to code for primary procedure)

►(Use 92974 in conjunction with 92920, 92924, 92928, 92933, 92937, 92941, 92943, 93454-93461)◄

(For intravascular radioelement application, see 77785-77787)

**# ⊙ 92975** Thrombolysis, coronary; by intracoronary infusion, including selective coronary angiography

**# 92977** by intravenous infusion

---

⊘=Modifier 51 Exempt  ⊙=Moderate Sedation  ✚=Add-on Code  ⌀=FDA approval pending

▶(For thrombolysis of vessels other than coronary, see 37211-37214)◀

(For cerebral thrombolysis, use 37195)

**# ⊙ ✚ 92978** Intravascular ultrasound (coronary vessel or graft) during diagnostic evaluation and/or therapeutic intervention including imaging supervision, interpretation and report; initial vessel (List separately in addition to code for primary procedure)

▶(Use 92978 in conjunction with 92975, 92920, 92924, 92928, 92933, 92937, 92941, 92943, 93454-93461, 93563, 93564)◀

**# ⊙ ✚ 92979** each additional vessel (List separately in addition to code for primary procedure)

(Use 92979 in conjunction with 92978)

(Intravascular ultrasound services include all transducer manipulations and repositioning within the specific vessel being examined, both before and after therapeutic intervention [eg, stent placement])

(For intravascular spectroscopy, use 0205T)

▶(For intravascular optical coherence tomography, see 0291T, 0292T)◀

 **Rationale**

Percutaneous coronary intervention codes 92980-92984, 92995, and 92996 were deleted, and 13 new codes were established to report these procedures. New guidelines were added to instruct users on the appropriate use of these new codes. The new codes and guidelines are listed under a new subsection within the Medicine/Cardiovascular/Therapeutic Services and Procedures section titled, **Coronary Therapeutic Services and Procedures**. In order to distinguish these coronary procedures from the noncoronary procedure codes in the Therapeutic Services and Procedures section, a separate subsection was created for noncoronary codes, titled, **Other Therapeutic Services and Procedures**. The resequencing principle was applied to the new codes, ie, they are out of numerical sequence.

The coronary intervention procedure coding changes were made because the old codes did not adequately reflect the complexity involved in current percutaneous coronary stent placement and angioplasty procedures. Deleted codes 92980 and 92981, which described the placement of intracoronary stent(s), included other therapeutic procedure performed. New codes 92928 and 92929 describe percutaneous placement of intracoronary stents and with angioplasty, when performed. However, they do not include other therapeutic interventions performed in the same vessel. In the new coding structure, codes 92920 and 92921 describe percutaneous coronary angioplasty only. These codes should be reported when only angioplasty is performed. The remaining new codes in the new section describe percutaneous coronary interventions in various combinations, and all of them include angioplasty when performed.

The new guidelines provide definitions of major coronary arteries, coronary artery branches, and coronary artery bypass grafts. They provide instructions on when diagnostic coronary angiography should and should not be reported. They also provide instructions on how to report percutaneous coronary intervention procedures using the new coding structure. There are several revised and new parenthetical notes that provide instruction on the appropriate use of the new codes.

In support of the addition of codes 37211-37214 to describe combined transcatheter thrombolytic therapy services, the cross-reference note following intraveous infusion code 92977 was updated to include reference to these new services.

A parenthetical note was added following the intravascular ultrasound code 92979 to reference the new optical coherence tomography (OCT) codes to distinguish between the two different technologies. See Rationale for codes 0291T and 0292T.

## Clinical Example (92920)

A 65-year-old female presents with progressive unstable angina. Stress testing shows anterior ischemia. Coronary arteriography demonstrates diffusely diseased diabetic-appearing coronary arteries with a 90% calcified lesion in the distal part of a tortuous left anterior descending coronary artery. The size of the vessel is less than the size of the smallest available stent. The patient is transferred to a percutaneous coronary intervention (PCI) center for percutaneous coronary balloon angioplasty on the following day. This is the first lesion in this coronary territory to be treated.

### Description of Procedure (92920)

A "time out" occurs during which confirmation of critical information is ensured, such as the patient's identity, planned procedure, access route, allergies, completion of the consent process, availability of proper equipment, and any unusual circumstances that might influence the procedure. Conscious sedation is administered and adequate conscious sedation monitoring is verified. Percutaneous arterial access is obtained, typically through the femoral artery or radial artery. A thin-walled needle is inserted percutaneously into the peripheral artery through which a flexible guidewire is inserted. The needle is removed over the wire, a sheath/dilator system is inserted over the guidewire, the dilator is removed, and the side-arm of the sheath is flushed to remove any clot or air. Intra-arterial vasodilators are administered to prevent arterial spasm for radial artery access. An appropriate guiding catheter is inserted over the wire through the sheath into the arterial system under fluoroscopic guidance throughout the procedure. The catheter is advanced retrograde through the arterial system to the ascending aorta. The wire is removed and the catheter is attached to the pressure manifold. The guide is aspirated to remove any air, atheroma, or thrombus. Pressure is measured in the aortic root. The catheter is then manipulated using fluoroscopic guidance into the ostium of a coronary artery. Typically, the guide must be manipulated to avoid aortic atheroma and adjusted substantially to engage the artery based on the anatomy of the aorta. The arterial pressure and waveform are then checked to be sure there is no evidence of catheter malposition or impairment of coronary flow due to an ostial stenosis. Frequently, several guide catheters are required to achieve a safe catheter engagement of the artery. Test contrast injections under fluoroscopy are performed to check catheter position.

Appropriate antiplatelet therapy pretreatment is confirmed, and additional anti-platelet therapy is administered as needed. Direct thrombin inhibitors or heparin is administered for anticoagulation. Therapeutic anticoagulation is confirmed by drawing blood from the guide and testing an activated clotting time (ACT). Additional anticoagulation is administered as needed to achieve a therapeutic ACT. Intracoronary vasodilators are administered. Multiple coronary injections are performed, each with the imaging system aligned in a different orientation, with simultaneous panning (moving the table) to assess the stenoses.

A coronary guidewire is then manipulated through the guide and down the coronary artery and carefully used to cross the target lesion. Typically, this requires manipulation of the wire in several angiographic views and often requires additional guidewires if the first wire is not successful. Guidewire position across the lesion is confirmed angiographically. The wire is adjusted as needed to ensure it is not lodged in a small distal vessel that might result in perforation or dissection. Multiple coronary injections are performed, each with the imaging system aligned in a different orientation, with simultaneous panning (moving the table) to assess the stenoses. An appropriate-sized balloon is selected. The balloon is de-aired and the lumen is allowed to fill passively with contrast. A balloon inflation device is prepared and filled with dilute contrast. The balloon is advanced over the coronary guidewire to the lesion. Balloon position is confirmed by angiography. The balloon is inflated gradually, observing for clinical and angiographic signs of ischemia, and watching for balloon deformation and appropriate balloon expansion. Typically, the patient develops chest pain and/or electrocardiographic changes that limit the duration of balloon inflation, and the balloon is quickly deflated. The balloon is reinflated several times to progressively higher atmospheres and for longer periods of time up to several minutes. The balloon is then exchanged back over the guidewire into the guide. Intracoronary vasodilators are again administered. Angiography is performed in multiple views. The lesion is not fully expanded and the angioplasty procedure is repeated multiple times with progressively larger balloons. Once an adequate expansion is achieved, the balloon is again exchanged out of the coronary artery into the guide. Completion angiography is performed after repeat administration of intracoronary vasodilators. Inspection of the images is performed for signs of vessel dissection, perforation, or impaired coronary flow. The coronary wire is then withdrawn back into the guide. Completion angiography is again performed after repeat administration of intracoronary vasodilators. Inspection of the images is again performed for signs of vessel dissection, perforation, or impaired coronary flow. The guide catheter is disengaged from the coronary ostium and then removed over a guidewire from the body. Anticoagulation infusions are stopped.

Angiography of the access site is often performed through the access sheath to assess for any complications and suitability for a percutaneous closure device. The catheter and sheath are removed and hemostasis is achieved by appropriate means by the physician or technician under the physician's supervision. Observation of the site is performed to ensure no immediate bleeding, if a vascular closure device is deployed. Manual pressure is required for a short time to achieve complete hemostasis. If manual pressure is used, the sheath is typically sewn in for subsequent removal, once the ACT level falls to a safe level.

 **Clinical Example (92921)**

A 65-year-old female presents with progressive unstable angina. Stress testing shows anterior ischemia. Coronary arteriography demonstrates diffusely diseased diabetic-appearing coronary arteries with a 90% calcified lesion in the distal part of a tortuous left anterior descending coronary artery. An additional 80% calcific lesion is noted in the first diagonal artery. The size of the vessels is less than the size of the smallest available stent. The patient is transferred to a percutaneous coronary intervention (PCI) center for percutaneous coronary balloon angioplasty on the following day. The first lesion has been treated. Now an additional lesion is to be treated.

**Description of Procedure (92921)**

The indwelling guide catheter from the first coronary intervention is removed over a guidewire. A new guide is selected to engage the second vessel. An appropriate guiding catheter is inserted over the wire through the sheath into the arterial system under fluoroscopic guidance throughout the procedure. The catheter is advanced retrograde through the arterial system to the ascending aorta. The wire is removed and the catheter is attached to the pressure manifold. The guide is aspirated to remove any air, atheroma, or thrombus. Pressure is measured in the aortic root. The catheter is then manipulated using fluoroscopic guidance into the ostium of a coronary artery. Typically, the guide must be manipulated to avoid aortic atheroma and adjusted substantially to engage the artery based on the anatomy of the aorta. The arterial pressure and waveform are then checked to be sure there is no evidence of catheter malposition or impairment of coronary flow due to an ostial stenosis. Frequently, several guide catheters are required to achieve a safe catheter engagement of the artery. Test contrast injections under fluoroscopy are performed to check catheter position.

A coronary guidewire is then manipulated through the guide and down the coronary artery and carefully used to cross the target lesion. Typically, this requires manipulation of the wire in several angiographic views and often requires additional guidewires if the first wire is not successful. Guidewire position across the lesion is confirmed angiographically. The wire is adjusted as needed to ensure it is not lodged in a small distal vessel that might result in perforation or dissection. Multiple coronary injections are performed, each with the imaging system aligned in a different orientation, with simultaneous panning (moving the table) to assess the stenoses.

An appropriate-sized balloon is selected. The balloon is de-aired and the lumen is allowed to fill passively with contrast. A balloon inflation device is prepared and filled with dilute contrast. The balloon is advanced over the coronary guidewire to the lesion. Balloon position is confirmed by angiography. The balloon is inflated gradually, observing for clinical and angiographic signs of ischemia, and watching for balloon deformation and appropriate balloon expansion. Typically, the patient develops chest pain and/or electrocardiographic changes that limit the duration of balloon inflation, and the balloon is quickly deflated. The balloon is reinflated

⊘=Modifier 51 Exempt   ⊙=Moderate Sedation   ✚=Add-on Code   ✗=FDA approval pending

several times to progressively higher atmospheres and for longer periods of time up to several minutes. The balloon is then exchanged back over the guidewire into the guide. Intracoronary vasodilators are again administered. Angiography is performed in multiple views. The lesion is not fully expanded and the angioplasty procedure is repeated multiple times with progressively larger balloons. Once an adequate expansion is achieved, the balloon is again exchanged out of the coronary artery into the guide. Completion angiography is performed after repeat administration of intracoronary vasodilators. Inspection of the images is performed for signs of vessel dissection, perforation, or impaired coronary flow. The coronary wire is then withdrawn back into the guide. Completion angiography is again performed after repeat administration of intracoronary vasodilators. Inspection of the images is again performed for signs of vessel dissection, perforation, or impaired coronary flow. The guide catheter is disengaged from the coronary ostium and then removed over a guidewire from the body. Anticoagulation infusions are stopped.

Angiography of the access site is often performed through the access sheath to assess for any complications and suitability for a percutaneous closure device. The catheter and sheath are removed, and hemostasis is achieved by appropriate means by the physician or technician under the physician's supervision. Observation of the site is performed to ensure no immediate bleeding if a vascular closure device is deployed. Manual pressure is required for a short time to achieve complete hemostasis. If manual pressure is used, the sheath is typically sewn in for subsequent removal, once the activated clotting time (ACT) level falls to a safe level.

 ## Clinical Example (92924)

A 64-year-old male with diffuse peripheral vascular disease presents with chronic stable angina refractory to medical therapy. Stress testing shows inferior ischemia at a low level of cardiac stress. Coronary arteriography demonstrates heavily calcified coronary arteries. The left anterior descending and circumflex coronary arteries are relatively free of occlusive disease but the right coronary artery has a long heavily calcified lesion that is 50% stenotic throughout and 80% stenotic at the worst point. The patient is transferred to a percutaneous coronary intervention (PCI) center for percutaneous coronary rotational atherectomy on the following day. The result after rotational atherectomy and angioplasty is "stent-like," and passage of a stent would be difficult due to proximal calcification and tortuosity so stenting is not performed. This is the first lesion in this coronary territory to be treated.

### Description of Procedure (92924)

A "time out" occurs during which confirmation of critical information is ensured, such as the patient's identity, planned procedure, access route, allergies, completion of the consent process, availability of proper equipment, and any unusual circumstances that might influence the procedure. Conscious sedation is administered and adequate conscious sedation monitoring is verified. Percutaneous arterial access is obtained, typically through the femoral artery or radial artery. A thin-walled needle is inserted percutaneously into the peripheral artery, through which a flexible guidewire is inserted. The needle is removed over the wire, a sheath/

dilator system is inserted over the guidewire, the dilator is removed, and the side-arm of the sheath is flushed to remove any clot or air. Intra-arterial vasodilators are administered to prevent arterial spasm for radial artery access. An appropriate guiding catheter is inserted over the wire through the sheath into the arterial system under fluoroscopic guidance throughout the procedure. The catheter is advanced retrograde through the arterial system to the ascending aorta. The wire is removed and the catheter is attached to the pressure manifold. The guide is aspirated to remove any air, atheroma, or thrombus. Pressure is measured in the aortic root. The catheter is then manipulated using fluoroscopic guidance into the ostium of a coronary artery. Typically, the guide must be manipulated to avoid aortic atheroma and adjusted substantially to engage the artery based on the anatomy of the aorta. The arterial pressure and waveform are then checked to be sure there is no evidence of catheter malposition or impairment of coronary flow due to an ostial stenosis. Frequently, several guide catheters are required to achieve a safe catheter engagement of the artery. Test contrast injections under fluoroscopy are performed to check catheter position.

Appropriate antiplatelet therapy pretreatment is confirmed, and additional antiplatelet therapy is administered as needed. Direct thrombin inhibitors or heparin is administered for anticoagulation. Therapeutic anticoagulation is confirmed by drawing blood from the guide and testing an activated clotting time (ACT). Additional anticoagulation is administered as needed to achieve a therapeutic ACT. Intracoronary vasodilators are administered. Multiple coronary injections are performed, each with the imaging system aligned in a different orientation, with simultaneous panning (moving the table) to assess the stenoses.

A coronary guidewire is then manipulated through the guide and down the coronary artery and carefully used to cross the target lesion. Typically, this requires manipulation of the wire in several angiographic views and often requires additional guidewires if the first wire is not successful. Guidewire position across the lesion is confirmed angiographically. The wire is adjusted as needed to ensure it is not lodged in a small distal vessel that might result in perforation or dissection. Multiple coronary injections are performed, each with the imaging system aligned in a different orientation, with simultaneous panning (moving the table) to assess the stenoses.

An appropriate-sized balloon is selected. The balloon is de-aired and the lumen is allowed to fill passively with contrast. The coronary guidewire is then removed through the balloon lumen and replaced with a wire specifically designed for rotational atherectomy. The balloon is removed over the wire. Balloon position is confirmed by angiography.

An appropriate-sized rotational atherectomy burr is selected and the rotational atherectomy system is assembled. A foot pedal is positioned under the table. The burr delivery unit is loaded with extreme care over the wire, as the latter is very susceptible to kinking. If kinked, the wire must be removed from the coronary and the entire process up to this point is redone. A continuous infusion to prevent no-reflow is administered. The burr is activated outside the body to test the rotational speed, and the console is used to adjust the speed to a proper level.

⃠=Modifier 51 Exempt   ⊙=Moderate Sedation   ✚=Add-on Code   ☏=FDA approval pending

The burr is advanced over the wire to the coronary artery proximal to the lesion. This typically requires carefully coordinated pulling of the wire during burr advancement to overcome resistance. The burr is adjusted to remove tension from the system. The device is activated to test the rotational speed in the body and adjusted as needed. Careful monitoring of the rhythm and blood pressure is performed as bradycardia and hypotension frequently occur. Once the test is complete, the burr is activated and advanced in a gradual back and forth motion to ablate calcific plaque. Typically, the patient develops chest pain and/or electrocardiographic changes during these "runs," which are kept short to avoid severe hypotension, bradycardia, and even heart block. Angiography is performed in between runs to assess coronary flow and to ensure no dissection or perforation. The operator must wait up to several minutes between runs to allow resolution of ischemia. Multiple runs are performed with the burr until it is able to progress through the resistant lesion. Polishing runs are then performed. The burr is exchanged out over the wire. A larger burr is then selected to enlarge the lumen more optimally. The same procedure is then performed with the larger burr. After several progressively larger burrs and successful enlargement of the lumen, balloon angioplasty is typically performed to smooth out irregularities and seal any atheromatous flaps up against the vessel wall to try to prevent abrupt vessel closure.

An appropriate-sized balloon is selected. The balloon is de-aired and the lumen is allowed to fill passively with contrast. A balloon inflation device is prepared and filled with dilute contrast. The balloon is advanced over the coronary guidewire to the lesion. Balloon position is confirmed by angiography. The balloon is inflated gradually, observing for clinical and angiographic signs of ischemia, and watching for balloon deformation and appropriate balloon expansion. Typically, the patient develops chest pain and/or electrocardiographic changes that limit the duration of balloon inflation, and the balloon is quickly deflated. The balloon is reinflated several times to progressively higher atmospheres and for longer periods of time up to several minutes. The balloon is then exchanged back over the guidewire into the guide. Intracoronary vasodilators are again administered. Angiography is performed in multiple views. Once an adequate expansion is achieved, the balloon is again exchanged out of the coronary artery into the guide. Completion angiography is performed after repeat administration of intracoronary vasodilators. Inspection of the images is performed for signs of vessel dissection, perforation, or impaired coronary flow. The coronary wire is then withdrawn back into the guide. Completion angiography is again performed after repeat administration of intracoronary vasodilators. Inspection of the images is again performed for signs of vessel dissection, perforation, or impaired coronary flow. The guide catheter is disengaged from the coronary ostium and then removed over a guidewire from the body. Anticoagulation infusions are stopped.

Angiography of the access site is often performed through the access sheath to assess for any complications and suitability for a percutaneous closure device. The catheter and sheath are removed and hemostasis is achieved by appropriate means by the physician or technician under the physician's supervision. Observation of the site is performed to ensure no immediate bleeding, if a vascular closure device is deployed. Manual pressure is required for a short time to achieve complete hemostasis. If manual pressure is used, the sheath is typically sewn in for subsequent removal once, the ACT level falls to a safe level.

 ### Clinical Example (92925)

A 64-year-old male with diffuse peripheral vascular disease presents with chronic stable angina refractory to medical therapy. Stress testing shows inferior ischemia at a low level of cardiac stress. Coronary arteriography demonstrates heavily calcified coronary arteries. The left anterior descending and circumflex coronary arteries are relatively free of occlusive disease but the right coronary artery has a long heavily calcified lesion that is 50% stenotic throughout and 80% stenotic at the worst point. The posterior descending artery has a long heavily calcified lesion that is 50% stenotic throughout and 80% stenotic at the worst point. The patient is transferred to a percutaneous coronary intervention (PCI) center for percutaneous coronary rotational atherectomy on the following day. The result after rotational atherectomy and angioplasty is "stent-like," and passage of a stent would be difficult due to proximal calcification and tortuosity so stenting is not performed. The first lesion has been treated. Now an additional lesion is to be treated.

### Description of Procedure (92925)

The indwelling guide catheter from the first coronary intervention is removed over a guidewire. A new guide is selected to engage the second vessel. An appropriate guiding catheter is inserted over the wire through the sheath into the arterial system under fluoroscopic guidance throughout the procedure. The catheter is advanced retrograde through the arterial system to the ascending aorta. The wire is removed and the catheter is attached to the pressure manifold. The guide is aspirated to remove any air, atheroma, or thrombus. Pressure is measured in the aortic root. The catheter is then manipulated using fluoroscopic guidance into the ostium of a coronary artery. Typically, the guide must be manipulated to avoid aortic atheroma and adjusted substantially to engage the artery based on the anatomy of the aorta. The arterial pressure and waveform are then checked to be sure there is no evidence of catheter malposition or impairment of coronary flow due to an ostial stenosis. Frequently, several guide catheters are required to achieve a safe catheter engagement of the artery. Test contrast injections under fluoroscopy are performed to check catheter position.

A coronary guidewire is then manipulated through the guide and down the coronary artery and carefully used to cross the target lesion. Typically, this requires manipulation of the wire in several angiographic views and often requires additional guidewires if the first wire is not successful. Guidewire position across the lesion is confirmed angiographically. The wire is adjusted as needed to ensure it is not lodged in a small distal vessel that might result in perforation or dissection. Multiple coronary injections are performed, each with the imaging system aligned in a different orientation, with simultaneous panning (moving the table) to assess the stenoses.

An appropriate-sized balloon is selected. The balloon is de-aired and the lumen is allowed to fill passively with contrast. The coronary guidewire is then removed through the balloon lumen and replaced with a wire specifically designed for

⊘=Modifier 51 Exempt  ⊙=Moderate Sedation  ✚=Add-on Code  ✗=FDA approval pending

rotational atherectomy. The balloon is removed over the wire. Balloon position is confirmed by angiography.

An appropriate-sized rotational atherectomy burr is selected and the rotational atherectomy system is assembled. A foot pedal is positioned under the table. The burr delivery unit is loaded with extreme care over the wire, as the latter is very susceptible to kinking. If kinked, the wire must be removed from the coronary and the entire process to this point is redone. A continuous infusion to prevent no-reflow is administered. The burr is activated outside the body to test the rotational speed, and the console is used to adjust the speed to a proper level.

The burr is advanced over the wire to the coronary artery proximal to the lesion. This typically requires carefully coordinated pulling of the wire during burr advancement to overcome resistance. The burr is adjusted to remove tension from the system. The device is activated to test the rotational speed in the body and adjusted as needed. Careful monitoring of the rhythm and blood pressure is performed as bradycardia and hypotension frequently occur. Once the test is complete, the burr is activated and advanced in a gradual back and forth motion to ablate calcific plaque. Typically, the patient develops chest pain and/or electro-cardiographic changes during these "runs," which are kept short to avoid severe hypotension, bradycardia, and even heart block. Angiography is performed in between runs to assess coronary flow and to ensure no dissection or perforation. The operator must wait up to several minutes between runs to allow resolution of ischemia. Multiple runs are performed with the burr until it is able to prog-ress through the resistant lesion. Polishing runs are then performed. The burr is exchanged out over the wire. A larger burr is then selected to enlarge the lumen more optimally. The same procedure is then performed with the larger burr. After several progressively larger burrs and successful enlargement of the lumen, balloon angioplasty is typically performed to smooth out irregularities and seal any atheromatous flaps up against the vessel wall to try to prevent abrupt vessel closure.

An appropriate-sized balloon is selected. The balloon is de-aired and the lumen is allowed to fill passively with contrast. A balloon inflation device is prepared and filled with dilute contrast. The balloon is advanced over the coronary guidewire to the lesion. Balloon position is confirmed by angiography. The balloon is inflated gradually, observing for clinical and angiographic signs of ischemia, and watching for balloon deformation and appropriate balloon expansion. Typically, the patient develops chest pain and/or electrocardiographic changes that limit the duration of balloon inflation, and the balloon is quickly deflated. The balloon is reinflated several times to progressively higher atmospheres and for longer periods of time up to several minutes. The balloon is then exchanged back over the guidewire into the guide. Intracoronary vasodilators are again administered. Angiography is performed in multiple views. Once an adequate expansion is achieved, the bal-loon is again exchanged out of the coronary artery into the guide. Completion angiography is performed after repeat administration of intracoronary vasodilators. Inspection of the images is performed for signs of vessel dissection, perforation, or impaired coronary flow. The coronary wire is then withdrawn back into the guide. Completion angiography is again performed after repeat administration of intracoronary vasodilators. Inspection of the images is again performed for signs of vessel dissection, perforation, or impaired coronary flow. The guide catheter is disengaged from the coronary ostium and then removed over a guidewire from the body. Anticoagulation infusions are stopped.

Angiography of the access site is often performed through the access sheath to assess for any complications and suitability for a percutaneous closure device. The catheter and sheath are removed and hemostasis is achieved by appropriate means by the physician or technician under the physician's supervision. Observation of the site is performed to ensure no immediate bleeding, if a vascular closure device is deployed. Manual pressure is required for a short time to achieve complete hemostasis. If manual pressure is used, the sheath is typically sewn in for subsequent removal, once the activated clotting time (ACT) level falls to a safe level.

###  Clinical Example (92928)

A 76-year-old obese male presents with unstable angina consistent with acute coronary syndrome. Coronary arteriography demonstrates a 22-mm long hazy 80% lesion in the circumflex coronary artery. The patient is transferred to a percutaneous coronary intervention (PCI) center for percutaneous coronary intervention on the following day. This is the first lesion in this coronary territory to be treated.

### Description of Procedure (92928)

A "time out" occurs during which confirmation of critical information is ensured, such as the patient's identity, planned procedure, access route, allergies, completion of the consent process, availability of proper equipment, and any unusual circumstances that might influence the procedure. Conscious sedation is administered and adequate conscious sedation monitoring is verified. Percutaneous arterial access is obtained, typically through the femoral artery or radial artery. A thin-walled needle is inserted percutaneously into the peripheral artery, through which a flexible guidewire is inserted. The needle is removed over the wire, a sheath/dilator system is inserted over the guidewire, the dilator is removed, and the side-arm of the sheath is flushed to remove any clot or air. Intra-arterial vasodilators are administered to prevent arterial spasm for radial artery access. An appropriate guiding catheter is inserted over the wire through the sheath into the arterial system under fluoroscopic guidance throughout the procedure. The catheter is advanced retrograde through the arterial system to the ascending aorta. The wire is removed and the catheter is attached to the pressure manifold. The guide is aspirated to remove any air, atheroma, or thrombus. Pressure is measured in the aortic root. The catheter is then manipulated using fluoroscopic guidance into the ostium of a coronary artery. Typically, the guide must be manipulated to avoid aortic atheroma and adjusted substantially to engage the artery based on the anatomy of the aorta. The arterial pressure and waveform are then checked to be sure there is no evidence of catheter malposition or impairment of coronary flow due to an ostial stenosis. Frequently, several guide catheters are required to achieve a safe catheter engagement of the artery. Test contrast injections under fluoroscopy are performed to check catheter position.

Appropriate antiplatelet therapy pretreatment is confirmed, and additional antiplatelet therapy is administered as needed. Direct thrombin inhibitors or heparin is administered for anticoagulation. Therapeutic anticoagulation is confirmed

⊘=Modifier 51 Exempt   ⊙=Moderate Sedation   ✚=Add-on Code   ✏=FDA approval pending

by drawing blood from the guide and testing an activated clotting time (ACT). Additional anticoagulation is administered as needed to achieve a therapeutic ACT. Intracoronary vasodilators are administered. Multiple coronary injections are performed, each with the imaging system aligned in a different orientation, with simultaneous panning (moving the table) to assess the stenoses.

A coronary guidewire is then manipulated through the guide and down the coronary artery and carefully used to cross the target lesion. Typically, this requires manipulation of the wire in several angiographic views and often requires additional guidewires if the first wire is not successful. Guidewire position across the lesion is confirmed angiographically. The wire is adjusted as needed to ensure it is not lodged in a small distal vessel that might result in perforation or dissection. Multiple coronary injections are performed, each with the imaging system aligned in a different orientation, with simultaneous panning (moving the table) to assess the stenoses.

An appropriate-sized balloon is selected. The balloon is de-aired and the lumen is allowed to fill passively with contrast. A balloon inflation device is prepared and filled with dilute contrast. The balloon is advanced over the coronary guidewire to the lesion. Balloon position is confirmed by angiography. The balloon is inflated gradually, observing for clinical and angiographic signs of ischemia, and watching for balloon deformation and appropriate balloon expansion. Typically, the patient develops chest pain and/or electrocardiographic changes that limit the duration of balloon inflation, and the balloon is quickly deflated. The balloon is reinflated several times to progressively higher atmospheres and for longer periods of time up to several minutes. The balloon is then exchanged back over the guidewire into the guide. Intracoronary vasodilators are again administered. Angiography is performed in multiple views. The lesion is not fully expanded and the angioplasty procedure is repeated multiple times with progressively larger balloons. Once an adequate expansion is achieved to allow stent deployment, the balloon is again exchanged out of the coronary artery into the guide. Completion angiography is performed after repeat administration of intracoronary vasodilators. Inspection of the images is performed for signs of vessel dissection, perforation, or impaired coronary flow.

The patient's ability to tolerate long-term dual antiplatelet therapy and to comply with this therapy is again confirmed. A stent of appropriate diameter and length is selected. The stent is advanced over the wire to the target lesion and carefully positioned. This may require placing additional coronary guidewires down the vessel to allow the stent to pass. The stent is deployed at high pressure. The original stent frequently does not cover the entire diseased segment and additional stents are then placed as needed using the same techniques. Next, a high-pressure, non-compliant balloon is advanced over the coronary guidewire into the stented segment, and this is inflated at high pressure to ensure stent expansion. Frequently, more than one balloon of different sizes is required. The balloon is then exchanged back over the guidewire into the guide. Intracoronary vasodilators are again administered. Angiography is performed in multiple views. If the result is acceptable, the coronary wire is then withdrawn back into the guide. Completion angiography is again performed after repeat administration of intracoronary vasodilators. Inspection of the images is again performed for signs of vessel dissection, perforation, or impaired coronary flow. The guide catheter is disengaged from the coronary ostium and then removed over a guidewire from the body. Anticoagulation infusions are stopped.

Angiography of the access site is often performed through the access sheath to assess for any complications and suitability for a percutaneous closure device. The catheter and sheath are removed and hemostasis is achieved by appropriate means by the physician or technician under the physician's supervision. Observation of the site is performed to ensure no immediate bleeding if a vascular closure device is deployed. Manual pressure is required for a short time to achieve complete hemostasis. If manual pressure is used, the sheath is typically sewn in for subsequent removal, once the ACT level falls to a safe level.

## Clinical Example (92929)

A 76-year-old obese male presents with unstable angina consistent with acute coronary syndrome. Coronary arteriography demonstrates a 22-mm long hazy 80% lesion in the circumflex coronary artery. An additional 22-mm long hazy 80% lesion is noted in the large first obtuse marginal branch. The patient is transferred to a percutaneous coronary intervention (PCI) center for percutaneous coronary intervention on the following day. The first lesion has been treated. Now an additional lesion is to be treated.

### Description of Procedure (92929)

The indwelling guide catheter from the first coronary intervention is removed over a guidewire. A new guide is selected to engage the second vessel. An appropriate guiding catheter is inserted over the wire through the sheath into the arterial system under fluoroscopic guidance throughout the procedure. The catheter is advanced retrograde through the arterial system to the ascending aorta. The wire is removed and the catheter is attached to the pressure manifold. The guide is aspirated to remove any air, atheroma, or thrombus. Pressure is measured in the aortic root. The catheter is then manipulated using fluoroscopic guidance into the ostium of a coronary artery. Typically, the guide must be manipulated to avoid aortic atheroma and adjusted substantially to engage the artery based on the anatomy of the aorta. The arterial pressure and waveform are then checked to be sure there is no evidence of catheter malposition or impairment of coronary flow due to an ostial stenosis. Frequently, several guide catheters are required to achieve a safe catheter engagement of the artery. Test contrast injections under fluoroscopy are performed to check catheter position.

A coronary guidewire is then manipulated through the guide and down the coronary artery and carefully used to cross the target lesion. Typically, this requires manipulation of the wire in several angiographic views and often requires additional guidewires if the first wire is not successful. Guidewire position across the lesion is confirmed angiographically. The wire is adjusted as needed to ensure it is not lodged in a small distal vessel that might result in perforation or dissection. Multiple coronary injections are performed, each with the imaging system aligned in a different orientation, with simultaneous panning (moving the table) to assess the stenoses.

⊘=Modifier 51 Exempt   ⊙=Moderate Sedation   ✚=Add-on Code   ✔=FDA approval pending

An appropriate-sized balloon is selected. The balloon is de-aired and the lumen is allowed to fill passively with contrast. A balloon inflation device is prepared and filled with dilute contrast. The balloon is advanced over the coronary guidewire to the lesion. Balloon position is confirmed by angiography. The balloon is inflated gradually, observing for clinical and angiographic signs of ischemia, and watching for balloon deformation and appropriate balloon expansion. Typically, the patient develops chest pain and/or electrocardiographic changes that limit the duration of balloon inflation, and the balloon is quickly deflated. The balloon is reinflated several times to progressively higher atmospheres and for longer periods of time up to several minutes. The balloon is then exchanged back over the guidewire into the guide. Intracoronary vasodilators are again administered. Angiography is performed in multiple views. The lesion is not fully expanded and the angioplasty procedure is repeated multiple times with progressively larger balloons. Once an adequate expansion is achieved to allow stent deployment, the balloon is again exchanged out of the coronary artery into the guide. Completion angiography is performed after repeat administration of intracoronary vasodilators. Inspection of the images is performed for signs of vessel dissection, perforation, or impaired coronary flow.

A stent of appropriate diameter and length is selected. The stent is advanced over the wire to the target lesion and carefully positioned. This may require placing additional coronary guidewires down the vessel to allow the stent to pass. The stent is deployed at high pressure. The original stent frequently does not cover the entire diseased segment and additional stents are then placed as needed using the same techniques. Next, a high-pressure, non-compliant balloon is advanced over the coronary guidewire into the stented segment and this is inflated at high pressure to ensure stent expansion. Frequently, more than one balloon of different sizes is required. The balloon is then exchanged back over the guidewire into the guide. Intracoronary vasodilators are again administered. Angiography is performed in multiple views. If the result is acceptable, the coronary wire is then withdrawn back into the guide. Completion angiography is again performed after repeat administration of intracoronary vasodilators. Inspection of the images is again performed for signs of vessel dissection, perforation, or impaired coronary flow. The guide catheter is disengaged from the coronary ostium and then removed over a guidewire from the body. Anticoagulation infusions are stopped.

Angiography of the access site is often performed through the access sheath to assess for any complications and suitability for a percutaneous closure device. The catheter and sheath are removed and hemostasis is achieved by appropriate means by the physician or technician under the physician's supervision. Observation of the site is performed to ensure no immediate bleeding if a vascular closure device is deployed. Manual pressure is required for a short time to achieve complete hemostasis. If manual pressure is used, the sheath is typically sewn in for subsequent removal, once the activated clotting time (ACT) level falls to a safe level.

###  Clinical Example (92933)

A 72-year-old male presents with progressive angina and pharmacologic stress testing showing lateral ischemia. Coronary arteriography shows 50% lesions in the left and right coronary arteries and an 80%, 12-mm long left circumflex coronary artery lesion. The vessels are extremely heavily calcified. After discussion with the patient and the patient's family regarding therapeutic options, the patient requests coronary intervention, which is scheduled for the next day. This is the first lesion in this coronary territory to be treated.

### Description of Procedure (92933)

A "time out" occurs during which confirmation of critical information is ensured, such as the patient's identity, planned procedure, access route, allergies, completion of the consent process, availability of proper equipment, and any unusual circumstances which might influence the procedure. Conscious sedation is administered and adequate conscious sedation monitoring is verified. Percutaneous arterial access is obtained, typically through the femoral artery or radial artery. A thin-walled needle is inserted percutaneously into the peripheral artery, through which a flexible guidewire is inserted. The needle is removed over the wire, a sheath/dilator system is inserted over the guidewire, the dilator is removed, and the sidearm of the sheath is flushed to remove any clot or air. Intra-arterial vasodilators are administered to prevent arterial spasm for radial artery access. An appropriate guiding catheter is inserted over the wire through the sheath into the arterial system under fluoroscopic guidance throughout the procedure. The catheter is advanced retrograde through the arterial system to the ascending aorta. The wire is removed and the catheter is attached to the pressure manifold. The guide is aspirated to remove any air, atheroma, or thrombus. Pressure is measured in the aortic root. The catheter is then manipulated using fluoroscopic guidance into the ostium of a coronary artery. Typically, the guide must be manipulated to avoid aortic atheroma and adjusted substantially to engage the artery based on the anatomy of the aorta. The arterial pressure and waveform are then checked to be sure there is no evidence of catheter malposition or impairment of coronary flow due to an ostial stenosis. Frequently, several guide catheters are required to achieve a safe catheter engagement of the artery. Test contrast injections under fluoroscopy are performed to check catheter position.

Appropriate antiplatelet therapy pretreatment is confirmed, and additional antiplatelet therapy is administered as needed. Direct thrombin inhibitors or heparin is administered for anticoagulation. Therapeutic anticoagulation is confirmed by drawing blood from the guide and testing an activated clotting time (ACT). Additional anticoagulation is administered as needed to achieve a therapeutic ACT. Intracoronary vasodilators are administered. Multiple coronary injections are performed, each with the imaging system aligned in a different orientation, with simultaneous panning (moving the table) to assess the stenoses.

A coronary guidewire is then manipulated through the guide and down the coronary artery and carefully used to cross the target lesion. Typically, this requires manipulation of the wire in several angiographic views and often requires additional guidewires, if the first wire is not successful. Guidewire position across the lesion is confirmed angiographically. The wire is adjusted as needed to ensure it is not lodged in a small distal vessel that might result in perforation or dissection. Multiple coronary injections are performed, each with the imaging system aligned

⊘=Modifier 51 Exempt  ⊙=Moderate Sedation  ✚=Add-on Code  ⋏=FDA approval pending

in a different orientation, with simultaneous panning (moving the table) to assess the stenoses.

An appropriate-sized balloon is selected. The balloon is de-aired and the lumen is allowed to fill passively with contrast. The coronary guidewire is then removed through the balloon lumen and replaced with a wire specifically designed for rotational atherectomy. The balloon is removed over the wire. Balloon position is confirmed by angiography.

An appropriate-sized rotational atherectomy burr is selected and the rotational atherectomy system is assembled. A foot pedal is positioned under the table. The burr delivery unit is loaded with extreme care over the wire, as the latter is very susceptible to kinking. If kinked, the wire must be removed from the coronary and the entire process up to this point is redone. A continuous infusion to prevent no-reflow is administered. The burr is activated outside the body to test the rotational speed, and the console is used to adjust the speed to a proper level.

The burr is advanced over the wire to the coronary artery proximal to the lesion. This typically requires carefully coordinated pulling of the wire during burr advancement to overcome resistance. The burr is adjusted to remove tension from the system. The device is activated to test the rotational speed in the body and adjusted as needed. Careful monitoring of the rhythm and blood pressure is performed as bradycardia and hypotension frequently occur. Once the test is complete, the burr is activated and advanced in a gradual back and forth motion to ablate calcific plaque. Typically, the patient develops chest pain and/or electro-cardiographic changes during these "runs," which are kept short to avoid severe hypotension, bradycardia, and even heart block. Angiography is performed in between runs to assess coronary flow and to ensure no dissection or perforation. The operator must wait up to several minutes between runs to allow resolution of ischemia. Multiple runs are performed with the burr until it is able to prog-ress through the resistant lesion. Polishing runs are then performed. The burr is exchanged out over the wire. A larger burr is then selected to enlarge the lumen more optimally. The same procedure is then performed with the larger burr. After several progressively larger burrs and successful enlargement of the lumen, balloon angioplasty is typically performed to smooth out irregularities and seal any athero-matous flaps up against the vessel wall to try to prevent abrupt vessel closure.

The vessel over the course of the atherectomy procedure is irregular, hazy, with slightly impaired flow, and there is concern for dissection. A stent of appropriate diameter and length is selected. The stent is advanced over the wire to the tar-get lesion and carefully positioned. This may require placing additional coronary guidewires down the vessel to allow the stent to pass. Often the stents will not pass through the calcific vessel and additional dilation with balloon angioplasty is required.

An appropriate-sized balloon is selected. The balloon is de-aired and the lumen is allowed to fill passively with contrast. A balloon inflation device is prepared and filled with dilute contrast. The balloon is advanced over the coronary guidewire to the lesion. Balloon position is confirmed by angiography. The balloon is inflated gradually, observing for clinical and angiographic signs of ischemia, and watching for balloon deformation and appropriate balloon expansion. Typically, the patient develops chest pain and/or electrocardiographic changes that limit the duration of balloon inflation, and the balloon is quickly deflated. The balloon is reinflated several times to progressively higher atmospheres and for longer periods of time up to several minutes. The balloon is then exchanged back over the guidewire into the guide. Intracoronary vasodilators are again administered. Angiography is performed in multiple views. Once an adequate expansion is achieved, the balloon is again exchanged out of the coronary artery into the guide. Completion angiography is performed after repeat administration of intracoronary vasodilators. Inspection of the images is performed for signs of vessel dissection, perforation, or impaired coronary flow.

Now a stent can be passed through the vessel to the target lesion. The stent is deployed at high pressure. The original stent frequently does not cover the entire diseased segment and additional stents are then placed as needed using the same techniques. Next, a high-pressure, non-compliant balloon is advanced over the coronary guidewire into the stented segment and this is inflated at high pressure to ensure stent expansion. Frequently, more than one balloon of different sizes is required. The balloon is then exchanged back over the guidewire into the guide. Intracoronary vasodilators are again administered. Angiography is performed in multiple views. If the result is acceptable, the coronary wire is then withdrawn back into the guide. Completion angiography is again performed after repeat administration of intracoronary vasodilators. Inspection of the images is again performed for signs of vessel dissection, perforation, or impaired coronary flow. The guide catheter is disengaged from the coronary ostium and then removed over a guidewire from the body. Anticoagulation infusions are stopped.

Angiography of the access site is often performed through the access sheath to assess for any complications and suitability for a percutaneous closure device. The catheter and sheath are removed and hemostasis is achieved by appropriate means by the physician or technician under the physician's supervision. Observation of the site is performed to ensure no immediate bleeding, if a vascular closure device is deployed. Manual pressure is required for a short time to achieve complete hemostasis. If manual pressure is used, the sheath is typically sewn in for subsequent removal, once the ACT level falls to a safe level.

###  Clinical Example (92934)

A 72-year-old male presents with progressive angina and pharmacologic stress testing showing lateral ischemia. Coronary arteriography shows 50% lesions in the left and right coronary arteries and an 80%, 12-mm long left circumflex coronary artery lesion. An additional 12-mm long 80% lesion is noted in the large first obtuse marginal branch. The vessels are extremely heavily calcified. After discussion with the patient and the patient's family regarding therapeutic options, the patient requests coronary intervention, which is scheduled for the next day. The first lesion has been treated. Now an additional lesion is to be treated.

### Description of Procedure (92934)

The indwelling guide catheter from the first coronary intervention is removed over a guidewire. A new guide is selected to engage the second vessel. An appropriate

⊘=Modifier 51 Exempt   ⊙=Moderate Sedation   ✚=Add-on Code   𝒩=FDA approval pending

guiding catheter is inserted over the wire through the sheath into the arterial system under fluoroscopic guidance throughout the procedure. The catheter is advanced retrograde through the arterial system to the ascending aorta. The wire is removed and the catheter is attached to the pressure manifold. The guide is aspirated to remove any air, atheroma, or thrombus. Pressure is measured in the aortic root. The catheter is then manipulated using fluoroscopic guidance into the ostium of a coronary artery. Typically, the guide must be manipulated to avoid aortic atheroma and adjusted substantially to engage the artery based on the anatomy of the aorta. The arterial pressure and waveform are then checked to be sure there is no evidence of catheter malposition or impairment of coronary flow due to an ostial stenosis. Frequently, several guide catheters are required to achieve a safe catheter engagement of the artery. Test contrast injections under fluoroscopy are performed to check catheter position.

A coronary guidewire is then manipulated through the guide and down the coronary artery and carefully used to cross the target lesion. Typically, this requires manipulation of the wire in several angiographic views and often requires additional guidewires if the first wire is not successful. Guidewire position across the lesion is confirmed angiographically. The wire is adjusted as needed to ensure it is not lodged in a small distal vessel that might result in perforation or dissection. Multiple coronary injections are performed, each with the imaging system aligned in a different orientation, with simultaneous panning (moving the table) to assess the stenoses.

An appropriate-sized balloon is selected. The balloon is de-aired and the lumen is allowed to fill passively with contrast. The coronary guidewire is then removed through the balloon lumen and replaced with a wire specifically designed for rotational atherectomy. The balloon is removed over the wire. Balloon position is confirmed by angiography.

An appropriate-sized rotational atherectomy burr is selected and the rotational atherectomy system is assembled. A foot pedal is positioned under the table. The burr delivery unit is loaded with extreme care over the wire, as the latter is very susceptible to kinking. If kinked, the wire must be removed from the coronary and the entire process up to this point is redone. A continuous infusion to prevent no-reflow is administered. The burr is activated outside the body to test the rotational speed and the console is used to adjust the speed to a proper level.

The burr is advanced over the wire to the coronary artery proximal to the lesion. This typically requires carefully coordinated pulling of the wire during burr advancement to overcome resistance. The burr is adjusted to remove tension from the system. The device is activated to test the rotational speed in the body and adjusted as needed. Careful monitoring of the rhythm and blood pressure is performed as bradycardia and hypotension frequently occur. Once the test is complete, the burr is activated and advanced in a gradual back and forth motion to ablate calcific plaque. Typically, the patient develops chest pain and/or electrocardiographic changes during these "runs," which are kept short to avoid severe hypotension, bradycardia, and even heart block. Angiography is performed in between runs to assess coronary flow and to ensure no dissection or perforation.

The operator must wait up to several minutes between runs to allow resolution of ischemia. Multiple runs are performed with the burr until it is able to progress through the resistant lesion. Polishing runs are then performed. The burr is exchanged out over the wire. A larger burr is then selected to enlarge the lumen more optimally. The same procedure is then performed with the larger burr. After several progressively larger burrs and successful enlargement of the lumen, balloon angioplasty is typically performed to smooth out irregularities and seal any atheromatous flaps up against the vessel wall to try to prevent abrupt vessel closure.

The vessel over the course of the atherectomy procedure is irregular, hazy, with slightly impaired flow, and there is concern for dissection. A stent of appropriate diameter and length is selected. The stent is advanced over the wire to the target lesion and carefully positioned. This may require placing additional coronary guidewires down the vessel to allow the stent to pass. Often the stents will not pass through the calcific vessel and additional dilation with balloon angioplasty is required.

An appropriate-sized balloon is selected. The balloon is de-aired and the lumen is allowed to fill passively with contrast. A balloon inflation device is prepared and filled with dilute contrast. The balloon is advanced over the coronary guidewire to the lesion. Balloon position is confirmed by angiography. The balloon is inflated gradually, observing for clinical and angiographic signs of ischemia, and watching for balloon deformation and appropriate balloon expansion. Typically, the patient develops chest pain and/or electrocardiographic changes that limit the duration of balloon inflation, and the balloon is quickly deflated. The balloon is reinflated several times to progressively higher atmospheres and for longer periods of time up to several minutes. The balloon is then exchanged back over the guidewire into the guide. Intracoronary vasodilators are again administered. Angiography is performed in multiple views. Once an adequate expansion is achieved, the balloon is again exchanged out of the coronary artery into the guide. Completion angiography is performed after repeat administration of intracoronary vasodilators. Inspection of the images is performed for signs of vessel dissection, perforation, or impaired coronary flow.

Now a stent can be passed through the vessel to the target lesion. The stent is deployed at high pressure. The original stent frequently does not cover the entire diseased segment and additional stents are then placed as needed using the same techniques. Next, a high-pressure, non-compliant balloon is advanced over the coronary guidewire into the stented segment, and this is inflated at high pressure to ensure stent expansion. Frequently, more than one balloon of different sizes is required. The balloon is then exchanged back over the guidewire into the guide. Intracoronary vasodilators are again administered. Angiography is performed in multiple views. If the result is acceptable, the coronary wire is then withdrawn back into the guide. Completion angiography is again performed after repeat administration of intracoronary vasodilators. Inspection of the images is again performed for signs of vessel dissection, perforation, or impaired coronary flow. The guide catheter is disengaged from the coronary ostium and then removed over a guidewire from the body. Anticoagulation infusions are stopped.

⊘=Modifier 51 Exempt   ⊙=Moderate Sedation   ✚=Add-on Code   ✔=FDA approval pending

Angiography of the access site is often performed through the access sheath to assess for any complications and suitability for a percutaneous closure device. The catheter and sheath are removed and hemostasis is achieved by appropriate means by the physician or technician under the physician's supervision. Observation of the site is performed to ensure no immediate bleeding if a vascular closure device is deployed. Manual pressure is required for a short time to achieve complete hemostasis. If manual pressure is used, the sheath is typically sewn in for subsequent removal, once the activated clotting time (ACT) level falls to a safe level.

 **Clinical Example (92937)**

A 79-year-old female who had bypass surgery 10 years ago presents with unstable angina consistent with an acute coronary syndrome. Coronary arteriography demonstrates that the culprit is a saphenous vein graft to a large left circumflex coronary artery. The vein graft is diffusely diseased and has subtotal occlusion by a 3-mm long thrombus. The patient is transferred to a percutaneous coronary intervention (PCI) center for percutaneous coronary intervention on the following day. This is the first lesion in this coronary territory to be treated.

**Description of Procedure (92937)**

A "time out" occurs during which confirmation of critical information is ensured, such as the patient's identity, planned procedure, access route, allergies, completion of the consent process, availability of proper equipment, and any unusual circumstances that might influence the procedure. Conscious sedation is administered and adequate conscious sedation monitoring is verified. Percutaneous arterial access is obtained, typically through the femoral artery or radial artery. A thin-walled needle is inserted percutaneously into the peripheral artery, through which a flexible guidewire is inserted. The needle is removed over the wire, a sheath/dilator system is inserted over the guidewire, the dilator is removed, and the side-arm of the sheath is flushed to remove any clot or air. Intra-arterial vasodilators are administered to prevent arterial spasm for radial artery access. An appropriate guiding catheter is inserted over the wire through the sheath into the arterial system under fluoroscopic guidance throughout the procedure. The catheter is advanced retrograde through the arterial system to the ascending aorta. The wire is removed and the catheter is attached to the pressure manifold. The guide is aspirated to remove any air, atheroma, or thrombus. Pressure is measured in the aortic root. The catheter is then manipulated using fluoroscopic guidance into the ostium of a bypass graft. Typically, the guide must be manipulated to avoid aortic atheroma and adjusted substantially to engage the artery based on the anatomy of the aorta. The arterial pressure and waveform are then checked to be sure there is no evidence of catheter malposition or impairment of coronary flow due to an ostial stenosis. Frequently, several guide catheters are required to achieve a safe catheter engagement of the artery. Test contrast injections under fluoroscopy are performed to check catheter position.

Appropriate antiplatelet therapy pretreatment is confirmed, and additional antiplatelet therapy is administered as needed. Direct thrombin inhibitors or heparin is administered for anticoagulation. Therapeutic anticoagulation is confirmed by drawing blood from the guide and testing an activated clotting time (ACT).

Additional anticoagulation is administered as needed to achieve a therapeutic ACT. Intracoronary vasodilators are administered. Multiple coronary injections are performed, each with the imaging system aligned in a different orientation, with simultaneous panning (moving the table) to assess the stenoses.

A coronary guidewire is then manipulated through the guide and down the bypass graft and carefully used to cross the target lesion. Typically, this requires manipulation of the wire in several angiographic views and often requires additional guidewires if the first wire is not successful. Guidewire position across the lesion is confirmed angiographically. The wire is adjusted as needed to ensure it is not lodged in a small distal vessel that might result in perforation or dissection. A proximal or distal protection device is then advanced down the graft over the coronary guidewire to capture embolic debris and help prevent no-reflow. The device is carefully positioned to avoid vessel disruption and to avoid interference with intervention at the target lesion. Microvascular vasodilators are administered through the graft to help prevent no-reflow. Multiple injections are performed, each with the imaging system aligned in a different orientation, with simultaneous panning (moving the table) to assess the stenoses.

The patient's ability to tolerate long-term dual antiplatelet therapy and to comply with this therapy is again confirmed. A stent of appropriate diameter and length is selected. The stent is advanced over the wire to the target lesion and carefully positioned. This may require placing additional coronary guidewires down the vessel to allow the stent to pass. As the lesion has generally not been predilated (so as to avoid embolization) positioning of the stent across the lesion often precipitates severe ischemia requiring therapy. If the stent cannot be advanced across the lesion, then the stent is removed, the lesion is predilated with angioplasty, and the stent is repositioned. The stent is deployed at high pressure. The original stent frequently does not cover the entire diseased segment and additional stents are then placed as needed using the same techniques. There is no-reflow characterized by severe ischemia, slow flow down the vessel, and electrocardiographic changes. Microvascular vasodilators are administered again, and if there is no resolution, an aspiration catheter is advanced down into the graft and debris is aspirated to restore flow. Once adequate flow is restored, assessment for the need for further balloon expansion is performed.

If needed, an appropriate-sized balloon is selected. The balloon is de-aired and the lumen is allowed to fill passively with contrast. A balloon inflation device is prepared and filled with dilute contrast. The balloon is advanced over the coronary guidewire to the lesion. Balloon position is confirmed by angiography. The balloon is inflated gradually, observing for clinical and angiographic signs of ischemia, and watching for balloon deformation and appropriate balloon expansion. Typically, the patient develops chest pain and/or electrocardiographic changes that limit the duration of balloon inflation, and the balloon is quickly deflated. The balloon is reinflated several times to progressively higher atmospheres and for longer periods of time up to several minutes. The balloon is then exchanged back over the guidewire into the guide. Intracoronary vasodilators are again administered. If the result is acceptable, the proximal or distal protection device is then removed. Often the removal catheter must be manipulated by multiple passes to cross through the stents to reach the protection device in the case of a distal protection device. Completion angiography is again performed after repeat administration of intracoronary vasodilators. Inspection of the images is again performed for signs of vessel dissection, perforation, or impaired coronary flow. The guide catheter is disengaged from the coronary ostium and then removed over a guidewire from the body. Anticoagulation infusions are stopped.

Angiography of the access site is often performed through the access sheath to assess for any complications and suitability for a percutaneous closure device. The catheter and sheath are removed and hemostasis is achieved by appropriate means by the physician or technician under the physician's supervision. Observation of the site is performed to ensure no immediate bleeding if a vascular closure device is deployed. Manual pressure is required for a short time to achieve complete hemostasis. If manual pressure is used, the sheath is typically sewn in for subsequent removal, once the ACT level falls to a safe level.

 **Clinical Example (92938)**

A 79-year-old female who had bypass surgery 10 years ago presents with unstable angina consistent with an acute coronary syndrome. Coronary arteriography demonstrates that the culprit is a saphenous vein graft to a large left circumflex coronary artery. The vein graft is diffusely diseased and has subtotal occlusion by a 3-mm long thrombus. The subtended left circumflex coronary artery gives off a large obtuse marginal branch with a 90% hazy lesion that is 20 mm long. The patient is transferred to a percutaneous coronary intervention (PCI) center for percutaneous coronary intervention the following day. The first lesion has been treated. Now an additional lesion is to be treated.

### Description of Procedure (92938)

Therapeutic anticoagulation is confirmed by drawing blood from the guide and testing an activated clotting time (ACT). Additional anticoagulation is administered as needed to achieve a therapeutic ACT. Intracoronary vasodilators are administered. Multiple coronary injections are performed, each with the imaging system aligned in a different orientation, with simultaneous panning (moving the table) to assess the stenosis.

A coronary guidewire is manipulated from its initial position and across the target lesion. This may require entirely removing the wire and reshaping the tip, or starting with a new wire and passing it through the graft. Typically, this requires manipulation of the wire in several angiographic views and often requires additional guidewires if the first wire is not successful. Guidewire position across the lesion is confirmed angiographically. The wire is adjusted as needed to ensure it is not lodged in a small distal vessel that might result in perforation or dissection. If appropriate, a proximal or distal protection device is then advanced down the graft over the coronary guidewire to capture embolic debris and help prevent no-reflow. The device is carefully positioned to avoid vessel disruption and to avoid interference with intervention at the target lesion. Microvascular vasodilators are administered through the graft to help prevent no-reflow. Multiple injections are performed, each with the imaging system aligned in a different orientation, with simultaneous panning (moving the table) to assess the stenoses.

A stent of appropriate diameter and length is selected. The stent is advanced over the wire to the target lesion and carefully positioned. This may require placing additional coronary guidewires down the vessel to allow the stent to pass. As the lesion has generally not been predilated (so as to avoid embolization), positioning of the stent across the lesion often precipitates severe ischemia requiring therapy. If the stent cannot be advanced across the lesion, the stent is removed, the lesion is predilated with angioplasty, and the stent is repositioned. The stent is deployed at high pressure. The original stent frequently does not cover the entire diseased segment and additional stents are then placed as needed using the same techniques. There is no-reflow characterized by severe ischemia, slow flow down the vessel, and electrocardiographic changes. Microvascular vasodilators are administered again, and if there is no resolution, an aspiration catheter is advanced down into the graft and debris is aspirated to restore flow. Once adequate flow is restored, assessment for the need for further balloon expansion is performed. If needed, an appropriate-sized balloon is selected. The balloon is de-aired and the lumen is allowed to fill passively with contrast. A balloon inflation device is prepared and filled with dilute contrast. The balloon is advanced over the coronary guidewire to the lesion. Balloon position is confirmed by angiography. The balloon is inflated gradually, observing for clinical and angiographic signs of ischemia, and watching for balloon deformation and appropriate balloon expansion. Typically, the patient develops chest pain and/or electrocardiographic changes that limit the duration of balloon inflation, and the balloon is quickly deflated. The balloon is reinflated several times to progressively higher atmospheres and for longer periods of time up to several minutes. The balloon is then exchanged back over the guidewire into the guide. Intracoronary vasodilators are again administered. If the result is acceptable, the proximal or distal protection device is then removed. Often the removal catheter must be manipulated by multiple passes to cross through the stents to reach the protection device in the case of a distal protection device. Completion angiography is again performed after repeat administration of intracoronary vasodilators. Inspection of the images is again performed for signs of vessel dissection, perforation, or impaired coronary flow. The guide catheter is disengaged from the coronary ostium and then removed over a guidewire from the body. Anticoagulation infusions are stopped.

Angiography of the access site is often performed through the access sheath to assess for any complications and suitability for a percutaneous closure device. The catheter and sheath are removed and hemostasis is achieved by appropriate means by the physician or technician under the physician's supervision. Observation of the site is performed to ensure no immediate bleeding if a vascular closure device is deployed. Manual pressure is required for a short time to achieve complete hemostasis. If manual pressure is used, the sheath is typically sewn in for subsequent removal, once the ACT level falls to a safe level.

 **Clinical Example (92941)**

A 56-year-old male calls 911 for sudden onset of crushing substernal chest pain. Pre-hospital 12-lead electrocardiography in the ambulance demonstrates acute anterior myocardial infarction with ST elevation in leads V2-V5. The heart attack alert system is activated. The emergency medical personnel bypass the emergency

⊘=Modifier 51 Exempt  ⊙=Moderate Sedation  ✚=Add-on Code  𝑵=FDA approval pending

department and take the patient directly to the cardiac catheterization laboratory, arriving within 50 minutes of symptom onset. After rapid assessment, immediate coronary angiography is performed (reported separately), demonstrating 100% occlusion by a large thrombus in the middle segment of the left anterior descending artery. The patient demonstrates runs of non-sustained ventricular tachycardia. Percutaneous coronary intervention is planned immediately with the goal of achieving first medical contact-to-balloon time of under 90 minutes. This is the first lesion in this coronary territory to be treated.

### Description of Procedure (92941)

A "time out" is rapidly performed and confirmation of critical information is ensured, such as the patient's identity, planned procedure, access route, allergies, completion of the consent process, availability of proper equipment, and any unusual circumstances that might influence the procedure. Conscious sedation is administered and adequate conscious sedation monitoring is verified. Percutaneous arterial access is rapidly obtained, typically through the femoral artery or radial artery. Often the pulse is rapid and thread in the setting of hypotension and access is frequently difficult as a result. A thin-walled needle is inserted percutaneously into the peripheral artery, through which a flexible guidewire is inserted. The needle is removed over the wire, a sheath/dilator system is inserted over the guidewire, the dilator is removed, and the sidearm of the sheath is flushed to remove any clot or air. Intra-arterial vasodilators are administered to prevent arterial spasm for radial artery access.

After diagnostic coronary angiography to identify the culprit lesion (reported separately), an appropriate guiding catheter is inserted over the wire through the sheath into the arterial system under fluoroscopic guidance throughout the procedure. The catheter is advanced retrograde through the arterial system to the ascending aorta. The wire is removed and the catheter is attached to the pressure manifold. The guide is aspirated to remove any air, atheroma, or thrombus. Pressure is measured in the aortic root. The catheter is then manipulated using fluoroscopic guidance into the ostium of a coronary artery. Typically, the guide must be manipulated to avoid aortic atheroma and adjusted substantially to engage the artery based on the anatomy of the aorta. The arterial pressure and waveform are then checked to be sure there is no evidence of catheter malposition or impairment of coronary flow due to an ostial stenosis. Frequently, several guide catheters are required to achieve a safe catheter engagement of the artery. Test contrast injections under fluoroscopy are performed to check catheter position.

Appropriate antiplatelet therapy pretreatment is confirmed, and additional antiplatelet therapy is administered as needed. Direct thrombin inhibitors or heparin is administered for anticoagulation. Therapeutic anticoagulation is confirmed by drawing blood from the guide and testing an activated clotting time (ACT). Additional anticoagulation is administered as needed to achieve a therapeutic ACT. Intracoronary vasodilators are administered.

A coronary guidewire is then manipulated through the guide and down the coronary artery and carefully used to cross the target lesion. Typically, this requires manipulation of the wire in several angiographic views and often requires additional guidewires, if the first wire is not successful. Guidewire position across the lesion is confirmed angiographically. The wire is adjusted as needed to ensure it is not lodged in a small distal vessel that might result in perforation or dissection. Brief angiography confirms intraluminal position of the guidewire. There is no flow down the vessel and the patient is typically in severe pain. An appropriate aspiration catheter is selected and rapidly advanced to the occluded vessel and thrombus is aspirated. Multiple rounds of intracoronary microvascular vasodilators are administered. Frequently, reperfusion arrhythmias occur, requiring additional pharmacologic management. Hypotension frequently requires titration of pressor agents. Antegrade coronary flow is restored, but there is globular thrombus superimposed on a critical residual lesion. Intracoronary antiplatelet agents are infused to help resolve the thrombus.

An appropriate-sized balloon is selected. The balloon is de-aired and the lumen is allowed to fill passively with contrast. A balloon inflation device is prepared and filled with dilute contrast. The balloon is advanced over the coronary guidewire to the lesion. Balloon position is confirmed by angiography. The balloon is inflated gradually, observing for clinical and angiographic signs of ischemia, and watching for balloon deformation and appropriate balloon expansion. Typically, the patient develops chest pain and/or electrocardiographic changes that limit the duration of balloon inflation, and the balloon is quickly deflated. The balloon is reinflated several times to progressively higher atmospheres and for longer periods of time up to several minutes. The balloon is then exchanged back over the guidewire into the guide. Intracoronary vasodilators are again administered. Angiography is performed in multiple views. The lesion is not fully expanded and the angioplasty procedure is repeated multiple times with progressively larger balloons. Once an adequate expansion is achieved to allow stent deployment, the balloon is again exchanged out of the coronary artery into the guide. Completion angiography is performed after repeat administration of intracoronary vasodilators. Inspection of the images is performed for signs of vessel dissection, perforation, or impaired coronary flow.

The patient's ability to tolerate long-term dual antiplatelet therapy and to comply with this therapy is again confirmed. A stent of appropriate diameter and length is selected. The stent is advanced over the wire to the target lesion and carefully positioned. This may require placing additional coronary guidewires down the vessel to allow the stent to pass. The stent is deployed at high pressure. The original stent frequently does not cover the entire diseased segment, and additional stents are then placed as needed using the same techniques. Next, a high-pressure, non-compliant balloon is advanced over the coronary guidewire into the stented segment, and this is inflated at high pressure to ensure stent expansion. Frequently, more than one balloon of different sizes is required. Frequently, there is some degree of no-reflow requiring additional microvascular vasodilators to resolve. Frequently, there is evidence of thrombotic embolization to distal vessels beyond the original lesion. This requires additional balloon dilation and aspiration thrombectomy at the site of the thrombus to resolve. Frequently, there is ongoing hemodynamic instability and electrical instability requiring additional pharmacologic therapy. The balloon is then exchanged back over the guidewire into the guide. Intracoronary vasodilators are again administered. Angiography is performed in multiple views. If the result is acceptable, the coronary wire is then withdrawn back into the guide. Completion angiography is again performed after repeat administration of intracoronary vasodilators. Inspection of the images is again performed for signs of vessel dissection, perforation, or impaired coronary flow. The guide catheter is disengaged from the coronary ostium and then removed over a guidewire from the body. Anticoagulation infusions are stopped.

Angiography of the access site is often performed through the access sheath to assess for any complications and suitability for a percutaneous closure device. The catheter and sheath are removed and hemostasis is achieved by appropriate means by the physician or technician under the physician's supervision. Observation of the site is performed to ensure no immediate bleeding if a vascular closure device is deployed. Manual pressure is required for a short time to achieve complete hemostasis. If manual pressure is used, the sheath is typically sewn in for subsequent removal, once the ACT level falls to a safe level.

 **Clinical Example (92943)**

A 72-year-old female presents with six months of exertional angina. Coronary angiography shows 100% left circumflex coronary stenosis. The lesion is on a bend in the circumflex coronary artery with focal calcification at the site and has antegrade bridging collaterals to the distal vessel, consistent with a chronic total occlusion. After a two-week trial of two antianginal agents, the patient is not satisfied with her quality of life and requests coronary intervention. This is the first lesion in this coronary territory to be treated.

**Description of Procedure (92943)**

A "time out" occurs during which confirmation of critical information is ensured, such as the patient's identity, planned procedure, access route, allergies, completion of the consent process, availability of proper equipment, and any unusual circumstances that might influence the procedure. Conscious sedation is administered and adequate conscious sedation monitoring is verified. Percutaneous arterial access is obtained, typically through the femoral artery or radial artery. A thin-walled needle is inserted percutaneously into the peripheral artery, through which a flexible guidewire is inserted. The needle is removed over the wire, a sheath/ dilator system is inserted over the guidewire, the dilator is removed, and the side-arm of the sheath is flushed to remove any clot or air. Intra-arterial vasodilators are administered to prevent arterial spasm for radial artery access. An appropriate guiding catheter is inserted over the wire through the sheath into the arterial system under fluoroscopic guidance throughout the procedure. The catheter is advanced retrograde through the arterial system to the ascending aorta. The wire is removed and the catheter is attached to the pressure manifold. The guide is aspirated to remove any air, atheroma, or thrombus. Pressure is measured in the aortic root. The catheter is then manipulated using fluoroscopic guidance into the ostium of a coronary artery. Typically, the guide must be manipulated to avoid aortic atheroma and adjusted substantially to engage the artery based on the anatomy of the aorta. The arterial pressure and waveform are then checked to be sure there is no evidence of catheter malposition or impairment of coronary flow due to an ostial stenosis. Frequently, several guide catheters are required to achieve a safe catheter engagement of the artery. Test contrast injections under fluoroscopy are performed to check catheter position.

Appropriate antiplatelet therapy pretreatment is confirmed, and additional antiplatelet therapy is administered as needed. Direct thrombin inhibitors or heparin is administered for anticoagulation. Therapeutic anticoagulation is confirmed by drawing blood from the guide and testing an activated clotting time (ACT). Additional anticoagulation is administered as needed to achieve a therapeutic ACT. Intracoronary vasodilators are administered. Multiple coronary injections are performed, each with the imaging system aligned in a different orientation, with simultaneous panning (moving the table) to assess the stenoses.

A coronary guidewire is then manipulated through the guide and down the coronary artery and carefully used to attempt to cross the target lesion. Typically, this requires manipulation of the wire in several angiographic views. Typically, crossing of the total occlusion with generic guidewires is unsuccessful. Typically, the operator uses additional guidewires progressing to increasingly stiff, guidewires in order to puncture through the chronic total occlusion, or more lubricious or tapered tip are used to engage and cross a microchannel. Guidewire position across the lesion is confirmed angiographically. Frequently, the wire is extraluminal and left in position while additional are used to reattempt crossing of the total occlusion. If crossing of the total occlusion is eventually achieved successfully, and the wire is intraluminal distally, the wire is adjusted as needed to ensure it is not lodged in a small distal vessel that might result in perforation or dissection. Multiple coronary injections are performed, each with the imaging system aligned in a different orientation, with simultaneous panning (moving the table) to assess the stenoses.

An appropriate-sized balloon is selected. The balloon is de-aired and the lumen is allowed to fill passively with contrast. A balloon inflation device is prepared and filled with dilute contrast. The balloon is advanced over the coronary guidewire to the lesion. Often no balloon will cross the rigid total occlusion. Specialty devices may be employed to screw or "Dotter" through the rigid total occlusion. Rotational atherectomy may be attempted to ablate the rigid material at the total occlusion site. If crossing is eventually achieved, an angioplasty balloon position is confirmed by angiography. The balloon is inflated gradually, observing for clinical and angiographic signs of ischemia, and watching for balloon deformation and appropriate balloon expansion. The patient may develop chest pain and/or electrocardiographic changes that limit the duration of balloon inflation, and the balloon is quickly deflated. The balloon is reinflated several times to progressively higher atmospheres and for longer periods of time up to several minutes. The balloon is then exchanged back over the guidewire into the guide. Intracoronary vasodilators are again administered. Angiography is performed in multiple views. The lesion is not fully expanded and the angioplasty procedure is repeated multiple times with progressively larger balloons. Once an adequate expansion is achieved to allow stent deployment, the balloon is again exchanged out of the coronary artery into the guide. Completion angiography is performed after repeat administration of intracoronary vasodilators. Inspection of the images is performed for signs of vessel dissection, perforation, or impaired coronary flow. Frequently, there is evidence of

Ⓢ=Modifier 51 Exempt   ⊙=Moderate Sedation   ✚=Add-on Code   𝑵=FDA approval pending

dissection from the recanalization of the total occlusion, and frequently, additional lesions are now evident in the vessel. In the event of a vessel perforation, emergent echocardiogram may be requested and pericardiocentesis, volume resuscitation, and vasopressors may be required to stabilize the patient.

The patient's ability to tolerate long-term dual antiplatelet therapy and to comply with this therapy is again confirmed. A stent of appropriate diameter and length is selected. The stent is advanced over the wire to the target lesion and carefully positioned. Frequently, the stent will not cross due to rigidity of the lesion. This may require placing additional coronary guidewires down the vessel, placement of a more aggressive guiding catheter, or more balloon dilation to allow the stent to pass. The stent is deployed at high pressure. The original stent frequently does not cover the entire diseased/dissected segment and additional stents are then placed as needed using the same techniques. Next, a high-pressure, non-compliant balloon is advanced over the coronary guidewire into the stented segment and this is inflated at high pressure to ensure stent expansion. Frequently, more than one balloon of different sizes is required. The balloon is then exchanged back over the guidewire into the guide. Intracoronary vasodilators are again administered. Angiography is performed in multiple views. If the result is acceptable, the coronary wire is then withdrawn back into the guide. Completion angiography is again performed after repeat administration of intracoronary vasodilators. Inspection of the images is again performed for signs of vessel dissection, perforation, or impaired coronary flow. The guide catheter is disengaged from the coronary ostium and then removed over a guidewire from the body. Anticoagulation infusions are stopped.

Angiography of the access site is often performed through the access sheath to assess for any complications and suitability for a percutaneous closure device. The catheter and sheath are removed and hemostasis is achieved by appropriate means by the physician or technician under the physician's supervision. Observation of the site is performed to ensure no immediate bleeding if a vascular closure device is deployed. Manual pressure is required for a short time to achieve complete hemostasis. If manual pressure is used, the sheath is typically sewn in for subsequent removal, once the ACT level falls to a safe level.

 **Clinical Example (92944)**

A 68-year-old male presents with a three-year history of stable angina. Stress testing shows inferior ischemia but no myocardial infarction. Coronary arteriography demonstrates 100% mid-right coronary occlusion with left-to-right collaterals to the distal vessel. The occluded segment is about 20 mm long and appears straight with focal calcification at the lesion site consistent with a chronic total occlusion. In the posterior descending, there is an additional occluded segment that is about 20 mm long and appears straight with focal calcification at the lesion site consistent with a chronic total occlusion. After a two-week trial of two antianginal agents, the patient is not satisfied with his quality of life and requests coronary intervention. The first lesion has been treated. Now an additional lesion is to be treated.

**Description of Procedure (92944)**

A "time out" occurs during which confirmation of critical information is ensured, such as the patient's identity, planned procedure, access route, allergies, completion of the consent process, availability of proper equipment, and any unusual circumstances that might influence the procedure. Conscious sedation is administered and adequate conscious sedation monitoring is verified. Percutaneous arterial access is obtained, typically through the femoral artery or radial artery. A thin-walled needle is inserted percutaneously into the peripheral artery, through which a flexible guidewire is inserted. The needle is removed over the wire, a sheath/dilator system is inserted over the guidewire, the dilator is removed, and the side-arm of the sheath is flushed to remove any clot or air. Intra-arterial vasodilators are administered to prevent arterial spasm for radial artery access. An appropriate guiding catheter is inserted over the wire through the sheath into the arterial system under fluoroscopic guidance throughout the procedure. The catheter is advanced retrograde through the arterial system to the ascending aorta. The wire is removed and the catheter is attached to the pressure manifold. The guide is aspirated to remove any air, atheroma, or thrombus. Pressure is measured in the aortic root. The catheter is then manipulated using fluoroscopic guidance into the ostium of a coronary artery. Typically, the guide must be manipulated to avoid aortic atheroma and adjusted substantially to engage the artery based on the anatomy of the aorta. The arterial pressure and waveform are then checked to be sure there is no evidence of catheter malposition or impairment of coronary flow due to an ostial stenosis. Frequently, several guide catheters are required to achieve a safe catheter engagement of the artery. Test contrast injections under fluoroscopy are performed to check catheter position.

Appropriate antiplatelet therapy pretreatment is confirmed, and additional antiplatelet therapy is administered as needed. Direct thrombin inhibitors or heparin is administered for anticoagulation. Therapeutic anticoagulation is confirmed by drawing blood from the guide and testing an activated clotting time (ACT). Additional anticoagulation is administered as needed to achieve a therapeutic ACT. Intracoronary vasodilators are administered. Multiple coronary injections are performed, each with the imaging system aligned in a different orientation, with simultaneous panning (moving the table) to assess the stenoses.

A coronary guidewire is then manipulated through the guide and down the coronary artery and carefully used to attempt to cross the target lesion. Typically, this requires manipulation of the wire in several angiographic views. Typically, crossing of the total occlusion with generic guidewires is unsuccessful. Typically, the operator uses additional guidewires progressing to increasingly stiffer guidewires in order to puncture through the chronic total occlusion, or more lubricious or tapered tips are used to engage and cross a microchannel. Guidewire position across the lesion is confirmed angiographically. Frequently, the wire is extraluminal and left in position while additional guidewires are used to reattempt crossing of the total occlusion. If crossing of the total occlusion is eventually achieved successfully, and the wire is intraluminal distally, the wire is adjusted as needed to ensure it is not lodged in a small distal vessel that might result in perforation or dissection. Multiple coronary injections are performed, each with the imaging system aligned in a different orientation, with simultaneous panning (moving the table) to assess the stenoses.

An appropriate-sized balloon is selected. The balloon is de-aired and the lumen is allowed to fill passively with contrast. A balloon inflation device is prepared and filled with dilute contrast. The balloon is advanced over the coronary guidewire to the lesion. Often no balloon will cross the rigid total occlusion. Specialty devices may be employed to screw or "Dotter" through the rigid total occlusion. Rotational atherectomy may be attempted to ablate the rigid material at the total occlusion site. If crossing is eventually achieved, an angioplasty balloon position is confirmed by angiography. The balloon is inflated gradually, observing for clinical and angiographic signs of ischemia, and watching for balloon deformation and appropriate balloon expansion. The patient may develop chest pain and/or electrocardiographic changes that limit the duration of balloon inflation, and the balloon is quickly deflated. The balloon is reinflated several times to progressively higher atmospheres and for longer periods of time up to several minutes. The balloon is then exchanged back over the guidewire into the guide. Intracoronary vasodilators are again administered. Angiography is performed in multiple views. The lesion is not fully expanded and the angioplasty procedure is repeated multiple times with progressively larger balloons. Once an adequate expansion is achieved to allow stent deployment, the balloon is again exchanged out of the coronary artery into the guide. Completion angiography is performed after repeat administration of intracoronary vasodilators. Inspection of the images is performed for signs of vessel dissection, perforation, or impaired coronary flow. Frequently, there is evidence of dissection from the recanalization of the total occlusion, and frequently, additional lesions are now evident in the vessel. In the event of a vessel perforation, emergent echocardiogram may be requested and pericardiocentesis, volume resuscitation, and vasopressors may be required to stabilize the patient.

The patient's ability to tolerate long-term dual antiplatelet therapy and to comply with this therapy is again confirmed. A stent of appropriate diameter and length is selected. The stent is advanced over the wire to the target lesion and carefully positioned. Frequently, the stent will not cross due to rigidity of the lesion. This may require placing additional coronary guidewires down the vessel, placement of a more aggressive guiding catheter, or more balloon dilation to allow the stent to pass. The stent is deployed at high pressure. The original stent frequently does not cover the entire diseased/dissected segment, and additional stents are then placed as needed using the same techniques. Next, a high-pressure, non-compliant balloon is advanced over the coronary guidewire into the stented segment, and this is inflated at high pressure to ensure stent expansion. Frequently, more than one balloon of different sizes is required. The balloon is then exchanged back over the guidewire into the guide. Intracoronary vasodilators are again administered. Angiography is performed in multiple views. If the result is acceptable, the coronary wire is then withdrawn back into the guide. Completion angiography is again performed after repeat administration of intracoronary vasodilators. Inspection of the images is again performed for signs of vessel dissection, perforation, or impaired coronary flow. The guide catheter is disengaged from the coronary ostium and then removed over a guidewire from the body. Anticoagulation infusions are stopped.

Angiography of the access site is often performed through the access sheath to assess for any complications and suitability for a percutaneous closure device. The catheter and sheath are removed and hemostasis is achieved by appropriate means by the physician or technician under the physician's supervision. Observation of the site is performed to ensure no immediate bleeding if a vascular closure device is deployed. Manual pressure is required for a short time to achieve complete hemostasis. If manual pressure is used, the sheath is typically sewn in for subsequent removal, once the ACT level falls to a safe level.

## Cardiography

Codes 93040-93042 are appropriate when an order for the test is triggered by an event, the rhythm strip is used to help diagnose the presence or absence of an arrhythmia, and a report is generated. There must be a specific order for an electrocardiogram or rhythm strip followed by a separate, signed, written, and retrievable report. It is not appropriate to use these codes for reviewing the telemetry monitor strips taken from a monitoring system. The need for an electrocardiogram or rhythm strip should be supported by documentation in the patient medical record.

(For echocardiography, see 93303-93350)

▶(For electrocardiogram, 64 leads or greater, with graphic presentation and analysis, use 93799)◀

 **Rationale**

The second parenthetical note following the Cardiography-head was inadvertently revised to include code 93799. This parenthetical note should have retained codes 0178T-0180T as the appropriate codes to use to report an electrocardiogram, 64 leads or greater, with graphic presentation and analysis. This correction will be included in the 2013 CPT errata document and posted to the AMA CPT Web site (www.ama-assn.org/ama/pub/physician-resources/solutions-managing-your-practice/coding-billing-insurance/cpt/about-cpt/errata.page).

## Cardiovascular Monitoring Services

▲93224 External electrocardiographic recording up to 48 hours by continuous rhythm recording and storage; includes recording, scanning analysis with report, review and interpretation by a physician or other qualified health care professional

93225  recording (includes connection, recording, and disconnection)

93226  scanning analysis with report

  ⊘=Modifier 51 Exempt ⊙=Moderate Sedation ✦=Add-on Code 𝒩=FDA approval pending

▲93227        review and interpretation by a physician or other qualified health care professional

(For less than 12 hours of continuous recording, use modifier 52)

▶(For greater than 48 hours of monitoring, see Category III codes 0295T-0298T)◀

 **Rationale**

In support of the new Category III codes 0295T-0298T for reporting external electrocardiographic recording for more than 48 hours up to 21 days, a cross-reference parenthetical note was added following codes 93224-93227 to direct users to codes 0295T-0298T for monitoring of more than 48 hours (See Category III Section). See also discussion on CPT nomenclature reporting neutrality.

## Cardiac Catheterization

Cardiac catheterization is a diagnostic medical procedure which includes introduction, positioning and repositioning, when necessary, of catheter(s), within the vascular system, recording of intracardiac and/or intravascular pressure(s), and final evaluation and report of procedure. There are two code families for cardiac catheterization: one for congenital heart disease and one for all other conditions. Anomalous coronary arteries, patent foramen ovale, mitral valve prolapse, and bicuspid aortic valve are to be reported with 93451-93464, 93566-93568.

▶Right heart catheterization includes catheter placement in one or more right-sided cardiac chamber(s) or structures (ie, the right atrium, right ventricle, pulmonary artery, pulmonary wedge), obtaining blood samples for measurement of blood gases, and cardiac output measurements (Fick or other method), when performed. Left heart catheterization involves catheter placement in a left-sided (systemic) cardiac chamber(s) (left ventricle or left atrium) and includes left ventricular injection(s) when performed. Do not report 93503 in conjunction with other diagnostic cardiac catheterization codes. When right heart catheterization is performed in conjunction with other cardiac catheterization services, report 93453, 93456, 93457, 93460, or 93461. For placement of a flow directed catheter (eg, Swan-Ganz) performed for hemodynamic monitoring purposes not in conjunction with other catheterization services, use 93503. Right heart catheterization does not include right ventricular or right atrial angiography (93566). When left heart catheterization is performed using either transapical puncture of the left ventricle or transseptal puncture of an intact septum, report 93462 in conjunction with 93452, 93453, 93458-93461, 93653, 93654. Catheter placement(s) in coronary artery(ies) involves selective engagement of the origins of the native coronary artery(ies) for the purpose of coronary angiography. Catheter placement(s) in bypass graft(s) (venous, internal mammary, free arterial graft[s]) involve selective engagement of the origins of the graft(s) for the purpose of bypass angiography. It is typically performed only in conjunction with coronary angiography of native vessels.◀

The cardiac catheterization codes (93452-93461), other than those for congenital heart disease, include contrast injection(s), imaging supervision, interpretation, and report for imaging typically performed. Codes for left heart catheterization (93452, 93453, 93458-93461), other than those for congenital heart disease, include intraprocedural injection(s) for left ventricular/left atrial angiography, imaging supervision, and interpretation, when performed. Codes for coronary catheter placement(s) (93454-93461), other than those for congenital heart disease, include intraprocedural injection(s) for coronary angiography, imaging supervision, and interpretation. Codes for catheter placement(s) in bypass graft(s) (93455, 93457, 93459, 93461), other than those for congenital heart disease, include intraprocedural injection(s) for bypass graft angiography, imaging supervision, and interpretation. Do not report 93563-93565 in conjunction with 93452-93461.

For cardiac catheterization for congenital cardiac anomalies, see 93530-93533. When contrast injection(s) are performed in conjunction with cardiac catheterization for congenital anomalies, see 93563-93568.

Cardiac catheterization (93451-93461) includes all roadmapping angiography in order to place the catheters, including any injections and imaging supervision, interpretation, and report. It does not include contrast injection(s) and imaging supervision, interpretation, and report for imaging that is separately identified by specific procedure code(s). For right ventricular or right atrial angiography performed in conjunction with cardiac catheterization for congenital or noncongenital heart disease (93451-93461, 93530-93533), use 93566. For aortography, use 93567. For pulmonary angiography, use 93568. For angiography of noncoronary arteries and veins, performed as a distinct service, use appropriate codes from the Radiology section and the Vascular Injection Procedures section.

►When cardiac catheterization is combined with pharmacologic agent administration with the specific purpose of repeating hemodynamic measurements to evaluate hemodynamic response, use 93463 in conjunction with 93451-93453 and 93456-93461. Do not report 93463 for intracoronary administration of pharmacologic agents during percutaneous coronary interventional procedures, during intracoronary assessment of coronary pressure, flow or resistance, or during intracoronary imaging procedures. Do not report 93463 in conjunction with 92920-92944, 92975, 92977.◄

When cardiac catheterization is combined with exercise (eg, walking or arm or leg ergometry protocol) with the specific purpose of repeating hemodynamic measurements to evaluate hemodynamic response, report 93464 in conjunction with 93451-93453, 93456-93461, and 93530-93533.

⊙+ **93462**   Left heart catheterization by transseptal puncture through intact septum or by transapical puncture (List separately in addition to code for primary procedure)

►(Use 93462 in conjunction with 93452, 93453, 93458-93461, 93653, 93654)◄

►(Do not report 93462 in conjunction with 93656)◄

⊙+ **93463**   Pharmacologic agent administration (eg, inhaled nitric oxide, intravenous infusion of nitroprusside, dobutamine, milrinone, or other agent) including assessing hemodynamic measurements before, during, after and repeat pharmacologic agent administration, when performed (List separately in addition to code for primary procedure)

►(Use 93463 in conjunction with 93451-93453, 93456-93461, 93563, 93564, 93580, 93581)◄

(Report 93463 only once per catheterization procedure)

►(Do not report 93463 for pharmacologic agent administration in conjunction with coronary interventional procedure codes 92920-92944, 92975, 92977)◄

 **Rationale**

In support of the percutaneous coronary intervention changes, the Cardiac Catheterization guidelines have been revised to instruct users not to report pharmacologic agent administration code 93463 with codes 92920-92944. The third parenthetical note following code 93463 has also been revised by replacing the deleted codes 92980, 92982, and 92995 with new codes 92920-92944. Another revision occurred in the second paragraph of the guidelines with the removal of

⊘=Modifier 51 Exempt   ⊙=Moderate Sedation   ✚=Add-on Code   ✚=FDA approval pending

deleted codes 93651 and 93652 and replaced with new codes 93653 and 93654 in the list of codes that can be reported in conjunction with code 93462, when left heart catheterization is performed using either transapical puncture of the left ventricle or transseptal puncture of an intact septum

In support of the changes to the Intracardiac Electrophysiological Procedures/ Studies section, the Cardiac Catheterization guidelines and the parenthetical note following code 93462 have been revised: codes 93561 and 93652 have been removed, and codes 93653 and 93654 have been added. In addition, an exclusionary parenthetical note was added restricting the use of code 93462 with code 93656.

Lastly, the parenthetical note following pharmacologic agent administration code 93463 has been revised with the addition of percutaneous transcatheter congenital defect closure codes 93580 and 93581.

## ►INJECTION PROCEDURES◄

⊙+ **93563**    Injection procedure during cardiac catheterization including imaging supervision, interpretation, and report; for selective coronary angiography during congenital heart catheterization (List separately in addition to code for primary procedure)

⊙+ **93564**    for selective opacification of aortocoronary venous or arterial bypass graft(s) (eg, aortocoronary saphenous vein, free radial artery, or free mammary artery graft) to one or more coronary arteries and in situ arterial conduits (eg, internal mammary), whether native or used for bypass to one or more coronary arteries during congenital heart catheterization, when performed (List separately in addition to code for primary procedure)

⊙+ **93565**    for selective left ventricular or left atrial angiography (List separately in addition to code for primary procedure)

(Do not report 93563-93565 in conjunction with 93452-93461)

(Use 93563-93565 in conjunction with 93530-93533)

⊙+ **93566**    for selective right ventricular or right atrial angiography (List separately in addition to code for primary procedure)

►(Use 93566 in conjunction with 93451, 93453, 93456, 93457, 93460, 93461, 93530-93533)◄

⊙+ **93567**    for supravalvular aortography (List separately in addition to code for primary procedure)

►(Use 93567 in conjunction with 93451-93461, 93530-93533)◄

►(For non-supravalvular thoracic aortography or abdominal aortography performed at the time of cardiac catheterization, use the appropriate radiological supervision and interpretation codes [36221, 75600-75630])◄

⊙+ **93568**    for pulmonary angiography (List separately in addition to code for primary procedure)

►(Use 93568 in conjunction with 93451, 93453, 93456, 93457, 93460, 93461, 93530-93533)◄

⊙**+93571**    Intravascular Doppler velocity and/or pressure derived coronary flow reserve measurement (coronary vessel or graft) during coronary angiography including pharmacologically induced stress; initial vessel (List separately in addition to code for primary procedure)

▶(Use 93571 in conjunction with 92920, 92924, 92928, 92933, 92937, 92941, 92943, 92975, 93454-93461, 93563, 93564)◀

⊙**+93572**    each additional vessel (List separately in addition to code for primary procedure)

▶(Use 93572 in conjunction with 93571)◀

(Intravascular distal coronary blood flow velocity measurements include all Doppler transducer manipulations and repositioning within the specific vessel being examined, during coronary angiography or therapeutic intervention [eg, angioplasty])

(For unlisted cardiac catheterization procedure, use 93799)

### ✍ Rationale

In the CPT 2011 code set, the diagnostic catheterization codes in the Medicine section were restructured to include imaging supervision, interpretation, and report. This was the result of a RUC screening for codes reported together more than 95% of the time. For 2013, parenthetical notes in the Medicine/Cardiovascular/Injection Procedures section that instruct users on how to report injection procedures were added and revised to make the instructions consistent with the 2011 diagnostic cardiac catheterization changes.

Specifically, two parenthetical notes were added following supravalvular aortography injection procedure code 93567. The first note instructs users to report code 93567 with cardiac catheterization codes 93451-93461 and 93530-93533. The second note directs users to codes 75600-75630 and 36221 for nonsupravalvular thoracic aortography or abdominal aortography performed at the time of cardiac catheterization. The note following pulmonary angiography injection procedure code 93568 has been revised by removing codes 93452, 93454, 93455, 93458, and 93459.

A parenthetical note was added following code 93566 stating that it may be reported in conjunction with codes 93451, 93453, 93456, 93457, 93460, 93461, and 93530-93533. A new parenthetical note was added following intravascular measurement code 93571 instructing users to report code 93571 with coronary intervention codes 92975, 92920, 92924, 92928, 92933, 92937, 92941, 92943; coronary catheterization codes 93454-93461; and injection procedure codes 93563 and 93564. To provide consistency with CPT add-on code convention, a parenthetical note was added following code 93572, instructing its use with code 93571.

# Intracardiac Electrophysiological Procedures/Studies

▶Intracardiac electrophysiologic studies (EPS) are invasive diagnostic medical procedures which include the insertion and repositioning of electrode catheters, recording of electrograms before and during pacing, programmed stimulation of multiple locations in the heart, analysis of recorded information, and report of the procedure. In many circumstances, patients with arrhythmias are evaluated and treated at the same encounter. In this situation, a diagnostic *electrophysiologic study* is performed, induced tachycardia(s) are *mapped*, and on the basis of the diagnostic and mapping information, the tissue is *ablated*.◀

▶***Arrhythmia Induction:*** In most electrophysiologic studies, an attempt is made to induce arrhythmia(s) from single or multiple sites within the heart. Arrhythmia induction may be achieved by multiple techniques, eg, by performing pacing at different rates or programmed stimulation (introduction of critically timed electrical impulses). Because arrhythmia induction occurs via the same catheter(s) inserted for the electrophysiologic study(ies), catheter insertion and temporary pacemaker codes are not additionally reported. Codes 93600-93603, 93610, 93612, and 93618 are used to describe unusual situations where there may be recording, pacing, or an attempt at arrhythmia induction from only one site in the heart. Code 93619 describes only evaluation of the sinus node, atrioventricular node, and His-Purkinje conduction system, without arrhythmia induction. Codes 93620-93624, 93640-93642, 93653, 93654, and 93656 all include recording, pacing, and attempted arrhythmia induction from one or more site(s) in the heart.

***Mapping:*** When a tachycardia is induced, the site of tachycardia origination or its electrical path through the heart is often defined by mapping. Mapping creates a multidimensional depiction of a tachycardia by recording multiple electrograms obtained sequentially or simultaneously from multiple catheter sites in the heart. Depending upon the technique, certain types of mapping catheters may be repositioned from point-to-point within the heart, allowing sequential recording from the various sites to construct maps. Other types of mapping catheters allow mapping without a point-to-point technique by allowing simultaneous recording from many electrodes on the same catheter and computer-assisted three-dimensional reconstruction of the tachycardia activation sequence.

Mapping is a distinct procedure performed in addition to a diagnostic electrophysiologic study or ablation procedure and may be separately reported using 93609 or 93613. Do not report standard mapping (93609) in addition to 3-dimensional mapping (93613).

***Ablation:*** Once the part of the heart involved in the tachycardia is localized, the tachycardia may be treated by ablation (the delivery of a radiofrequency or cryo-energy to the area to selectively destroy cardiac tissue). Ablation procedures (93653-93657) are performed at the same session as electrophysiology studies and therefore represent a combined code description. When reporting ablation therapy codes (93653-93657), the single site electrophysiology studies (93600-93603, 93610, 93612, 93618) and the comprehensive electrophysiology studies (93619, 93620) may not be reported separately. Codes 93622 and 93623 may be reported separately with 93656 for treatment of atrial fibrillation. However, 93621 for left atrial pacing and recording from coronary sinus or left atrium should not be reported in conjunction with 93656 as this is a component of 93656.

The differences in the techniques involved for ablation of supraventricular arrhythmias, ventricular arrhythmias, and atrial fibrillation are reflected within the descriptions for 93653-93657. Code 93653 is a primary code for catheter ablation for treatment of supraventricular tachycardia caused by dual atrioventricular nodal pathways, accessory atrioventricular connections, or other atrial foci. Code 93654 describes catheter ablation for treatment of ventricular tachycardia or focus of ventricular ectopy. Code 93656 is a primary code for reporting treatment of atrial fibrillation by ablation to achieve complete pulmonary vein electrical isolation. Codes 93653, 93654, and 93656 are distinct primary procedure codes and may not be reported together.

Codes 93655 and 93657 are add-on codes listed in addition to the primary ablation code to report ablation of sites distinct from the primary ablation site. After ablation of the primary target site, post-ablation electrophysiologic evaluation is performed as part of those ablation services (93653, 93654, 93656) and additional mechanisms of tachycardia may be identified. For example, if the primary tachycardia ablated was atrioventricular nodal reentrant tachycardia and during post-ablation testing an atrial tachycardia, atrial flutter, or accessory pathway with orthodromic reentry tachycardia was identified, this would be considered a separate mechanism of tachycardia. Pacing maneuvers are performed to define the mechanism(s) of the new tachycardia(s). Catheter ablation of this distinct mechanism of tachycardia is then performed at the newly discovered atrial or ventricular origin. Appropriate post-ablation attempts at re-induction and observation are again performed. Code 93655 is listed in conjunction with 93653 when repeat ablation is for treatment of an additional supraventricular tachycardia mechanism and with 93654 when the repeat ablation is for treatment of an additional ventricular tachycardia mechanism. Code 93655 may be reported with 93656 when an additional non-atrial fibrillation tachycardia is separately diagnosed after pulmonary vein isolation. Code 93657 is reported in conjunction with 93656 when successful pulmonary vein isolation is achieved, attempts at re-induction of atrial fibrillation identify an additional left or right atrial focus for atrial fibrillation, and further ablation of this new focus is performed.

In certain circumstances, depending on the chamber of origin, a catheter or catheters may be maneuvered into the left ventricle to facilitate arrhythmia diagnosis. This may be accomplished via a retrograde aortic approach by means of the arterial access or through a transseptal puncture. For ablation treatment of supraventricular tachycardia (93653) and ventricular tachycardia (93654), the left heart catheterization by transseptal puncture through intact septum (93462) may be reported separately as an add-on code. However, for ablation treatment of atrial fibrillation (93656), the transseptal puncture (93462) is a standard component of the procedure and may not be reported separately. Do not report 93462 in conjunction with 93656.◄

Modifier 51 should not be appended to 93600-93603, 93610, 93612, 93615-93618, 93631.

⊙+ **93609**   Intraventricular and/or intra-atrial mapping of tachycardia site(s) with catheter manipulation to record from multiple sites to identify origin of tachycardia (List separately in addition to code for primary procedure)

▶(Use 93609 in conjunction with 93620, 93653)◄

▶(Do not report 93609 in conjunction with 93613, 93654)◄

⊙+ **93613**   Intracardiac electrophysiologic 3-dimensional mapping (List separately in addition to code for primary procedure)

▶(Use 93613 in conjunction with 93620, 93653)◄

▶(Do not report 93613 in conjunction with 93609, 93654)◄

⊙**93620**  Comprehensive electrophysiologic evaluation including insertion and repositioning of multiple electrode catheters with induction or attempted induction of arrhythmia; with right atrial pacing and recording, right ventricular pacing and recording, His bundle recording

(Do not report 93620 in conjunction with 93600, 93602, 93610, 93612, 93618 or 93619)

⊙**+93621**    with left atrial pacing and recording from coronary sinus or left atrium (List separately in addition to code for primary procedure)

(Use 93621 in conjunction with 93620)

►(Do not report 93621 in conjunction with 93656)◄

⊘**93631**  Intra-operative epicardial and endocardial pacing and mapping to localize the site of tachycardia or zone of slow conduction for surgical correction

►(For operative ablation of an arrhythmogenic focus or pathway by a separate individual, see 33250-33261)◄

►(93651, 93652 have been deleted. To report, see 93653-93657)◄

⊙●**93653**  Comprehensive electrophysiologic evaluation including insertion and repositioning of multiple electrode catheters with induction or attempted induction of an arrhythmia with right atrial pacing and recording, right ventricular pacing and recording, His recording with intracardiac catheter ablation of arrhythmogenic focus; with treatment of supraventricular tachycardia by ablation of fast or slow atrioventricular pathway, accessory atrioventricular connection, cavo-tricuspid isthmus or other single atrial focus or source of atrial re-entry

►(Do not report 93653 in conjunction with 93600-93603, 93610, 93612, 93618-93620, 93642, 93654)◄

⊙●**93654**    with treatment of ventricular tachycardia or focus of ventricular ectopy including intracardiac electrophysiologic 3D mapping, when performed, and left ventricular pacing and recording, when performed

►(Do not report 93654 in conjunction with 93279-93284, 93286-93289, 93600-93603, 93609, 93610, 93612, 93613, 93618-93620, 93622, 93642, 93653)◄

⊙+●**93655**  Intracardiac catheter ablation of a discrete mechanism of arrhythmia which is distinct from the primary ablated mechanism, including repeat diagnostic maneuvers, to treat a spontaneous or induced arrhythmia (List separately in addition to code for primary procedure)

►(Use 93655 in conjunction with 93653, 93654, 93656)◄

⊙●**93656**  Comprehensive electrophysiologic evaluation including transseptal catheterizations, insertion and repositioning of multiple electrode catheters with induction or attempted induction of an arrhythmia with atrial recording and pacing, when possible, right ventricular pacing and recording, His bundle recording with intracardiac catheter ablation of arrhythmogenic focus, with treatment of atrial fibrillation by ablation by pulmonary vein isolation

►(Do not report 93656 in conjunction with 93279-93284, 93286-93289, 93462, 93600, 93602, 93603, 93610, 93612, 93618, 93619, 93620, 93621, 93653, 93654)◄

⊙+●**93657**  Additional linear or focal intracardiac catheter ablation of the left or right atrium for treatment of atrial fibrillation remaining after completion of pulmonary vein isolation (List separately in addition to code for primary procedure)

►(Use 93657 in conjunction with 93656)◄

**93660** Evaluation of cardiovascular function with tilt table evaluation, with continuous ECG monitoring and intermittent blood pressure monitoring, with or without pharmacological intervention

▶(For testing of autonomic nervous system function, see 95921, 95924, 95943)◀

**+93662** Intracardiac echocardiography during therapeutic/diagnostic intervention, including imaging supervision and interpretation (List separately in addition to code for primary procedure)

▶(Use 93662 in conjunction with 92987, 93453, 93460-93462, 93532, 93580, 93581, 93621, 93622, 93653, 93654, 93656 as appropriate)◀

### Rationale

As a result of the Joint CPT/RUC screen for procedures inherently performed together, several changes have been made to bundle electrophysiological (EP) evaluation and intracardiac ablation procedures. Intracardiac catheter ablation codes 93651 and 93652 were deleted, and three new codes (93653, 93654, 93656) were established, which combine comprehensive electrophysiologic evaluation with intracardiac catheter ablation of arrhythmogenic focus services.

Two codes were established to report intracardiac catheter ablation of a discrete mechanism of arrhythmia, which is distinct from the primary ablated mechanism (93655) and additional linear or focal intracardiac catheter ablation of the left or right atrium (93657).

Instructional parenthetical notes were revised and added to instruct users on the proper use of the new codes. The Intracardiac Electrophysiological Procedures/Studies guidelines were revised so that they no longer indicate that EP evaluation and catheter ablation are reported separately. The guidelines were revised to clarify that ablation procedures and EP studies are performed at the same session, and they no longer state that these are performed on different dates. The guidelines also state that comprehensive EP studies with left ventricular pacing and recording (93622) may be reported with comprehensive EP studies with right ventricular pacing and recording (93656) for treatment of atrial fibrillation.

Additional text was added to the guidelines that describe the types of arrhythmias that codes 93653-93657 are intended to be used with, as well as the appropriate use of these codes in certain circumstances. See also CPT nomenclature reporting neutrality.

In correlation with the changes made to the Autonomic Function Tests subsection, the parenthetical note following code 93660 was revised by deleting codes 95922 and 95923 and adding new codes 95924 and 95943.

### Clinical Example (93653)

A 64-year-old female has recurrent palpitations. An event monitor has documented supraventricular tachycardia.

#### Description of Procedure (93653)

The patient is brought to the electrophysiology lab. Direct current cardioversion/defibrillation and electrophysiology (EP) testing/ablation equipment is confirmed present and in proper working order. Fluoroscopic equipment that will be used

Ⓢ=Modifier 51 Exempt  ☉=Moderate Sedation  ✚=Add-on Code  𝒩=FDA approval pending

to visualize catheter movements and location is tested. Local analgesia is administered along with anesthesia appropriate to the patient including moderate sedation. Venous access is obtained. Arterial access to monitor blood pressure and to facilitate retrograde aortic access to the left ventricle is obtained. Multi-electrode catheters are advanced from the access sheaths and into the respective cardiac chambers where they will be used to pace and record. Pacing and sensing is performed in the right atrium and right ventricle. His bundle recording is obtained. Refractory periods are measured. Attempts at arrhythmia induction are performed via maneuvers that include burst pacing and premature pacing using programmed electrical stimulation at multiple drive cycle lengths from multiple atrial and ventricular sites. Once the SVT is induced, pacing maneuvers are performed to elucidate the mechanism of the tachycardia.

Once the combination of both diagnostic maneuvers and mapping is complete, catheter ablation may be performed. An ablation catheter is maneuvered from the sites of vascular access to the appropriate cardiac location to facilitate delivery of ablative energy. Multiple lesions are delivered to ensure eradication of the arrhythmia focus and to provide consolidation lesions in the surrounding tissue. Throughout the ablation, the patient is monitored for hemodynamic compromise due to cardiac perforation, bradyarrhythmias, or tachyarrhythmias, embolic phenomena, or damage to cardiac or vascular structures. Following the ablation portion of the procedure, further electrophysiologic testing is performed to assess the outcome of ablation using decremental, burst, and premature pacing maneuvers. These are repeated following a 30-minute period following the conclusion of the final ablation lesion. Sheaths are removed, appropriate hemostasis is achieved, and follow-up assessment of the patient for any complications is performed.

## Clinical Example (93654)

A 73-year-old male with a history of New York Heart Association Class III heart failure due to ischemic dilated cardiomyopathy (EF 25%) and prior myocardial infarction presents with recurrent implantable cardioverter-defibrillator (ICD) therapies for drug-refractory ventricular tachycardia.

### Description of Procedure (93654)

The patient is brought to the electrophysiology laboratory. Direct current cardioversion/defibrillation, electrophysiology (EP), and ablation equipment is confirmed present and in proper working order. Fluoroscopic equipment that will be used to visualize catheter movements and location is tested. Three-dimensional mapping equipment is tested and confirmed to be functioning normally. Local analgesia is administered. Patients with implantable cardioverter-defibrillators will have their devices reprogrammed and/or transiently deactivated at the start of the case to minimize adverse consequences resulting from electromagnetic interference from radiofrequency current application.

Venous access is obtained. Arterial access to monitor blood pressure and to facilitate retrograde aortic access to the left ventricle is obtained. Multi-electrode catheters are advanced from the access sheaths and into the respective cardiac chambers where they will be used to pace and record. An intracardiac echo probe is placed via a femoral venous access approach. The intracardiac echo is used in conjunction with the three-dimensional mapping system to create a three-dimensional shell of the right or left ventricle, including the aortic root, aortic valve leaflets, coronary, and mitral valve annulus. Papillary muscles are also recorded in the three-dimensional anatomical ultrasound map. Pacing and sensing is performed in the right atrium and right ventricle. His bundle recording is obtained. Refractory periods are measured. Attempts at ventricular tachycardia induction are performed via burst pacing, decremental pacing, and premature pacing using programmed electrical stimulation at multiple drive cycle lengths from multiple ventricular sites.

Once an arrhythmia is induced, pacing maneuvers are performed to elucidate the mechanism of the ventricular tachycardia. The electrical activation sequence is mapped with the three-dimensional electroanatomical mapping system and activation timing is superimposed upon the three-dimensional echo image previously obtained. Anticoagulation is administered once catheters have been placed on the left side of the heart. Once the ventricular tachycardia circuit is localized, a catheter is moved to the appropriate location or region of abnormal myocardium to deliver ablative energy. Multiple lesions are delivered to ensure eradication of the arrhythmia focus and to provide consolidation lesions in the surrounding tissue. Throughout the ablation the patient is monitored for hemodynamic compromise due to cardiac perforation, bradyarrhythmias, or tachyarrhythmias, embolic phenomena, or damage to cardiac or vascular structures.

Following the ablation portion of the procedure, further electrophysiologic testing is performed to assess the outcome of ablation using decremental, burst, and premature pacing maneuvers. These are repeated after a 30-minute period following the conclusion of the final ablation lesion. Anticoagulation is reversed. Sheaths are removed, appropriate hemostasis is achieved, and follow-up assessment of the patient for any complications is performed. Patients with implantable cardioverter-defibrillators will have their devices reprogrammed to an active configuration with rates reprogrammed as necessary to treat any remaining arrhythmias.

 ## Clinical Example (93655)

A 64-year-old female has undergone successful ablation of her atrial supraventricular tachycardia (SVT) focus (reported separately). Attempts to re-induce that arrhythmia reveal an additional atrial focus (also reported separately). A decision is made to ablate this additional focus, following its discovery.

### Description of Procedure (93655)

A full electrophysiologic study and ablation procedure has been performed. Diagnostic and ablative electrophysiology (EP) catheters are in cardiac chambers. During the course of the post-ablation electrophysiologic evaluation, a second (or greater) mechanism of tachycardia is identified. For example, if the primary tachycardia that is ablated was atrioventricular (AV) nodal reentrant tachycardia, and during post-ablation testing, an atrial tachycardia, atrial flutter, or accessory pathway with orthotropic reentry tachycardia is identified, this would be considered a separate mechanism of tachycardia. Pacing maneuvers are performed to define the mechanism(s) of the new tachycardia(s). Mapping is performed to define the optimal ablation site(s) that is distinct from the initial ablation site(s). Catheter

⊘=Modifier 51 Exempt  ⊙=Moderate Sedation  ✦=Add-on Code  𝒩=FDA approval pending

ablation of this distinct mechanism of tachycardia is performed at its origin. Multiple lesions are delivered to ensure eradication of the arrhythmia focus, and to provide consolidation lesions in the surrounding tissue. Appropriate post-ablation attempts at re-education and observation for 30 minutes are performed.

 **Clinical Example** (93656)

A 62-year-old man with a history of hypertension has recurrent atrial fibrillation. Despite rate or rhythm control with antiarrhythmic drugs, he remains symptomatic.

**Description of Procedure (93656)**

The patient is brought to the electrophysiology laboratory. Direct current cardioversion/defibrillation, electrophysiology (EP), and ablative equipment is confirmed present and in proper working order. Fluoroscopic equipment that will be used to visualize catheter movements and location is tested. Local analgesia is administered. Venous access is obtained. Arterial access to monitor blood pressure and to retrograde aortic access to the left ventricle is be obtained. By means of the venous access sites, multi-electrode catheters are positioned in specific cardiac chambers. Two transseptal catheterizations are performed to achieve access and facilitate placement of both a circular mapping catheter and an ablation catheter in the left atrium. Additional anticoagulation is administered. Conduction intervals and refractory periods are measured and arrhythmia induction attempted. His bundle recording and ventricular pacing and sensing are performed. A circular mapping catheter is passed into the left atrium, and pulmonary vein conduction is assessed and recorded. Selective venography of the pulmonary veins is performed to define anatomy. Catheter ablation is then performed to achieve pulmonary vein isolation. Point lesions encircling the pulmonary vein region are created, which are guided by anatomical mapping and electrical signals provided by a circular mapping catheter. Pulmonary vein isolation, as measured by the circular mapping catheter as well as loss of tissue voltage and tissue pacing capture are the measured endpoints. Throughout the ablation, the patient is monitored for hemodynamic compromise due to cardiac perforation, bradyarrhythmias, or tachyarrhythmias, embolic phenomena, thrombus formation, or damage to cardiac or vascular structures, including meticulous monitoring for lesion delivery within the pulmonary vein or close to the esophagus. Following the ablation portion of the procedure, further electrophysiologic testing is performed to assess the outcome of ablation over a 30-minute period following the last ablation lesion. Once electrophysiology testing and ablation are completed, anticoagulation is reversed. Post-procedure, sheaths are removed, appropriate hemostasis is achieved, and follow-up assessment of the patient for any complications is performed.

 **Clinical Example** (93657)

A 72-year-old male has symptomatic atrial fibrillation refractory to medical therapy. An electrophysiology (EP) study and ablation are performed to achieve pulmonary vein isolation (reported separately). Despite demonstration of electrical isolation of the pulmonary veins, atrial fibrillation continues.

### Description of Procedure (93657)

A full electrophysiologic study and ablation procedure has been performed for atrial fibrillation. Diagnostic and ablation catheters are present in cardiac chambers. Pulmonary vein isolation has been accomplished. Due to the presence of non-pulmonary vein sources of atrial fibrillation, additional non-pulmonary vein ablation lesions are created. Regions of fractionated potentials are mapped and ablated outside the pulmonary vein area. In addition, linear lesions are attempted along the roof, mitral isthmus, or septal aspect of the left atrium. Non-pulmonary vein focal sources of atrial fibrillation induction are induced, localized, and ablated. These lesion locations are distinct from the pulmonary vein lesions performed in the main EP study/atrial fibrillation ablation procedure. During the delivery of ablation energy, continuous monitoring for hemodynamic instability, arrhythmias, embolic events, and injury to the esophagus is performed. Following restoration of sinus rhythm, conduction intervals are measured and arrhythmia induction is re-attempted over a 30-minute period following the last ablation lesion.

## Pulmonary

### Pulmonary Diagnostic Testing and Therapies

**94770**  Carbon dioxide, expired gas determination by infrared analyzer

►(For bronchoscopy, see 31622-31646)◄

 **Rationale**

To maintain consistency and uniformity in the CPT code set, the cross-reference note following code 94770 has been updated to direct users to the appropriate range of bronchoscopy codes.

►(For thoracentesis, use 32554, 32555)◄

 **Rationale**

In support of the deletion of code 32421, *Thoracentesis, puncture of pleural cavity for aspiration, initial or subsequent*, and the establishment of new codes 32554 and 32555, the cross-reference note following code 94770 was revised to include codes 32554 and 32555 for reporting thoracentesis.

## Allergy and Clinical Immunology

### Allergy Testing

(For allergy laboratory tests, see 86000-86999)

►(For administration of medications [eg, epinephrine, steroidal agents, antihistamines] for therapy for severe or intractable allergic reaction, use 96372)◄

⊘=Modifier 51 Exempt   ⊙=Moderate Sedation   ✚=Add-on Code   𝒩=FDA approval pending

### ✍️ Rationale

The parenthetical note above code 95004 was revised to specify instructions for administration of medications for severe or intractable allergic reactions, and to provide examples of types of medications administered.

**95012**   Nitric oxide expired gas determination

▶(95010 and 95015 have been deleted. To report, see 95017 and 95018)◀

●**95017**   Allergy testing, any combination of percutaneous (scratch, puncture, prick) and intracutaneous (intradermal), sequential and incremental, with venoms, immediate type reaction, including test interpretation and report, specify number of tests

●**95018**   Allergy testing, any combination of percutaneous (scratch, puncture, prick) and intracutaneous (intradermal), sequential and incremental, with drugs or biologicals, immediate type reaction, including test interpretation and report, specify number of tests

### ✍️ Rationale

Codes 95010 and 95015 were deleted and replaced by codes 95017 and 95018. The new codes 95017 and 95018 are used to report percutaneous and intracutaneous allergy testing. The codes are differentiated based on whether the testing procedure utilizes venoms (identified by code 95017) or drugs/biologicals (identified by code 95018), rather than differentiating primarily based on the technique used as with the old codes (95010 and 95015). This change was made because there is very little difference in the work needed to provide percutaneous versus intracutaneous allergy testing. However, the cost of the supplies varies greatly (supply of venoms differs significantly from the supply of drugs/biologicals). As a result, development of the new codes (95017 and 95018) and deletion of the codes previously used for allergy testing (95010 and 95015) allows for more specific identification of the effort and materials that are included as part of these procedures. To exemplify this, a parenthetical cross-reference was included following the deletion of codes 95010 and 95015 to direct users to the correct codes to use to identify these procedures.

### 🩺 Clinical Example (95017)

A 42-year-old male with a history of being stung by an insect followed by generalized urticaria and mild chest discomfort requires venom allergy testing. The allergist performs 27 total tests, which include percutaneous and intracutaneous tests of venoms and appropriate positive and negative controls.

**Description of Procedure (95017)**

The first test includes five percutaneous venom tests and two percutaneous control tests (positive histamine and negative diluent). After 15 to 20 minutes, the physician interprets this initial test by viewing the skin reaction at the venom-test sites compared to control-sites, and determines whether intracutaneous testing can proceed. Sequential and incremental intracutaneous testing is performed in four batches of five venoms. Fifteen to 20 minutes after each test, the physician interprets this test by viewing the skin reaction at the venom-test sites compared to control-sites. The physician is available in the office for the entire intraservice period and checks the patient periodically and before administration of each test for local and systemic reactions.

 **Clinical Example (95018)**

A 48-year-old female with chronic sinusitis and a history of adverse reactions to multiple antibiotics requires drug allergy testing. The allergist performs a total of 9 tests, which includes percutaneous and intracutaneous tests of penicillin and appropriate positive and negative controls.

### Description of Procedure (95018)

The first test includes four percutaneous tests, including benzylpenicilloyl poly-lysine, penicillin G potassium, and two control tests (positive histamine and negative diluent). After 15 to 20 minutes, the physician interprets this initial test by viewing the skin reaction at the drug-test sites compared to control-test sites, and determines whether intracutaneous testing should proceed. Next, intracutaneous testing is performed, which includes five tests: benzylpenicilloyl polylysine in duplicate, penicillin G potassium in duplicate, and one negative-control test (diluent). After 15 to 20 minutes, the physician interprets the test by viewing the skin reaction at the drug-test sites compared to control-test sites. The physician is available in the office for the entire intraservice period and checks the patient periodically and before administration of each test for local and systemic reactions.

▶(95075 has been deleted. For ingestion challenge testing, see 95076, 95079)◀

## ▶Ingestion Challenge Testing◀

▶Codes 95076 and 95079 are used to report ingestion challenge testing. Report 95076 for initial 120 minutes of **testing** time (ie, not physician face-to-face time). Report 95079 for each additional 60 minutes of **testing** time (ie, not physician face-to-face time). For total **testing** time less than 61 minutes (eg, positive challenge resulting in cessation of testing), report an evaluation and management service, if appropriate. Patient assessment/monitoring activities for allergic reaction (eg, blood pressure testing, peak flow meter testing) are not separately reported. Intervention therapy (eg, injection of steroid or epinephrine) may be reported separately as appropriate.◀

▶For purposes of reporting testing times, if an evaluation and management service is required, then testing time ends.◀

●**95076** Ingestion challenge test (sequential and incremental ingestion of test items, eg, food, drug or other substance); initial 120 minutes of testing

+ ●**95079** each additional 60 minutes of testing (List separately in addition to code for primary procedure)

▶(Use 95079 in conjunction with 95076)◀

 **Rationale**

Codes 95076 and 95079 are used to report allergen ingestion challenge testing. These codes are intended to be used in place of code 95075 (which was deleted) to allow description of this service as a time-based service. A new section heading was also developed to facilitate placement of the new codes and to distinguish

⊘=Modifier 51 Exempt  ⊙=Moderate Sedation  ✚=Add-on Code  ⁄=FDA approval pending

the the use of these codes from other allergy testing procedures. Code 95076 is used to identify the first 120 minutes of allergen ingestion testing using food, drugs, or other substances, and code 95079 is intended to be used to identify each additional 60 minutes of testing. A deletion cross-reference has been inserted in place of deleted code 95075 to direct users to the new codes to identify ingestion challenge testing. A note has also been placed following code 95079 to provide instruction regarding the use of this add-on code.

A new guideline has also been added to further exemplify the intended use for these new codes. The guideline (1) identifies the appropriate amount of time needed to report these services (ie, total time less than 61 minutes is reported by Evaluation and Management [E/M] services); (2) excludes use of separate codes (such as blood pressure testing or peak flow meter testing) to identify patient assessment or monitoring activities needed to identify an allergic reaction; and (3) notes that intervention therapy (such as injections needed for steroid or epinephrine treatment) may be separately reported. The guideline also notes that provision of any E/M services ends the testing time.

###  Clinical Example (95076)

An 8-year-old with a history of an acute allergic reaction to peanut at age 2 years has been monitored by serial allergy skin and serum tests. She had no additional known exposures to peanut. The patient undergoes ingestion challenge testing to determine if her peanut allergy has resolved.

#### Description of Procedure (95076)

Ingestion challenge testing of peanut butter is conducted. This typically involves incremental peanut butter dosing from a minute amount placed on the philtrum, followed by a minute amount placed on the tongue, followed by sequential ingestion of one-eighth, one-quarter, one-half, one, and two teaspoon(s) of peanut butter. Between the doses, there is a period of close patient monitoring for reaction (eg, hives, angioedema, wheezing) and assessing patient status prior to the next dose. After the final dose, observation and monitoring are continued until the patient is considered clinically stable and a final physical examination is normal. The physician is available in the office for the entire intraservice period.

Patient assessment/monitoring activities for allergic reaction (eg, blood pressure testing, peak flow meter testing) are not reported separately. Intervention therapy (eg, injection of steroid or epinephrine) may be reported separately, as appropriate. For purposes of reporting testing time, if an evaluation and management service is required, testing time ends.

### Clinical Example (95079)

An 8-year-old with a history of an acute allergic reaction to peanut at age 2 years has been monitored by serial allergy skin and serum tests. She had no additional known exposures to peanuts. While undergoing ingestion challenge testing to determine if her peanut allergy has resolved (first 120 minutes reported separately as 95076), she had a potential reaction requiring extended testing and additional testing was performed.

**Description of Procedure (95079)**

The typical patient undergoing more than 120 minutes of ingestion challenge testing (reported separately with code 95076) will have had one or more "potential" reactions during testing, which requires additional/extended monitoring and assessment between doses. These reactions resolve, allowing testing to continue. Between the doses, there is a period of close patient monitoring for reaction (eg, hives, angioedema, wheezing) and assessing patient status prior to the next dose. After the final dose, observation and monitoring are continued until the patient is considered clinically stable and a final physical examination is normal. The physician is available in the office for the entire intraservice period.

Patient assessment/monitoring activities for allergic reaction (eg, blood pressure testing, peak flow meter testing) are not reported separately. Intervention therapy (eg, injection of steroid or epinephrine) may be reported separately as appropriate. For purposes of reporting testing time, if an evaluation and management service is required, testing time ends.

# Neurology and Neuromuscular Procedures

Neurologic services are typically consultative, and any of the levels of consultation (99241-99255) may be appropriate.

In addition, services and skills outlined under **Evaluation and Management** levels of service appropriate to neurologic illnesses should be reported similarly.

►Codes 95812-95822, 95950-95953 and 95956 use recording time as a basis for code use. Recording time is when the recording is underway and data is being collected. Recording time excludes set up and take down time. Codes 95961-95962 use physician or other qualified health care professional attendance time as a basis for code use.◄

(Do not report codes 95860-95875 in addition to 96000-96004)

 **Rationale**

In support of the deletion of code 95920, *Intraoperative neurophysiology testing, per hour (List separately in addition to code for primary procedure)*, the last paragraph of the Neurology and Neuromuscular Procedure guidelines was revised by deleting code 95920 from the list of codes that use recording time as a basis for code use.

## Sleep Medicine Testing

Sleep medicine services include procedures that evaluate adult and pediatric patients for a variety of sleep disorders. Sleep medicine testing services are diagnostic procedures using in-laboratory and portable technology to assess physiologic data and therapy.

►All sleep services (95800-95811) include recording, interpretation, and report. (Report with modifier 52 if less than 6 hours of recording for 95800, 95801 and 95806, 95807, 95810, 95811; if less than 7 hours of recording for 95782, 95783, or if less than four nap opportunities are recorded for 95805).◄

⃠=Modifier 51 Exempt   ⊙=Moderate Sedation   ✚=Add-on Code   ⚠=FDA approval pending

| | |
|---|---|
| **85782** | ▶Code is out of numerical sequence. See 95803-95783◀ |
| **85783** | ▶Code is out of numerical sequence. See 95803-95783◀ |
| ▲**95808** | Polysomnography; any age, sleep staging with 1-3 additional parameters of sleep, attended by a technologist |
| ▲**95810** | age 6 years or older, sleep staging with 4 or more additional parameters of sleep, attended by a technologist |
| ▲**95811** | age 6 years or older, sleep staging with 4 or more additional parameters of sleep, with initiation of continuous positive airway pressure therapy or bilevel ventilation, attended by a technologist |
| #●**95782** | younger than 6 years, sleep staging with 4 or more additional parameters of sleep, attended by a technologist |
| #●**95783** | younger than 6 years, sleep staging with 4 or more additional parameters of sleep, with initiation of continuous positive airway pressure therapy or bi-level ventilation, attended by a technologist |

### Rationale

Two codes, 95782 and 95783, were established to report pediatric polysomnography for children younger than 6 years of age. Polysomnography is performed on pediatric patients to assess for sleep disorders. Polysomnography with positive airway pressure titration is performed on pediatric patients to determine the appropriate pressure to use in treatment of obstructive sleep apnea. These patients are monitored for a longer period of time than adults (typically, 9 hours of recording is performed), which also typically require a 1:1 technologist to patient ratio. Additional channels of recording are typically used in pediatric studies, for example, breath-by-breath $CO_2$ monitoring. Because the recording is longer and there are more channels of data, pediatric studies are more complex to review. Therefore, new codes are required to accurately describe the work performed on children younger than 6 years of age. Codes 95782 and 95783 appear with the hash symbol (#) to indicate that these codes are out of numerical sequence. Two reference notes were added to instruct the user to the appropriate code range of 95803-95783 for the placement of codes 95782 and 95783.

In support of the establishment of codes 95782 and 95783, code 95808 was revised to include the terms "any age," and codes 95810 and 95811 were revised to include age specification "age 6 years or older." Codes 95810 and 95811 more accurately describe services performed on adults but not the extent of services provided for pediatric patients younger than 6 years of age.

The Sleep Medicine Testing introductory guidelines were also revised to include an instructional note indicating that modifier 52 should be appended if reporting less than 7 hours of sleep testing for pediatric polysomnography (95782, 95783).

### Clinical Example (95782)

A 5-year-old girl has enlarged tonsils and loud snoring. A polysomnogram is ordered.

**Description of Procedure (95782)**

The technologist's summary and notes as well as the patient's sleep logs and comments on the pre-, intra-, and post-sleep periods are reviewed. The sleep recording already downloaded to the reading station is opened. Analysis of the raw data at 30-second intervals (epoch by epoch) for adequacy of recording signals and marked sleep stages is performed. The technologist's preliminary evaluation of artifacts, sleep stages, and physiologic changes noted during the recording is analyzed. The recording for changes in respiration, electrocardiography (EKG), oxygen saturation, electromyography (EMG), periodic limb movements, sleep state, electroencephalography (EEG), and capnography is evaluated. The changes of all physiologic signals with the simultaneous video recording of the patient are correlated. The decision whether the total sleep time is adequate for interpretation, and determination whether the recording addresses the clinical question(s) are made.

 **Clinical Example (95783)**

A 4-year-old boy with obstructive sleep apnea presents with ongoing witnessed apneas and persistent daytime sleepiness after removal of tonsils and adenoids. A polysomnogram is ordered for continuous positive airway pressure titration.

**Description of Procedure (95783)**

The technologist's summary and notes are reviewed. The sleep recording already downloaded to the reading station is opened. Analysis of the raw data at 30-second intervals (epoch by epoch) for adequacy of recording signals and marked sleep stages is performed. The technologist's preliminary evaluation of artifacts, sleep stages, and physiologic changes noted during the recording is analyzed. The recording for changes in respiration, electrocardiography (EKG), oxygen saturation, electromyography (EMG), periodic limb movements, sleep state, electroencephalography (EEG), and capnography is evaluated. The changes of all physiologic signals with the simultaneous video recording of the patient are correlated. The recording for optimal positive airway pressure application (mask) is evaluated. The decision if the total sleep time is adequate for interpretation is made. The recording, including the identification and assessment of abnormal events in the recording, is analyzed. The determination whether the recording addresses the clinical question(s) is made.

# Electromyography

Needle electromyographic (EMG) procedures include the interpretation of electrical waveforms measured by equipment that produces both visible and audible components of electrical signals recorded from the muscle(s) studied by the needle electrode.

Use 95870 or 95885 when four or fewer muscles are tested in an extremity. Use 95860-95864 or 95886 when five or more muscles are tested in an extremity.

▶Use EMG codes (95860-95864 and 95867-95870) when no nerve conduction studies (95907-95913) are performed on that day. Use 95885, 95886, and 95887 for EMG services when nerve conduction studies (95907-95913) are performed in conjunction with EMG on the same day.◀

⊘=Modifier 51 Exempt   ⊙=Moderate Sedation   ✚=Add-on Code   ⫫=FDA approval pending

Report either 95885 or 95886 once per extremity. Codes 95885 and 95886 can be reported together up to a combined total of four units of service per patient when all four extremities are tested.

**95860**    Needle electromyography; 1 extremity with or without related paraspinal areas

**95872**    Needle electromyography using single fiber electrode, with quantitative measurement of jitter, blocking and/or fiber density, any/all sites of each muscle studied

**#+95885**    Needle electromyography, each extremity, with related paraspinal areas, when performed, done with nerve conduction, amplitude and latency/velocity study; limited (List separately in addition to code for primary procedure)

**#+95886**    complete, five or more muscles studied, innervated by three or more nerves or four or more spinal levels (List separately in addition to code for primary procedure)

▶(Use 95885, 95886 in conjunction with 95907-95913)◀

(Do not report 95885, 95886 in conjunction with 95860-95864, 95870, 95905)

**#+95887**    Needle electromyography, non-extremity (cranial nerve supplied or axial) muscle(s) done with nerve conduction, amplitude and latency/velocity study (List separately in addition to code for primary procedure)

▶(Use 95887 in conjunction with 95907-95913)◀

(Do not report 95887 in conjunction with 95867-95870, 95905)

### ✍ Rationale

In support of the changes to the Nerve Conduction Tests section, the Electromyography guidelines and the parenthetical notes following needle electromyography add-on codes 95886 and 95887 were revised to reflect the deletion of codes 95900, 95903, 95904, 95934, and 95936, and the establishment of codes 95907-95913.

## Nerve Conduction Tests

▶The following applies to nerve conduction tests (95907-95913): Codes 95907-95913 describe nerve conduction tests when performed with individually placed stimulating, recording, and ground electrodes. The stimulating, recording, and ground electrode placement and the test design must be individualized to the patient's unique anatomy. Nerves tested must be limited to the specific nerves and conduction studies needed for the particular clinical question being investigated. The stimulating electrode must be placed directly over the nerve to be tested, and stimulation parameters properly adjusted to avoid stimulating other nerves or nerve branches. In most motor nerve conduction studies, and in some sensory and mixed nerve conduction studies, both proximal and distal stimulation will be used. Motor nerve conduction study recordings must be made from electrodes placed directly over the motor point of the specific muscle to be tested. Sensory nerve conduction study recordings must be made from electrodes placed directly over the specific nerve to be tested. Waveforms must be reviewed on site in real time, and the technique (stimulus site, recording site, ground site, filter settings) must be adjusted, as appropriate, as the test proceeds in order to minimize artifact, and to minimize the chances of unintended stimulation of adjacent nerves and the unintended recording from adjacent muscles or nerves. Reports must be prepared on site by the examiner, and consist of the work product of the interpretation of numerous test results, using well-established techniques to assess the amplitude, latency, and configuration of waveforms elicited by stimulation at each site of each nerve tested. This includes the calculation of nerve conduction velocities, sometimes including specialized F-wave indices, along with comparison to normal values, summarization of clinical and electrodiagnostic data, and physician or other qualified health care professional interpretation. Codes 95907-95913 describe one or more nerve conduction studies. For the purposes of coding, a single conduction study is defined as a sensory conduction test, a motor conduction test with or without an F wave test, or an H-reflex test. Each type of study (sensory, motor with or without F wave, H-reflex) for each nerve includes all orthodromic and antidromic impulses associated with that nerve and constitutes a distinct study when determining the number of studies in each grouping (eg, 1-2 or 3-4 nerve conduction studies). Each type of nerve conduction study is counted only once when multiple sites on the same nerve are stimulated or recorded. The numbers of these separate tests should be added to determine which code to use. For a list of nerves, see Appendix J. Use 95885-95887 in conjunction with 95907-95913 when performing electromyography with nerve conduction studies.◄

Code 95905 describes nerve conduction tests when performed with preconfigured electrodes customized to a specific anatomic site.

▶(95900, 95903, 95904 have been deleted. For nerve conduction studies, see 95907-95913)◄

⊘ **95905**   Motor and/or sensory nerve conduction, using preconfigured electrode array(s), amplitude and latency/velocity study, each limb, includes F-wave study when performed, with interpretation and report;

(Report 95905 only once per limb studied)

▶(Do not report 95905 in conjunction with 95885, 95886, 95907-95913)◄

● **95907**   Nerve conduction studies; 1-2 studies

● **95908**      3-4 studies

● **95909**      5-6 studies

● **95910**      7-8 studies

● **95911**      9-10 studies

● **95912**      11-12 studies

● **95913**      13 or more studies

### ✐ Rationale

Nerve conduction study codes 95900, 95903, and 95904 were deleted, seven new nerve conduction codes (95907-95913) were established, and guidelines were revised. The unit of service in codes 95907-95913 refers to the number of nerve conduction studies performed; whereas the unit of service in the previous codes 95900-95904 referred to each nerve. These changes were made in an effort to address the overlap and number of codes reported for a typical neurological assessment.

⊘=Modifier 51 Exempt   ⊙=Moderate Sedation   ✛=Add-on Code   𝗡=FDA approval pending

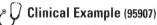
## Clinical Example (95907)

A 45-year-old female with a history of proximal median nerve injury secondary to IV line placement is referred back to the lab 6 months after initial study. Repeat testing is requested to evaluate recovery.

### Description of Procedure (95907)

The stimulating electrode is placed directly over the nerve to be tested, and the stimulation parameters are properly adjusted to avoid stimulating other nerves or nerve branches. In most motor nerve conduction studies, both proximal and distal stimulation are performed. Motor nerve conduction study recordings with or without F-wave testing, when performed, are made from electrodes placed directly over the motor point of the specific muscle to be tested. Sensory nerve conduction study recordings, when performed, must be made from electrodes placed directly over the specific nerve to be tested. H-reflex study recordings, when performed, must be made from electrodes placed directly over the specific nerve-muscle combination to be tested. Waveforms are reviewed on site in real time, and the technique (stimulus site, recording site, ground site, filter settings) is adjusted, as appropriate, as the test proceeds in order to minimize artifact and to minimize the chances of unintended stimulation of adjacent nerves and the unintended recording from adjacent muscles or nerves. Using well-established techniques, the amplitude, latency, and configuration of waveforms elicited by stimulation at each site of the nerve tested are assessed. This includes the calculation of nerve conduction velocities, sometimes including specialized F-wave indices, along with comparison to normal values. Test design changes during the course of the study in response to the information obtained. One to two nerve conduction studies are performed.

## Clinical Example (95908)

A 56-year-old female with nocturnal paresthesias is referred for evaluation of possible carpal tunnel syndrome. She is referred for nerve conduction testing.

### Description of Procedure (95908)

The stimulating electrode is placed directly over the nerve to be tested, and the stimulation parameters are properly adjusted to avoid stimulating other nerves or nerve branches. In most motor nerve conduction studies, both proximal and distal stimulation are performed. Motor nerve conduction study recordings with or without F-wave testing, when performed, are made from electrodes placed directly over the motor point of the specific muscle to be tested. Sensory nerve conduction study recordings, when performed, must be made from electrodes placed directly over the specific nerve to be tested. H-reflex study recordings, when performed, must be made from electrodes placed directly over the specific nerve-muscle combination to be tested. Waveforms are reviewed on site in real time, and the technique (stimulus site, recording site, ground site, filter settings) is adjusted, as appropriate, as the test proceeds in order to minimize artifact, and to minimize the chances of unintended stimulation of adjacent nerves and the unintended recording from adjacent muscles or nerves. Using well-established techniques, the amplitude, latency, and configuration of waveforms elicited by stimulation at each site of the nerve tested are assessed. This includes the calculation of nerve conduction velocities, sometimes including specialized F-wave indices, along with comparison to normal values. Test design changes during the course of the study in response to the information obtained. Three to four nerve conduction studies are performed.

###  Clinical Example (95909)

A 64-year-old diabetic male is referred for further evaluation of progressive numbness, tingling, and pain in the feet, worse at night, and progressive balance difficulties. Evaluation for peripheral neuropathy vs. polyradiculoneuropathy is requested.

#### Description of Procedure (95909)

The stimulating electrode is placed directly over the nerve to be tested, and the stimulation parameters are properly adjusted to avoid stimulating other nerves or nerve branches. In most motor nerve conduction studies, both proximal and distal stimulation are performed. Motor nerve conduction study recordings with or without F-wave testing, when performed, are made from electrodes placed directly over the motor point of the specific muscle to be tested. Sensory nerve conduction study recordings, when performed, must be made from electrodes placed directly over the specific nerve to be tested. H-reflex study recordings, when performed, must be made from electrodes placed directly over the specific nerve-muscle combination to be tested. Waveforms are reviewed on site in real time, and the technique (stimulus site, recording site, ground site, filter settings) is adjusted, as appropriate, as the test proceeds in order to minimize artifact, and to minimize the chances of unintended stimulation of adjacent nerves and the unintended recording from adjacent muscles or nerves. Using well-established techniques, the amplitude, latency, and configuration of waveforms elicited by stimulation at each site of the nerve tested are assessed. This includes the calculation of nerve conduction velocities, sometimes including specialized F-wave indices, along with comparison to normal values. Test design changes during the course of the study in response to the information obtained. Five to six nerve conduction studies are performed.

### Clinical Example (95910)

A 34-year-old female typist is referred for further evaluation of bilateral upper limb numbness and tingling that occurs during the day at work but can also wake her from sleep at times. The symptoms are described as affecting the entire hand and progressing up to the elbow when severe. Nerve conduction studies are indicated to evaluate for carpal tunnel syndrome versus neuropathy, brachial plexopathy, or cervical radiculopathy.

#### Description of Procedure (95910)

The stimulating electrode is placed directly over the nerve to be tested, and the stimulation parameters are properly adjusted to avoid stimulating other nerves or nerve branches. In most motor nerve conduction studies, both proximal and distal stimulation are performed. Motor nerve conduction study recordings with or without F-wave testing, when performed, are made from electrodes placed directly over the motor point of the specific muscle to be tested. Sensory nerve conduction

⊘=Modifier 51 Exempt   ⊙=Moderate Sedation   ✚=Add-on Code   𝒩=FDA approval pending

study recordings, when performed, must be made from electrodes placed directly over the specific nerve to be tested. H-reflex study recordings, when performed, must be made from electrodes placed directly over the specific nerve-muscle combination to be tested. Waveforms are reviewed on site in real time, and the technique (stimulus site, recording site, ground site, filter settings) is adjusted, as appropriate, as the test proceeds in order to minimize artifact, and to minimize the chances of unintended stimulation of adjacent nerves and the unintended recording from adjacent muscles or nerves. Using well-established techniques, the amplitude, latency, and configuration of waveforms elicited by stimulation at each site of the nerve tested are assessed. This includes the calculation of nerve conduction velocities, sometimes including specialized F-wave indices, along with comparison to normal values. Test design changes during the course of the study in response to the information obtained. Seven to eight nerve conduction studies are performed.

 **Clinical Example (95911)**

A 42-year-old male who was involved in a snowmobile accident 2 months earlier, and now has a flail right upper limb, is referred for further evaluation of traumatic brachial plexopathy.

**Description of Procedure (95911)**

The stimulating electrode is placed directly over the nerve to be tested, and the stimulation parameters are properly adjusted to avoid stimulating other nerves or nerve branches. In most motor nerve conduction studies, both proximal and distal stimulation are performed. Motor nerve conduction study recordings with or without F-wave testing, when performed, are made from electrodes placed directly over the motor point of the specific muscle to be tested. Sensory nerve conduction study recordings, when performed, must be made from electrodes placed directly over the specific nerve to be tested. H-reflex study recordings, when performed, must be made from electrodes placed directly over the specific nerve-muscle combination to be tested. Waveforms are reviewed on site in real time, and the technique (stimulus site, recording site, ground site, filter settings) is adjusted, as appropriate, as the test proceeds in order to minimize artifact, and to minimize the chances of unintended stimulation of adjacent nerves and the unintended recording from adjacent muscles or nerves. Using well-established techniques, the amplitude, latency, and configuration of waveforms elicited by stimulation at each site of the nerve tested are assessed. This includes the calculation of nerve conduction velocities, sometimes including specialized F-wave indices, along with comparison to normal values. Test design changes during the course of the study in response to the information obtained. Nine to 10 nerve conduction studies are performed.

 **Clinical Example (95912)**

A 75-year-old diabetic female with a three-month history of pain, numbness, and weakness progressively involving different peripheral nerve distributions is referred, with the question of mononeuritis multiplex secondary to vasculitis.

**Description of Procedure (95912)**

The stimulating electrode is placed directly over the nerve to be tested, and the stimulation parameters are properly adjusted to avoid stimulating other nerves or nerve branches. In most motor nerve conduction studies, both proximal and distal stimulation are performed. Motor nerve conduction study recordings with or without F-wave testing, when performed, are made from electrodes placed directly over the motor point of the specific muscle to be tested. Sensory nerve conduction study recordings, when performed, must be made from electrodes placed directly over the specific nerve to be tested. H-reflex study recordings, when performed, must be made from electrodes placed directly over the specific nerve-muscle combination to be tested. Waveforms are reviewed on site in real time, and the technique (stimulus site, recording site, ground site, filter settings) is adjusted, as appropriate, as the test proceeds in order to minimize artifact, and to minimize the chances of unintended stimulation of adjacent nerves and the unintended recording from adjacent muscles or nerves. Using well-established techniques, the amplitude, latency, and configuration of waveforms elicited by stimulation at each site of the nerve tested are assessed. This includes the calculation of nerve conduction velocities, sometimes including specialized F-wave indices, along with comparison to normal values. Test design changes during the course of the study in response to the information obtained. Eleven to 12 nerve conduction studies are performed.

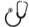 **Clinical Example (95913)**

A 61-year-old diabetic male presents with symptoms of bilateral carpal tunnel syndrome, which is severe on the right in which there is thenar wasting, as well as progressive numbness and tingling in the lower limbs. Evaluation for carpal tunnel syndrome vs neuropathy, as well as to rule out length-dependent peripheral neuropathy is performed.

**Description of Procedure (95913)**

The stimulating electrode is placed directly over the nerve to be tested, and the stimulation parameters are properly adjusted to avoid stimulating other nerves or nerve branches. In most motor nerve conduction studies, both proximal and distal stimulation are performed. Motor nerve conduction study recordings with or without F-wave testing, when performed, are made from electrodes placed directly over the motor point of the specific muscle to be tested. Sensory nerve conduction study recordings, when performed, must be made from electrodes placed directly over the specific nerve to be tested. H-reflex study recordings, when performed, must be made from electrodes placed directly over the specific nerve-muscle combination to be tested. Waveforms are reviewed on site in real time, and the technique (stimulus site, recording site, ground site, filter settings) is adjusted, as appropriate, as the test proceeds in order to minimize artifact, and to minimize the chances of unintended stimulation of adjacent nerves and the unintended recording from adjacent muscles or nerves. Using well-established techniques, the amplitude, latency, and configuration of waveforms elicited by stimulation at each site of the nerve tested are assessed. This includes the calculation of nerve conduction velocities, sometimes including specialized F-wave indices, along with comparison to normal values. Test design changes during the course of the study in response to the information obtained. Thirteen or more nerve conduction studies are performed.

## Intraoperative Neurophysiology

▶Codes 95940, 95941 describe ongoing neurophysiologic monitoring, testing, and data interpretation distinct from performance of specific type(s) of baseline neurophysiologic study(s) performed during surgical procedures. When the service is performed by the surgeon or anesthesiologist, the professional services are included in the surgeon's or anesthesiologist's primary service code(s) for the procedure and are not reported separately. Do not report these codes for automated monitoring devices that do not require continuous attendance by a professional qualified to interpret the testing and monitoring.

Recording and testing are performed either personally or by a technologist who is physically present with the patient during the service. Supervision is performed either in the operating room or by real time connection outside the operating room. The monitoring professional must be solely dedicated to performing the intraoperative neurophysiologic monitoring and must be available to intervene at all times during the service as necessary, for the reported time period(s). For any given period of time spent providing these services, the service takes full attention and, therefore, other clinical activities beyond providing and interpreting of monitoring cannot be provided during the same period of time.

Throughout the monitoring, there must be provisions for continuous and immediate communication directly with the operating room team in the surgical suite. One or more simultaneous cases may be reported (95941). When monitoring more than one procedure, there must be the immediate ability to transfer patient monitoring to another monitoring professional during the surgical procedure should that individual's exclusive attention be required for another procedure. Report 95941 for all remote or non-one-on-one monitoring time connected to each case regardless of overlap with other cases.

Codes 95940, 95941 include only the ongoing neurophysiologic monitoring time distinct from performance of specific type(s) of baseline neurophysiologic study(s), or other services such as intraoperative functional cortical or subcortical mapping. Codes 95940 and 95941 are reported based upon the time spent monitoring only, and not the number of baseline tests performed or parameters monitored. The time spent performing or interpreting the baseline neurophysiologic study(ies) should not be counted as intraoperative monitoring, but represents separately reportable procedures. When reporting 95940 and 95941, the same neurophysiologic study(ies) performed at baseline should be reported not more than once per operative session. Baseline study reporting is based upon the total unique studies performed. For example, if during the course of baseline testing and one-on-one monitoring, two separate nerves have motor testing performed in conjunction with limited single extremity EMG, then 95885 and 95907 would be reported in addition to 95940. For procedures that last beyond midnight, report services using the day on which the monitoring began and using the total time monitored.

Code 95940 is reported per 15 minutes of service. Code 95940 requires reporting only the portion of time the monitoring professional was physically present in the operating room providing one-on-one patient monitoring, and no other cases may be monitored at the same time. Report continuous intraoperative neurophysiologic monitoring in the operating room (95940) in addition to the services related to monitoring from outside the operating room (95941).

Code 95941 should be used once per hour even if multiple methods of neurophysiologic monitoring are used during the time. Code 95941 requires the monitoring of neurophysiological data that is collected from the operating room continuously on-line in real time via a secure data link. When reporting 95941, real-time ability must be available through sufficient data bandwidth transfer rates to view and interrogate the neurophysiologic data contemporaneously.

Report 95941 for all cases in which there was no physical presence by the monitoring professional in the operating room during the monitoring time or when monitoring more than one case in an operating room. It is also used to report the time of monitoring physically performed outside of the operating room in those cases where monitoring occurred both within and outside the operating room. Do not report 95941 if the monitoring lasts 30 minutes or less.

Intraoperative neurophysiology monitoring codes 95940 and 95941 are each used to report the total duration of respective time spent providing each service, even if that time is not in a single continuous block.◄

►(95920 has been deleted. To report, see 95940, 95941)◄

#+●95940   Continuous intraoperative neurophysiology monitoring in the operating room, one on one monitoring requiring personal attendance, each 15 minutes (List separately in addition to code for primary procedure)

►(Use 95940 in conjunction with the study performed, 92585, 95822, 95860-95870, 95907-95913, 95925, 95926, 95927, 95928, 95929, 95930-95937, 95938, 95939)◄

#+●95941   Continuous intraoperative neurophysiology monitoring, from outside the operating room (remote or nearby) or for monitoring of more than one case while in the operating room, per hour (List separately in addition to code for primary procedure)

►(Use 95941 in conjunction with the study performed, 92585, 95822, 95860-95870, 95907-95913, 95925, 95926, 95927, 95928, 95929, 95930-95937, 95938, 95939)◄

(For time spent waiting on standby before monitoring, use 99360)

(For electrocorticography, use 95829)

(For intraoperative EEG during nonintracranial surgery, use 95955)

(For intraoperative functional cortical or subcortical mapping, see 95961-95962)

(For intraoperative neurostimulator programming and analysis, see 95970-95975)

### ✍ Rationale

Intraoperative Neurophysiology testing code 95920 was deleted and replaced with two new codes, 95940 and 95941, which better capture the services provided by both physicians and other qualified health care professionals who perform neurophysiology monitoring, either dedicated to a single case (one-on-one monitoring) inside the operating room or outside the operating room (eg, remote facility site), or a case that is monitored simultaneously with other operative cases.

Codes 95940 and 95941 describe continuous neurophysiologic monitoring, testing, and data interpretation during surgical procedures by physicians and other qualified health care professionals, other than the operating surgeon or anesthesiologist. When the monitoring is performed by the surgeon or anesthesiologist, the

---

⊘=Modifier 51 Exempt   ⊙=Moderate Sedation   ✚=Add-on Code   𝑵=FDA approval pending

services are included in the surgeon's or anesthesiologist's primary service code(s) for the procedure and are not reported separately.

Codes 95940 and 95941 are not intended for reporting automated monitoring devices, which do not require continuous attendance by a professional qualified to interpret the testing and monitoring.

Throughout the monitoring described in codes 95940 and 95941, there must be provision for continuous and immediate communication directly with the operating room team in the surgical suite. One or more simultaneous cases may be reported separately with code 95941. When monitoring more than one procedure, there must be the immediate ability to transfer patient monitoring to another monitoring professional during the surgical procedure should the individual's exclusive attention be required for another procedure.

To report code 95940 requires the physical presence of the monitoring professional in the operating room providing one-on-one patient monitoring for 15-minutes. This code may be reported more than once based on 15-minute time increments. It also must be reported in conjunction with the study that is performed as described in codes 92585, 95822, 95860-95870, 95907-95913, 95925, 95926, 95927, 95928, 95929, 95930-95937, 95938, and 95939.

To report 95941 requires the individual to monitor neurophysiological data collected from the operating room continuously online in real time via a secure data link. To report code 95941, the individual must have the real-time ability to view and interrogate the data. This code may only be used if the monitoring extends beyond 30 minutes. It also must be reported in conjunction with the study that is performed as described in codes 92585, 95822, 95860-95870, 95907-95913, 95925, 95926, 95927, 95928, 95929, 95930-95937, 95938, and 95939.

For a single case in which supervision is conducted both inside and outside the operating room at different times, report code 95940 for that portion of the case monitored in the operating room, and report code 95941 for the portion of that same case monitored outside the operating room.

 ### Clinical Example (95940)

A 32-year-old female has new onset of seizures and MRI evidence of a mass in the right frontal lobe consistent with a glioma. A decision was made to resect the tumor. Intraoperative neurophysiologic testing and monitoring was ordered to avoid damaging or resecting motor pathways during surgery.

**Description of Procedure (95940)**

The physician personally performs the intraoperative monitoring or testing process during one or more aspects of the procedure and provides a diagnostic interpretation of these neurophysiologic tests in real time during the surgery. Data collection typically is from multiple data channels of electromyography (EMG), electroencephalography (EEG), or evoked potentials (EPs). Data are compared to a baseline diagnostic test recorded immediately prior to when the monitoring began. Data are reviewed on several screen displays either simultaneously or sequentially. This in-room service involves personal investigation and resolution of technical issues that may compromise the monitoring. The provider personally consults with the surgeon or anesthesiologist about the neurophysiologic status and the clinical implications as appropriate throughout the procedure. To accomplish this, the provider compares responses over time, actively tests structures to assess the integrity (ie, measures responses to electric stimulations of the extremities or brain), and interprets the findings in order to localize abnormalities and assess the potential implications. This information is communicated directly to the surgeon and anesthesiologist and adjustments in the procedure are recommended as necessary. The impact of adjustments are then monitored and communicated. Ongoing neurophysiologic diagnostic testing procedures typically involve averaging hundreds or thousands of individual trials of microvolt or nanovolt data collection in 16 to 32 channels, which are measured in millisecond or microsecond accuracies.

### Clinical Example (95941)

A 56-year-old male complains of 3 months of leg weakness and two episodes of falling. Neurologic exam showed increased lower extremity reflexes, an up-going right toe, and mildly decreased lower extremity sensation. Imaging showed cervical spondylosis producing severe spinal canal stenosis and cervical myelopathy. Surgery was scheduled for spinal cord decompression with cervical anterior and posterior instrumentation. Intraoperative neurophysiologic monitoring was ordered to monitor spinal cord integrity during the procedure.

### Description of Procedure (95941)

The physician or other qualified health care provider provides an interpretation of diagnostic neurophysiologic tests in real time during the surgery. The interpretations are made by viewing tracings on a remote computer screen similar to the screen used by the technologist in the operating room. Data collection typically is from 16 to 32 data channels of electromyography (EMG), electroencephalography (EEG), or evoked potentials (EPs). Data are compared to baseline EMG, EEG, or EPs recorded just prior to the intraoperative monitoring. This patient's data are typically reviewed on four to eight different screen-displays that can be viewed either simultaneously or sequentially. The physician supervises the direct electrical scalp stimulation of 200 to 600 volts, taking precautions to prevent injury or seizures. The physician screens for and identifies changes that occur during surgery and determines if they present a risk of clinical harm, as opposed to changes due to other causes. When investigating causes of change, the physician applies knowledge of the patient's medical history and physical findings, imaging findings, anesthetic changes, technical details of the testing, and what the surgeon is doing. The physician then arrives quickly at a diagnostic assessment of risk, severity, and location. The physician informs the surgeon and anesthesiologist of the risk. The physician may recommend clinical changes in anesthetic or surgical techniques to reduce risk of neurologic injury. The physician then measures the adequacy of response to interventions. To make these determinations, the physician supervises performance of and provides diagnostic interpretations of the ongoing results of neurophysiologic testing procedures. This typically involves averaging hundreds or thousands of individual trials of microvolt or nanovolt data collection in 16 to 32 channels, which are measured to millisecond or microsecond accuracies.

# Autonomic Function Tests

▶The purpose of autonomic nervous system function testing is to determine the presence of autonomic dysfunction, the site of autonomic dysfunction, and the various autonomic subsystems that may be disordered.

Code 95921 should be reported only when electrocardiographic monitoring of heart rate derived from the time elapsing between two consecutive R waves in the electrocardiogram, or the R-R interval, is displayed on a monitor and stored for subsequent analysis of waveforms. Testing is typically performed in the prone position. A tilt table may be used, but is not required equipment for testing of the parasympathetic function. At least two of the following components need to be included in testing:

1. Heart rate response to deep breathing derived from a visual quantitative analysis of recordings with subject breathing at a rate of 5-6 breaths per minute.

2. Valsalva ratio determined by dividing the maximum heart rate by the lowest heart rate. The initial heart rate responses to sustained oral pressure (blowing into a tube with an open glottis) consist of tachycardia followed by a bradycardia at 15-45 seconds after the Valsalva pressure has been released. A minimum of two Valsalva maneuvers are to be performed. The initial cardioacceleration is an exercise reflex while the subsequent tachycardia and bradycardia are baroreflex-mediated.

3. A 30:15 ratio (R-R interval at beat 30)/(R-R interval at beat 15) used as an index of cardiovascular function.

Code 95922 should be reported only when all of the following components are included in testing:

1. Continuous recording of beat-to-beat BP and heart rate. The heart rate needs to be derived from an electrocardiogram (ECG) unit such that an accurate quantitative graphical measurement of the R-R interval is obtained.

2. A period of supine rest of at least 20 minutes prior to testing.

3. The performance and recording of beat-to-beat blood pressure and heart rate during a minimum of two (2) Valsalva maneuvers.

4. The performance of passive head-up tilt with continuous recording of beat-to-beat blood pressure and heart rate for a minimum of five minutes, followed by passive tilt-back to the supine position. This must be performed using a tilt table.

Code 95924 should be reported only when both the parasympathetic function and the adrenergic function are tested together with the use of a tilt table.◀

▶(To report autonomic function testing that does not include beat-to-beat recording or for testing without use of a tilt table, use 95943)◀

**95921**    Testing of autonomic nervous system function; cardiovagal innervation (parasympathetic function), including 2 or more of the following: heart rate response to deep breathing with recorded R-R interval, Valsalva ratio, and 30:15 ratio

---

| 95922 | vasomotor adrenergic innervation (sympathetic adrenergic function), including beat-to-beat blood pressure and R-R interval changes during Valsalva maneuver and at least 5 minutes of passive tilt |

▶(Do not report 95922 in conjunction with 95921)◀

| 95923 | sudomotor, including 1 or more of the following: quantitative sudomotor axon reflex test (QSART), silastic sweat imprint, thermoregulatory sweat test, and changes in sympathetic skin potential |

| ●95924 | combined parasympathetic and sympathetic adrenergic function testing with at least 5 minutes of passive tilt |

▶(Do not report 95924 in conjunction with 95921 or 95922)◀

| #●95943 | Simultaneous, independent, quantitative measures of both parasympathetic function and sympathetic function, based on time-frequency analysis of heart rate variability concurrent with time-frequency analysis of continuous respiratory activity, with mean heart rate and blood pressure measures, during rest, paced (deep) breathing, Valsalva maneuvers, and head-up postural change |

▶(Do not report 95943 in conjunction with 93040, 95921, 95922, 95924)◀

## ✍ Rationale

As a result of the AMA/Specialty Society RVS Update Committee (RUC) analysis, a combined code was requested for instances when both parasympathetic and adrenergic function types of autonomic testing are performed together, and to ensure users who do not use tilt table during automatic testing report the appropriate code. In order to accommodate this request, code 95924 was established to report testing of a combined parasympathetic and adrenergic function testing with at least 5 minutes of passive tilt table during the same encounter. The purpose of autonomic nervous system function testing is to determine the presence of autonomic dysfunction, the site of autonomic dysfunction, and the various autonomic subsystems that may be disordered.

In order to exemplify the reporting of these services, new instructional guidelines were added to identify all types of autonomic function tests. The guidelines also instruct how to report the autonomic function testing codes and what components are specifically required in each test. When reporting code 95921, at least two of the following components need to be included when testing: (1) heart rate response to deep breathing derived from a visual quantitative analysis of recordings with subject breathing at a rate of 5-6 breaths per minute; (2) Valsalva ratio determined by dividing the maximum heart rate by the lowest heart rate. The guidelines further clarify that the initial heart rate responses to sustained oral pressure (blowing into a tube with an open glottis) consist of tachycardia followed by a bradycardia at 15-45 seconds after the Valsalva pressure has been released. Consequently, a minimum of two Valsalva maneuvers are to be performed. The initial cardioacceleration is an exercise reflex while the subsequent tachycardia and bradycardia are baroreflex-mediated; and (3) a 30:15 ratio (R-R interval at beat 30)/(R-R interval at beat 15) used as an index of cardiovascular function.

The guidelines further clarify that when reporting 95922, all of the following components should be included when testing: (1) Continuous recording of beat-to-beat BP and heart rate. The heart rate needs to be derived from an electrocardiogram (ECG) unit such that an accurate quantitative graphical measurement of the R-R interval is obtained; (2) A period of supine rest of at least 20 minutes prior to testing; (3) The performance and recording of beat-to-beat blood pressure and heart rate during a minimum of two Valsalva maneuvers; and (4) the performance of passive head-up tilt with continuous recording of beat-to-beat blood pressure and heart rate for a minimum of five minutes, followed by passive tilt-back to the supine position. This must be performed using a tilt table.

Code 95924 is intended to be reported only when both the parasympathetic function testing and the adrenergic function are tested together with the use of a tilt table. However, when an autonomic function testing does not include beat-to-beat recording or for testing without the use of a tilt table, it would be appropriate to report code 95943.

Two exclusionary parenthetical notes were also added to clarify the reporting of this service. The first note was added following code 95922 to preclude the reporting of code 95922 in addition to code 95921. The second note was added following code 95924 to preclude the reporting of a combined parasympathetic and adrenergic function testing (95924) in addition to autonomic function testing (95921 or 95922).

In further accommodating the request of the AMA/Specialty Society RVS Update Committee (RUC) analysis, code 95943 was established to report testing performed without the use of a tilt table. Code 95943 is intended to describe simultaneous, independent, quantitative measures of both parasympathetic function and sympathetic function, based on time-frequency analysis of heart rate variability concurrent with time-frequency analysis of continuous respiratory activity, with mean heart rate and blood pressure measures, during rest, paced (deep) breathing, Valsalva maneuvers, and head-up postural change, which allows for heart rate variability (HRV) with respiratory activity and blood pressure to be measured from a standing or sitting position.

An exclusionary parenthetical note was added following code 95943 to preclude the reporting of parasympathetic function and sympathetic function testing (95943), in addition to the rhythm strip (93040), autonomic function testing (95921, 95922), or the combined parasympathetic and adrenergic function testing procedures 95924.

 **Clinical Example (95924)**

A patient presents with repeated, unexplained episodes of fainting. Tests of cardiovascular function indicate severe cardiovagal impairment. Testing of the autonomic nervous system, specifically of parasympathetic function and vasomotor adrenergic function using a 5-minute tilt with a passive tilt table, is recommended.

**Description of Procedure (95924)**

Supervision of patient preparation and the performance of the test by the technician. The patient lays on a tilt table in a flat position. The patient is connected to an electrocardiography (EKG) machine and electrodes are attached to the chest, legs, and arms. If needed, an intravenous (IV) line is placed in the arm. The patient's blood pressure and heart rate are monitored while lying still and are constantly monitored during the procedure. Deep breathing and a series of Valsalva maneuvers are performed until reproducible arterial responses are obtained. EKG monitoring of the patient's heart rate derived from the R-R interval is displayed on a monitor and stored for analysis. Heart response to deep breathing is derived from an analysis of recordings with the patient breathing at a rate of five to six breaths per minute. This is a measure of cardiovagal or parasympathetic testing. Continuous beat-to-beat recording of blood pressure and heart rate in response to the Valsalva maneuver are captured and at least five minutes of passive tilt-up and tilt-back are performed. A series of Valsalva maneuvers are performed until reproducible arterial responses are obtained. These blood pressure responses are analyzed in order to assess cardiac and vascular adrenergic function. The Valsalva ratio is determined by dividing the maximum heart rate by the lowest heart rate. This is another measure of cardiovagal or parasympathetic function. The initial heart rate responses to standing consist of tachycardia at 3 and then at 12 to 15 seconds followed by a bradycardia at 20 seconds. The initial cardioacceleration is an exercise reflex while the subsequent tachycardia and bradycardia are baroreflex-medicated. The 30:15 ratio (R-R interval at beat 30)/(R-R interval at beat 15) is used as index of cardiovascular function. The physician reviews and analyzes this data.

After obtaining a baseline heart rate and blood pressure measurement, safety straps are applied across the patient's chest and legs to hold the patient in place. The patient is raised to the upright and lowered to the supine position several times. The duration of time spent in the supine and upright position can vary from 5 to 30 minutes. Medication may be administered and adjusted during the testing to increase the patient's heart rate and blood pressure. After completing the test, the patient remains flat or supine until the patient's heart rate and blood pressure return to normal. The patient is observed for 10 to 20 minutes and then disconnected from the equipment. The results of these measures are reviewed, data are interpreted, and a clinical correlation of the findings is done based on the patient's history.

 ### Clinical Example (95943)

A 63-year-old female with hypertension presents with complaints of dizziness and lightheadedness, mild depression, sleep disturbance, and frequent headaches for which common treatments are unsuccessful. Physical exam does not completely explain symptoms. Autonomic function testing is ordered.

### Description of Procedure (95943)

Patient sits in a chair. The tech or physician connects electrodes. Measurements are made while at rest seated in a chair, followed immediately by paced breathing, then rest, followed immediately by a series of short Valsalva maneuvers followed immediately by rest, followed immediately by a rapid head-up postural change, followed immediately by quiet standing. Throughout this study, EKG and continuous respiratory activity data are collected and analyzed and parasympathetic and sympathetic activity is computed, and mean HR and BP measures are recorded

⊘=Modifier 51 Exempt   ⊙=Moderate Sedation   ✦=Add-on Code   𝑵=FDA approval pending for each of the six phases of the clinical study. The patient is observed for any complications.

## Evoked Potentials and Reflex Tests

95930    Visual evoked potential (VEP) testing central nervous system, checkerboard or flash

▶(95934, 95936 have been deleted. To report H-reflex testing, see 95907-95913)◄

 **Rationale**

In support of the changes to the Nerve Conduction Tests section, H-reflex study codes 95934 and 95936 were deleted. These tests are now reported with new codes 95907-95913. A parenthetical note was added, directing users to the new codes to report H-reflex studies. Codes 95907-95913 describe one or more nerve conduction studies. For the purposes of coding, a single conduction study is defined as a sensory conduction test, a motor conduction test with or without an F-wave test, or an H-reflex test.

95937    Neuromuscular junction testing (repetitive stimulation, paired stimuli), each nerve, any 1 method

95940    ▶Code is out of numerical sequence. See 95921-95943◄

95941    ▶Code is out of numerical sequence. See 95921-95943◄

95943    ▶Code is out of numerical sequence. See 95921-95943◄

 **Rationale**

Continuous intraoperative neurophysiology monitoring codes 95940 and 95941 are out of numerical sequence and are located in the Intraoperative Neurophysiology subsection. Two reference notes were added, instructing users to the appropriate code range of 95921-95943 for the placement of these codes.

Quantitative measurement of parasympathetic function and sympathetic function code 95943 is out of numerical sequence and is now located in the Autonomic Function Tests subsection. A reference note was added, instructing users to the appropriate code range of 95921-95943 for the placement of this code.

## Neurostimulators, Analysis-Programming

95970    Electronic analysis of implanted neurostimulator pulse generator system (eg, rate, pulse amplitude, pulse duration, configuration of wave form, battery status, electrode selectability, output modulation, cycling, impedance and patient compliance measurements); simple or complex brain, spinal cord, or peripheral (ie, cranial nerve, peripheral nerve, sacral nerve, neuromuscular) neurostimulator pulse generator/transmitter, without reprogramming

+95975        complex cranial nerve neurostimulator pulse generator/transmitter, with intraoperative or subsequent programming, each additional 30 minutes after first hour (List separately in addition to code for primary procedure)

(Use 95975 in conjunction with 95974)

**95980** Electronic analysis of implanted neurostimulator pulse generator system (eg, rate, pulse amplitude and duration, configuration of wave form, battery status, electrode selectability, output modulation, cycling, impedance and patient measurements) gastric neurostimulator pulse generator/transmitter; intraoperative, with programming

**95981**     subsequent, without reprogramming

**95982**     subsequent, with reprogramming

▶(For intraoperative or subsequent analysis, with programming, when performed, of vagus nerve trunk stimulator used for blocking therapy [morbid obesity], see 0312T, 0317T)◀

 **Rationale**

To provide users with instructions regarding the appropriate codes to use to identify vagus nerve blocking therapy procedures, a parenthetical cross-reference was placed following code 95982. For additional information regarding the intended use for codes 0312T, 0317T, see the Rationale for these codes.

## Motion Analysis

Codes 96000-96004 describe services performed as part of a major therapeutic or diagnostic decision making process. Motion analysis is performed in a dedicated motion analysis laboratory (ie, a facility capable of performing videotaping from the front, back and both sides, computerized 3D kinematics, 3D kinetics, and dynamic electromyography). Code 96000 may include 3D kinetics and stride characteristics. Codes 96002-96003 describe dynamic electromyography.

Code 96004 should only be reported once regardless of the number of study(ies) reviewed/interpreted.

▶(For performance of needle electromyography procedures, see 95860-95870, 95872, 95885-95887)◀

(For gait training, use 97116)

**96000** Comprehensive computer-based motion analysis by video-taping and 3D kinematics;

**96001**     with dynamic plantar pressure measurements during walking

**96002** Dynamic surface electromyography, during walking or other functional activities, 1-12 muscles

**96003** Dynamic fine wire electromyography, during walking or other functional activities, 1 muscle

▶(Do not report 96002, 96003 in conjunction with 95860-95866, 95869-95872, 95885-95887)◀

 **Rationale**

In support of the changes to the Nerve Conduction Tests section, the parenthetical note following the Motion Analysis guidelines was revised: codes 95873, 95874, and 95875 were removed, and codes 95885-95887 were added. The parenthetical note following code 96003 was revised with the addition of codes 95865, 95866, and 95885-95887.

⊘=Modifier 51 Exempt   ⊙=Moderate Sedation   ✚=Add-on Code   ⫫=FDA approval pending

# Hydration, Therapeutic, Prophylactic, Diagnostic Injections and Infusions, and Chemotherapy and Other Highly Complex Drug or Highly Complex Biologic Agent Administration

▶Physician or other qualified health care professional work related to hydration, injection, and infusion services predominantly involves affirmation of treatment plan and direct supervision of staff.◀

Codes 96360-96379, 96401, 96402, 96409-96425, 96521-96523 are not intended to be reported by the physician in the facility setting. If a significant, separately identifiable office or other outpatient Evaluation and Management service is performed, the appropriate E/M service (99201-99215, 99241-99245, 99354-99355) should be reported using modifier 25 in addition to 96360-96549. For same day E/M service, a different diagnosis is not required.

When administering multiple infusions, injections or combinations, only one "initial" service code should be reported for a given date, unless protocol requires that two separate IV sites must be used. Do not report a second initial service on the same date due to an intravenous line requiring a re-start, an IV rate not being able to be reached without two lines, or for accessing a port of a multi-lumen catheter. If an injection or infusion is of a subsequent or concurrent nature, even if it is the first such service within that group of services, then a subsequent or concurrent code from the appropriate section should be reported (eg, the first IV push given subsequent to an initial one-hour infusion is reported using a subsequent IV push code).

▶*Initial infusion:* For physician or other qualified health care professional reporting, an initial infusion is the *key or primary reason for the encounter* reported irrespective of the temporal order in which the infusion(s) or injection(s) are administered. For facility reporting, an initial infusion is based using the hierarchy. For both physician or other qualified health care professional and facility reporting, only one *initial* service code (eg, 96365) should be reported unless the protocol or patient condition requires that two separate IV sites must be utilized. The difference in time and effort in providing this second IV site access is also reported using the *initial* service code with modifier 59 appended (eg, 96365, 96365-59).◀

*Sequential infusion:* A sequential infusion is an infusion or IV push of a new substance or drug following a primary or initial service. All sequential services require that there be a new substance or drug, except that facilities may report a sequential intravenous push of the same drug using 96376.

*Concurrent infusion:* A concurrent infusion is an infusion of a new substance or drug infused at the same time as another substance or drug. A concurrent infusion service is not time based and is only reported once per day regardless of whether an additional new drug or substance is administered concurrently. Hydration may not be reported concurrently with any other service. A separate subsequent concurrent administration of another new drug or substance (the third substance or drug) is not reported.

▶In order to determine which service should be reported as the initial service when there is more than one type of service, hierarchies have been created. These vary by whether the physician or other qualified health care professional or a facility is reporting. The order of selection for reporting is based upon the physician's or other qualified health care professional's knowledge of the clinical condition(s) and treatment(s). The hierarchy that facilities are to use is based upon a structural algorithm. When these codes are reported by the physician or other qualified health care professional, the "initial" code that best describes the key or primary reason for the encounter should always be reported irrespective of the order in which the infusions or injections occur.◄

When these codes are reported *by the facility*, the following instructions apply. The initial code should be selected using a hierarchy whereby chemotherapy services are primary to therapeutic, prophylactic, and diagnostic services which are primary to hydration services. Infusions are primary to pushes, which are primary to injections. This hierarchy is to be followed by facilities and supersedes parenthetical instructions for add-on codes that suggest an add-on of a higher hierarchical position may be reported in conjunction with a base code of a lower position. (For example, the hierarchy would not permit reporting 96376 with 96360, as 96376 is a higher order code. IV push is primary to hydration.)

When reporting multiple infusions of the same drug/substance on the same date of service, the initial code should be selected. The second and subsequent infusion(s) should be reported based on the individual time(s) of each additional infusion(s) of the same drug/substance using the appropriate add-on code.

***Example:*** In the outpatient observation setting, a patient receives one-hour intravenous infusions of the same antibiotic every 8 hours on the same date of service through the same IV access. The hierarchy for facility reporting permits the reporting of code 96365 for the first one-hour dose administered. Add-on 96366 would be reported twice (once for the second and third one-hour infusions of the same drug).

►When reporting codes for which infusion time is a factor, use the actual time over which the infusion is administered. Intravenous or intra-arterial push is defined as: (a) an injection in which the health care professional who administers the drug/substance is continuously present to administer the injection and observe the patient, or (b) an infusion of 15 minutes or less. If intravenous hydration (96360, 96361) is given from 11 PM to 2 AM, 96360 would be reported once and 96361 twice. For continuous services that last beyond midnight, use the date in which the service began and report the total units of time provided continuously. However, if instead of a continuous infusion, a medication was given by intravenous push at 10 PM and 2 AM, as the service was not continuous, the two administrations would be reported as an initial service (96374) and sequential (96376) as: 1) no other infusion services were performed; and 2) the push of the same drug was performed more than 30 minutes beyond the initial administration. A "keep open" infusion of any type is not separately reported.◄

## 📝 Rationale

The infusion and intravenous push administration facility reporting examples in the Hydration, Therapeutic, Prophylactic, Diagnostic Injections and Infusions, and Chemotherapy and Other Highly Complex Drug or Highly Complex Biologic Agent Administration guidelines were revised to reflect appropriate reporting occurring on a single date of service and over a range of dates. The CPT code set includes codes and modifiers to accommodate outpatient facility reporting of specific circumstances. Because hospital outpatient reporting represents services performed within either a given 24-hour period (single calendar date) or a range of dates, the infusion and intravenous push administration facility reporting examples were revised to reflect appropriate reporting. Previously, the example for outpatient facility reporting related to the IV-push coding instruction, namely, the reporting of two units of code 96374, *Therapeutic, prophylactic, or diagnostic injection (specify substance or drug); intravenous push, single or initial substance/drug, representing single date reporting.* For 2013, reporting should include one unit of code 96374 and one unit of add-on code 96376, *Therapeutic, prophylactic, or diagnostic injection (specify substance or drug); each additional sequential intravenous push of the same substance/drug provided in a facility (List separately in addition to code for primary procedure),* when facility reporting represents services occurring on a range of dates. See also discussion on CPT nomenclature reporting neutrality.

## Physical Medicine and Rehabilitation

### Tests and Measurements

Requires direct one-on-one patient contact.

▶(For muscle testing, manual or electrical, joint range of motion, electromyography, or nerve velocity determination, see 95831-95857, 95860-95872, 95885-95887, 95907-95913)◀

97750    Physical performance test or measurement (eg, musculoskeletal, functional capacity), with written report, each 15 minutes

 **Rationale**

In support of the changes to the Nerve Conduction Tests section, the parenthetical note above code 97750 in the Physical Medicine and Rehabilitation/Tests and Measurements section were revised: codes 95866, 95872-95875, and 95904 were removed and codes 95885-95887 and 95907-95913 were added.

## Non-Face-to-Face Nonphysician Services

### Telephone Services

98966    Telephone assessment and management service provided by a qualified nonphysician health care professional to an established patient, parent, or guardian not originating from a related assessment and management service provided within the previous 7 days nor leading to an assessment and management service or procedure within the next 24 hours or soonest available appointment; 5-10 minutes of medical discussion

98967      11-20 minutes of medical discussion

98968      21-30 minutes of medical discussion

▶(Do not report 98966-98968 during the same month with 99487-99489)◀

▶(Do not report 98966-98968 when performed during the service time of codes 99495, 99496)◀

## Rationale

To support the establishment of new Complex Chronic Care Coordination Services codes 99487-99489 and Transitional Care Management Services codes 99495 and 99496, two exclusionary parenthetical notes were added following Telephone Services codes 98966-98968 to instruct that these services should not be reported in conjunction with Complex Chronic Care Coordination Services codes 99487-99489 or Transitional Care Management Services codes 99495 and 99496.

## On-line Medical Evaluation

An on-line electronic medical evaluation is a non-face-to-face assessment and management service by a qualified health care professional to a patient using Internet resources in response to a patient's on-line inquiry. Reportable services involve the qualified health care professional's personal timely response to the patient's inquiry and must involve permanent storage (electronic or hard copy) of the encounter. This service is reported only once for the same episode of care during a seven-day period, although multiple qualified health care professionals could report their exchange with the same patient. If the on-line medical evaluation refers to an assessment and management service previously performed and reported by the qualified health care professional within the previous seven days (either qualified health care professional requested or unsolicited patient follow-up) or within the postoperative period of the previously completed procedure, then the service(s) are considered covered by the previous assessment and management office service or procedure. A reportable service encompasses the sum of communication (eg, related telephone calls, prescription provision, laboratory orders) pertaining to the on-line patient encounter.

▲98969    Online assessment and management service provided by a qualified nonphysician health care professional to an established patient or guardian, not originating from a related assessment and management service provided within the previous 7 days, using the Internet or similar electronic communications network

(Do not report 98969 when using 99339-99340, 99374-99380 for the same communication[s])

(Do not report 98969 for anticoagulation management when reporting 99363, 99364)

▶(Do not report 98969 during the same month with 99487-99489)◀

▶(Do not report 98969 when performed during the service time of codes 99495, 99496)◀

## Rationale

To support the establishment of new Complex Chronic Care Coordination services codes 99487-99489 and Transitional Care Management Services codes 99495, 99496, two exclusionary parenthetical notes were added following online medical evaluation services code 98969 to instruct that these services should not be reported in conjunction with Complex Chronic Care Coordination services codes 99487-99489 or Transitional Care Management Services codes 99495, 99496. See also discussion on CPT nomenclature reporting neutrality.

⊘=Modifier 51 Exempt  ⊙=Moderate Sedation  ✚=Add-on Code  𝒩=FDA approval pending

# Other Services and Procedures

▲**99174**  Instrument-based ocular screening (eg, photoscreening, automated-refraction), bilateral

(Do not report 99174 in conjunction with 92002-92014, 99172, 99173)

 **Rationale**

Code 99174 was revised to clarify that it is intended for reporting vision screening utilizing autorefractors and photoscreeners, and a combination of these devices for routine vision screening often performed in conjunction with well-child checkups for children ages 3-6, who cannot read vision charts. The instrumentation is non-invasive. The technology has changed since this methodology was employed and code 99174 first appeared in the CPT code set in 2008. Automated vision devices help to identify a variety of visual disturbances, including amblyopia, strabismus, refractive error, media opacity, etc. There is no physician work associated with the service represented in code 99174, and thus the phrase, "with interpretation and report" was omitted from the code descriptor for this code.

# Category II

Although not as extensive as in previous years, a number of changes have occurred in Category II. This includes the addition of 7 new codes, use of a number of existing Category II codes for new measures, and the addition of a new measure set for inflammatory bowel disease (IBD).

# Category II Codes

[10]American Gastroenterological Association (AGA), www.gastro.org/quality

 **Rationale**

A new measure developer has been included within the footnotes. The American Gastroenterological Association (AGA) has been added to the listing with the appropriate URL to allow users to locate the actual measures from the AGA's Web site. In addition, codes that are used within AGA-developed measures are numerically cited and referenced as number 10 to assist users to note and locate the measure from the AGA Web site.

## Patient History

**1036F**   Current tobacco non-user (CAD, CAP, COPD, PV)[1] (DM)[4] (IBD)[10]

 **Rationale**

Code 1036F is an existing code that is now being used within the inflammatory bowel disease (IBD) measure set. Used as one of two codes within the Screening and Cessation Intervention[10] measure, this code separates tobacco non-users from users and it prevents further reporting of this measure for non-users. The measure itself is used to identify whether a patient 18 years of age or older with a diagnosis od IBD was screened for tobacco use at least once during the one-year measurement period, and if confirmed as a current tobacco user, received cessation counseling intervention. As is noted in the **Alphabetical Clinical Topics Listing** on the CPT Web site, the counseling intervention includes either a brief counseling session of three minutes or less, pharmacotherapy, or both for patients who are confirmed users of any type of tobacco products. If identified as a tobacco user, code 4004F, *Tobacco use cessation intervention, counseling,* is used to identify compliance with the requirements of the measure, which includes: (1) identifying users of tobacco, and (2) provision of treatment as noted for those patients with IBD that are identified as tobacco users. If there are medical reasons that exist for exclusion from the measure (eg, exclusion from reporting for patients who have a limited life expectancy), reporting instructions have been included to use modifier 1P in addition to code 4004F.

Beacuse smoking has been linked to many adverse outcomes, all patients should be encouraged to quit smoking after surgery for Crohn's disease. This includes clinician screening of all adults for tobacco use and the provision of tobacco cessation interventions for those who use tobacco products. There is also a recommendation within the measure that all patients be asked if they use tobacco and have their tobacco-use status documented on a regular basis. Evidence has shown that clinical screening systems, such as expanding the vital signs to include tobacco status or the use of other reminder systems, such as chart stickers or computer prompts, significantly increase rates of clinician intervention. All physicians should strongly advise every patient who smokes to quit because evidence shows that physician advice to quit smoking increases abstinence rates.

●**1052F**    Type, anatomic location, and activity all assessed (IBD)[10]

### Rationale
Code 1052F is a new code that identifies the type, anatomic location, and activity assessed for a measure of the same name within the inflammatory bowel disease (IBD) measure set. This measure is used to determine whether a patient 18 years of age or older with a diagnosis of IBD was assessed for disease type, anatomic location, and activity at least once during the reporting year. The measure snapshot listed in the **Alphabetical Clinical Topics Listing** on the CPT Web site cites a number of factors that are important for identifying the appropriate patient population for whom the measure requirements should be met. This includes patients who have a documented assessment of: (1) an inflammatory bowel disease (such as Crohn's disease, Ulcerative Colitis, or some other unclassified inflammatory bowel disease); (2) the anatomic location of the disease based on current or historical endoscopic and/or radiologic data; and (3) an assessment of luminal disease activity (whether quiescent, mild, moderate, or severe) and presence of extraintestinal manifestations. The measure allows for documentation of exclusions when reporting this measure, which includes patient reasons for not completing the assessment. As a result, the reporting instructions note that modifier 2P may be used to report patient exclusions for providing the service.

## Diagnostic/Screening Processes or Results

**3095F**    Central dual-energy X-ray absorptiometry (DXA) results documented (OP)[5](IBD)[10]

**3096F**    Central dual-energy X-ray absorptiometry (DXA) ordered (OP)[5](IBD)[10]

### Rationale
Codes 3095F and 3096F are existing codes that have been included for reporting the Corticosteroid Related Iatrogenic Injury—Bone Loss Assessment[10] measure in the inflammatory bowel disease (IBD) measure set. Codes 3095F and 3096F identify compliance for this measure because the intent of the use of this measure is to determine whether a patient 18 years of age or older with a diagnosis of IBD, and is receiving corticosteroids beyond a specific treatment threshold (ie, corticosteroid administration that is equal to or greater than 10 mg per day or receiving corticosteroid treatment for 60 consecutive days or more) has a bone loss assessment once during the reporting year. Code 3095F is used to identify the documentation of the results of a dual-energy X-ray absorptiometry procedure. Code 3096F is used to identify the order for a central dual X-ray absorptiometry. There are two other codes that may be used to report this measure. Code 4005F is an existing code that identifies if a pharmacologic therapy regimen has been prescribed, if osteoporosis is noted for the patient. Code 3750F is used to identify patients who

⊘=Modifier 51 Exempt    ⊙=Moderate Sedation    ✚=Add-on Code    ⋏=FDA approval pending

should be excluded from consideration for the measure (those who are not receiving a dose of corticosteroids greater than or equal to 10 mg/day, or for 60 or more consecutive days).

Additional information is provided in the **Alphabetical Clinical Topics Listing** on the CPT Web site for the Corticosteroid Related Iatrogenic Injury—Bone Loss Assessment[10] measure. The information includes a list of thresholds for corticosteroid substances, which helps to further clarify the specific amount that require risk assessment for bone loss. The added notes also identify that documentation for the assessment for bone loss must be performed in order to comply with the measure's specifications.

**3216F**  Patient has documented immunity to Hepatitis B (HEP-C)[1] (IBD)[10]

### 🖎 Rationale

Code 3216F is used to report the Assessment of Hepatitis B Virus Before Initiating Anti-TNF Therapy[10] measure. This measure is included in the inflammatory bowel disease (IBD) measure set, and is used to determine whether a patient 18 years of age or older with a daignosis of IBD had a Hepatitis B virus (HBV) status assessment with interpretation of results within one year before receiving the first course of tumor necrosis factor (TNF) therapy. Code 3216F is used to separate the patient population for measurement because it excludes patients who have a documented immunity to Hepatitis and who are, therefore, not part of the targeted population of patients. Code 6150F is also used to identify patients who are not included as part of the targeted population because this code is used to identify patients who are not receiving the first course of anti-TNF (tumor necrosis factor) therapy. Codes 3517F and 4149F both identify different actions that note compliance for this measure. Code 3517F is used to identify compliance with the specific intent of the measure, ie, assessment of HBV status and interpretation of results within one year before the administration of an anti-TNF therapy. Code 4149F also notes compliance, but is used to note additional action that is needed. It identifies the administration or previous receipt of the Hepatitis B vaccine.

Additional information was also included to assist users with the intended use when reporting these codes. Information was included in the measure snapshot listed in the **Alphabetical Clinical Topics Listing** on the CPT Web site, which provides additional information regarding appropriate procedures (and CPT codes) for assessment. In addition, because there are medical and patient reasons that are noted as exclusions, reporting instructions noted the use of modifiers 1P and 2P when these exclusions exist.

**3510F**  Documentation that tuberculosis (TB) screening test performed and results interpreted (HIV)[5] (IBD)[10]

### 🖎 Rationale

Code 3510F is used for reporting in the Testing for Latent TB Before Initiating Anti-TNF Therapy[10] measure for the inflammatory bowel disease (IBD) measure set. The measure notes whether a patient 18 years of age or older with a diagnosis of IBD had a tuberculosis (TB) screening with interpretation of results within 6 months before receiving the first course of anti-TNF (tumor necrosis factor) therapy. Code 3510F notes compliance for the measure, denoting documentation that a tuberculosis screening has been performed with an interpretation of results. Code 6150F is also included for use in this measure, identifying patients who are not receiving the first course of anti-TNF (tumor necrosis factor) therapy, and who are, therefore, excluded from measurement. Medical and patient exclusions are allowed for reporting this measure. As a result, modifiers 1P and 2P may be used to report this measure when appropriate exclusions exist.

● **3517F**   Hepatitis B Virus (HBV) status assessed and results interpreted within one year prior to receiving a first course of anti-TNF (tumor necrosis factor) therapy (IBD)[10]

● **3520F**   Clostridium difficile testing performed (IBD)[10]

● **3750F**   Patient not receiving dose of corticosteroids greater than or equal to 10mg/day for 60 or greater consecutive days (IBD)[10]

### ✍ Rationale

Code 3517F is used to report the Assessment of Hepatitis B Virus Before Initiating Anti-TNF Therapy[10] measure within the inflammatory bowel disease (IBD) measure set. For more information regarding the use of this code to report this measure, see the Rationale for code 3216F.

Code 3520F is used in the Testing for Clostridium difficile—Inpatient Measure in the inflammatory bowel disease (IBD) measure set. This measure is used to determine whether testing for Clostridium difficile is provided for a patient 18 years of age or older with a diagnosis of IBD and is hospitalized (for any reason), and has refractory diarrhea at the time of hospitalization, or who develops diarrhea during hospitalization. Because medical reasons exist for use of this code for this measure, modifier 1P may be reported when appropriate medical circumstances exist.

Code 3750F is an existing code that has been included to report the Corticosteroid Related Iatrogenic Injury—Bone Loss Assessment[10] measure and the Corticosteroid Sparing Therapy[10] measure in the inflammatory bowel disease (IBD) measure set. For more information regarding the use of this code to report this measure, see the Rationale for codes 3095F, 3096F, and 4142F.

## Therapeutic, Preventive, or Other Interventions

**4004F**   Patient screened for tobacco use **and** received tobacco cessation intervention (counseling, pharmacotherapy, or both), if identified as a tobacco user (PV, CAD)[1]

### ✍ Rationale

Code 4004F is an existing code that is used to report the Screening and Cessation Intervention[10] measure in the inflammatory bowel disease (IBD) measure set. For more information regarding the use of this code to report this measure, see the Rationale for code 1036F.

⊘=Modifier 51 Exempt   ⊙=Moderate Sedation   ✛=Add-on Code   𝒩=FDA approval pending

**4005F** Pharmacologic therapy (other than minerals/vitamins) for osteoporosis prescribed (OP)[5] (IBD)[10]

 **Ratioanle**

Code 4005F is an existing code that has been included to report the Corticosteroid Related Iatrogenic Injury—Bone Loss Assessment[10] measure in the inflammatory bowel disease (IBD) measure set. For more information regarding the use of this code to report this measure, see the Rationale for codes 3095F and 3096F.

**4035F** Influenza immunization recommended (COPD)[1] (IBD)[10]

**4037F** Influenza immunization ordered or administered (COPD, PV, CKD, ESRD)[1] (IBD)[10]

 **Rationale**

Codes 4035F and 4037F are existing codes that have been included to report the Influenza Immunization[10] measure within the inflammatory bowel disease (IBD) measure set. This measure is included to identify whether a patient 18 years of age or older with a diagnosis of IBD had an influenza immunization recommended, administered, or previously received during the reporting year. Both codes are used to identify compliance for the measure: use code 4035F to identify the recommendation of an influenza administration and code 4037F to identify the administration or previous receipt of the immunization. Medical, patient, and system reasons exist as exclusions for this measure. As a result, modifiers 1P, 2P, and 3P may be appended to either code to identify existing exclusions for this measure. This includes the use of modifier 1P in addition to code 4037F to identify circumstances when the immunization was not ordered because it was previously received. To reflect this, the reporting instructions listed in the **Alphabetical Clinical Topics Listing** have been editorially revised to provide instructions regarding the appropriate method to report previous receipt of flu vaccine.

**4040F** Pneumococcal vaccine administered or previously received (COPD)[1] (PV)[1,2] (IBD)[10]

 **Rationale**

Code 4040F is an existing code that is used to report the Pneumoccal Immunization[10] measure in the inflammatory bowel disease (IBD) measure set. This measure identifies whether a patient 8 years of age or older with a diagnosis of IBD has received a pneumoccal vaccination administration. Code 4040F is used to note compliance for the measure and includes language similar to the title of this measure to specify the use of this code. Reporting instructions have also been included to identify exclusions that may be reported for the measure. As a result, modifiers 1P or 2P is noted in the instructions for reporting these modifiers for medical or patient reasons.

●**4069F** Venous thromboembolism (VTE) prophylaxis received (IBD)[10]

●**4142F** Corticosteroid sparing therapy prescribed (IBD)[10]

 **Rationale**

Code 4069F is used to report the Prophylaxis for Venous Thromboembolism—Inpatient Measure[10] in the inflammatory bowel disease (IBD) measure set. This code is used to identify whether a patient 18 years of age or older with a diagnosis of IBD and hospitalized for any reason has received prophylaxis for venous thromboembolism prevention. Code 4069F is used to note compliance for this measure and is the only code utilized for this measure. A definition of prophylaxis is included in the snapshot of the **Alphabetical Clinical Topics Listing**. It notes: "For purposes of this measure, DVT prophylaxis can include Low Molecular Weight Heparin (LMWH), Low-Dose Unfractionated Heparin (LDUH), intravenous heparin, low-dose subcutaneous heparin, or intermittent pneumatic compression devices when pharmacological prophylaxis is contraindicated. Mechanical prophylaxis does not include anti-embolism stockings such as TED hose. (See Category II code 4070F)." Because no exclusions are identified for this measure, modifiers 1P, 2P, and 3P may not be reported for this measure.

Code 4142F is a new code for the Corticosteroid Sparing Therapy[10] measure in the inflammatory bowel disease (IBD) measure set. This measure identifies whether a patient 18 years of age or older with a diagnosis of IBD, who has been managed by corticosteroids over a specified threshold-level was prescribed corticosteroid sparing therapy in the last measurement year. Code 4142F identifies compliance with the measure, noting that the corticosteroid therapy has been prescribed. Code 3750F is included to denote those patients who have not received a threshold amount of corticosteroids for treatment and who should, therefore, be excluded from measurement. Information is also included to assist in reporting this measure, including a list of thresholds for corticosteroid substances that further clarifies the specific amounts that requires attention. Reporting instructions have also been provided to report modifier 1P for medical exclusions for this measure.

**4149F**    Hepatitis B vaccine injection administered or previously received (HEP-C, HIV)[1] (IBD)[10]

 **Rationale**

Code 4149F is used to report the Assessment of Hepatitis B Virus Before Initiating Anti-TNF Therapy[10] measure in the inflammatory bowel disease (IBD) measure set. For more information regarding the use of this code to report this measure, see the Rationale for code 3216F.

## Patient Safety

●**6150F**    Patient not receiving a first course of anti-TNF (tumor necrosis factor) therapy (IBD)[10]

 **Rationale**

Code 6150F is used to report the Assessment of Hepatitis B Virus Before Initiating Anti-TNF Therapy[10] measure and in the Testing for Latent TB Before Initiating Anti-TNF Therapy[10] within the inflammatory bowel disease (IBD) measure set. For more information regarding the use of this code to report these measures, see the Rationale for codes 3216F and 3510F.

⊘=Modifier 51 Exempt   ⊙=Moderate Sedation   ✚=Add-on Code   ✈=FDA approval pending

# Category III

Changes that have been made to the Category III section include the addition of 28 codes, revision of 3 codes, and deletion of 12 codes.

The Category III code guidelines were revised and expanded to include references to the semi-annual publication of actions of the CPT Editorial Panel, which are related to both the revised and new Category III codes that are released semi-annually. The guidelines accurately describe the current practice for the publication of Category III codes and their descriptors to the CPT Web site.

In accordance with CPT guidelines for archiving Category III codes, 4 codes and related introductory guidelines and parenthetical notes have been deleted for 2013.

# Category III Codes

The following section contains a set of temporary codes for emerging technology, services, and procedures. Category III codes allow data collection for these services/procedures. Use of unlisted codes does not offer the opportunity for the collection of specific data. If a Category III code is available, this code must be reported instead of a Category I unlisted code. This is an activity that is critically important in the evaluation of health care delivery and the formation of public and private policy. The use of the codes in this section allow physicians and other qualified health care professionals, insurers, health services researchers, and health policy experts to identify emerging technology, services, and procedures for clinical efficacy, utilization and outcomes.

The inclusion of a service or procedure in this section neither implies nor endorses clinical efficacy, safety, or the applicability to clinical practice. The codes in this section may not conform to the usual requirements for CPT Category I codes established by the Editorial Panel. For Category I codes, the Panel requires that the service/procedure be performed by many health care professionals in clinical practice in multiple locations and that FDA approval, as appropriate, has already been received. The nature of emerging technology, services, and procedures is such that these requirements may not be met. For these reasons, temporary codes for emerging technology, services, and procedures have been placed in a separate section of the CPT codebook and the codes are differentiated from Category I CPT codes by the use of alphanumeric characters.

▶Services/procedures described in this section make use of alphanumeric characters. These codes have an alpha character as the 5th character in the string, preceded by four digits. The digits are not intended to reflect the placement of the code in the Category I section of CPT nomenclature. Codes in this section may or may not eventually receive a Category I CPT code. In either case, in general, a given Category III code will be archived five years from the date of initial publication or extension unless a modification of the archival date is specifically noted at the time of a revision or change to a code (eg, addition of parenthetical instructions, reinstatement). Services/procedures described by Category III codes which have been archived after five years, without conversion, must be reported using the Category I unlisted code unless another specific cross-reference is established at the time of archiving. New codes or revised codes in this section are released semi-annually via the AMA/CPT Internet site, to expedite dissemination for reporting. The full set of temporary codes for emerging technology, services, and procedures are published annually in the CPT codebook. Go to www.ama-assn.org/go/cpt for the most current listing.◀

## ✍ Rationale

The Category III guidelines were revised to include reference to the semi-annual publication of actions of the CPT Editorial Panel related to both revised and new Category III codes released semi-annually. The revised guidelines accurately describe the current practice for publication of Category III codes and descriptors to the CPT Web site. CPT Category III codes are released on the CPT Web site biannually on January 1 and July 1 of each year, to reflect the most recent actions of the CPT Editorial Panel. The Panel actions that are published on the Web site will include addition of any new codes and descriptors or descriptor revisions.

►(0030T has been deleted)◄

►(To report antiprothrombin [phospholipid cofactor] antibody, use 86849)◄

### 🖎 Rationale

In accordance with CPT guidelines for archiving Category III codes, code 0030T and related parenthetical notes have been deleted for CPT 2013.

Code 0030T was used to report antiprothrombin (phospholipid cofactor) antibody. A parenthetical note was added to instruct the use of Category I unlisted code 86849. The parenthetical note following 86148 was also updated to denote the appropriate Category I unlisted code 86849 to report.

►(0048T has been deleted. To report, use 33991)◄

►(0050T has been deleted. To report, see 33990-33993)?◄

### 🖎 Rationale

In accordance with the conversion of Category III codes 0048T and 0050T to Category I codes 33990-33993, two cross-reference notes have been added directing users to the new Category I codes for percutaneous ventricular assist device procedures.

**0101T**    Extracorporeal shock wave involving musculoskeletal system, not otherwise specified, high energy

(For application of low energy musculoskeletal system extracorporeal shock wave, use 0019T)

►(For extracorporeal shock wave therapy involving integumentary system not otherwise specified, see 0299T, 0300T)◄

►(Do not report 0101T in conjunction with 0299T, 0300T when treating same area)◄

**0102T**    Extracorporeal shock wave, high energy, performed by a physician, requiring anesthesia other than local, involving lateral humeral epicondyle

(For application of low energy musculoskeletal system extracorporeal shock wave, use 0019T)

### 🖎 Rationale

In support of the establishment of Category III codes 0299T and 0300T, an instructional parenthetical note was added following code 0101T directing the user to Category III codes 0299T and 0300T to report of extracorporeal shock wave therapy involving integumentary system not otherwise specified. An exclusionary parenthetical note was also added to preclude the reporting of extracorporeal shock wave including musculoskeletal (0101T) in addition to extracorporeal shock wave involving the integumentary system (Category III codes 0299T and 0300T) when treating the same area.

►(0173T has been deleted)◄

### 🖎 Rationale

In accordance with CPT guidelines for archiving Category III codes, code 0173T and related parenthetical notes were deleted for 2013. Code 0173T was used to report intraocular pressure monitoring during vitrectomy surgery.

▲0195T   Arthrodesis, pre-sacral interbody technique, disc space preparation, discectomy, without instrumentation, with image guidance, includes bone graft when performed; L5-S1 interspace

✚▲0196T   L4-L5 interspace (List separately in addition to code for primary procedure)

(Use 0196T in conjunction with 0195T)

▶(Do not report 0195T, 0196T in conjunction with 20930-20938, 22558, 22840, 22845, 22848, 22851, 72275, 76000, 76380, 76496, 76497, 77002, 77003, 77011, 77012)◀

### 🖎 Rationale

Codes 0195T and 0196T were revised to represent pre-sacral interbody fusion, excluding posterior instrumentation procedures. These codes identify the primary level of pre-sacral interbody fusion at L5-S1 (identified by use of code 0195T) and the additional level of fusion at L4-L5 (identified by use of add-on code 0196T). Code 0196T is intended to be used as an add-on code for code 0195T, and it includes descriptor language and a parenthetical note that specify this intent. Similar to notes included to identify the intended use of code 22586 (which identifies pre-sacral interbody fusion performed with posterior instrumentation), codes 0195T and 0196T are listed with exclusionary parenthetical notes that restrict the use of these code in conjunction with fusion (20930-20938), posterior instrumentation (22840-22848), and imaging (72275, 77002, 77003, 77011, 77012) procedures, which are inherently included as part of this service. For more information regarding the intended use of code 22586, see the Rationale for code 22586).

### 🩺 Clinical Example (0195T)

A 40-year-old male presents with a history of low back pain and radicular leg pain. The patient continues to have limitations to his activities both at home and at work, despite adequate physical therapy and other nonoperative interventions. Work-up shows degenerative disc disease with or without spondylolisthesis at L5-S1. The patient is a candidate for lumbar fusion and desires to proceed with a pre-sacral interbody fusion including a discectomy and bone graft.

#### Description of Procedure (0195T)

The patient undergoes an anterior L5-S1 lumbar discectomy and fusion via a pre-sacral approach. Bone grafting is performed and an anterior screw is inserted into S1, across the L5-S1 interspace, and into the L5 vertebral body.

### 🩺 Clinical Example (0196T)

A 45-year-old male presents with a history of low back pain unresponsive to nonoperative management for more than one year. Work-up and evaluation show a degenerative disc and/or annular tear at L4-L5 and L5-S1. The patient continues to have limitations to his activities both at home and at work, despite adequate physical therapy and other nonoperative interventions. Examination of the patient is consistent with lumbar annular tear with increased pain with forward bending and/or lifting. The patient is a candidate for a level 2 lumbar fusion and desires to proceed with surgery. At the completion of the first level, the second level procedure is performed.

**Description of Procedure (0196T)**
After a L5-S1 anterior pre-sacral discectomy and interbody arthrodesis have been performed, the surgeon performs a L4-L5 discectomy and arthrodesis through the same anterior, pre-sacral approach. Bone grafting is performed, and the screw across L5-S1 is advanced across the L4-L5 disc space.

**+ 0205T**   Intravascular catheter-based coronary vessel or graft spectroscopy (eg, infrared) during diagnostic evaluation and/or therapeutic intervention including imaging supervision, interpretation, and report, each vessel (List separately in addition to code for primary procedure)

▶(Use 0205T in conjunction with 92920, 92924, 92928, 92933, 92937, 92941, 92943, 92975, 93454-93461, 93563, 93564)◀

 **Rationale**
In support of the percutaneous coronary intervention changes in the Medicine section, the parenthetical note following Category III intravascular, procedure code 0205T was revised to reflect the appropriate new percutaneous coronary intervention and catheterization and injection procedure codes.

**▲0206T**   Computerized database analysis of multiple cycles of digitized cardiac electrical data from two or more ECG leads, including transmission to a remote center, application of multiple nonlinear mathematical transformations, with coronary artery obstruction severity assessment

(When a 12-lead ECG is performed, 93000-93010 may be reported, as appropriate)

 **Rationale**
Code 0206T was revised to more clearly reflect two or more lead digitized computational electrophysiologic analysis of cardiac signals.

 **Clinical Example (0206T)**
A 65-year-old male presents with chest pain, hypertension, and a left bundle branch block. A thallium stress test was nondiagnostic and coronary angiography is being considered. A computational analysis of digitized cardiac signals is performed to determine an ischemia severity score, which indicates whether the patient should undergo coronary angiography.

**Description of Procedure (0206T)**
Sources of signal interference or existing electronic noise are identified and an optimal location for obtaining the electric signals is found. The testing procedure is fully explained to the patient and care is taken to ensure the patient is in a comfortable supine position and that all jewelry and electronic equipment (eg, beepers, cell phones) are removed. Demographic and clinical data are entered into the computer. The patient's skin is prepared and two cardiac electrodes (which are hooked up to the computer) are placed on the patient in prespecified locations

⃠=Modifier 51 Exempt   ⊙=Moderate Sedation   ✚=Add-on Code   ✵=FDA approval pending

that are the same as the locations for the standard 12-lead electrocardiogram (EKG) leads II and V5. Three 82-second samples of cardiac electrical data are obtained from the two leads. The physician directly supervises the data collection and evaluates the quality of the tracings to ensure appropriate quality before initiating digital signal processing and transmission of data to the remote center. The electrical data is transmitted to the remote center via the Internet. At the remote center, the data is transformed using multiple nonlinear mathematic transformations. The resulting mathematic functions and clusters of the 166 indices are then compared to the index patterns in a large digital empirical patient database and analyzed to aid the physician in determining whether areas of local and/or global cardiac ischemia are present. The computer at the remote center generates diagnostic information, including a coronary artery obstruction severity assessment that is transmitted to the physician over the Internet. The physician downloads and prints the assessment and interprets the diagnostic information provided, including the coronary ischemia severity score.

**0232T**   Injection(s), platelet rich plasma, any site, including image guidance, harvesting and preparation when performed

(Do not report 0232T in conjunction with 20550, 20551, 20600-20610, 20926, 76942, 77002, 77012, 77021, 86965)

►(Do not report 38220-38230 for bone marrow aspiration for platelet rich stem cell injection. For bone marrow aspiration for platelet rich stem cell injection, use 0232T)◄

## ✍ Rationale

In support of parenthetical changes to codes 20938 and 38220, an instructional note following Category III code 0232T has been revised to clarify the reporting of code 0232T for the harvest, preparation, and injection of platelet-rich stem cells derived by bone marrow aspiration (in contrast to code 38220).

►(0242T has been deleted. To report, use 91112)◄

## ✍ Rationale

Code 0242T was deleted and replaced by code 91112. This code is used to report gastrointestinal tract transit and pressure measurements taken from the stomach to the colon via wireless capsule. A parenthetical cross-reference was inserted in place of deleted code 0242T to alert users to the appropriate code for this procedure. For more information regarding the intended use for code 91112, see the Rationale for code 91112.

►(0250T-0252T have been deleted. For airway sizing and insertion and removal of bronchial valve[s], see 31647-31649)◄

## ✍ Rationale

Category III codes 0250T-0252T were deleted. A parenthetical note was added directing users to the appropriate codes for bronchial valve placement and removal procedures via bronchoscopy. For more information regarding the use of codes 31647-31649 for airway sizing and insertion of bronchial valve(s), see the Rationale for these Category I codes.

▶(0256T has been deleted. To report, see 33361-33364)◀

▶(0257T has been deleted. To report, see 33365, 0318T)◀

▶(0258T has been deleted. To report, see 33365, 33366)◀

▶(0259T has been deleted. To report, see 33365-33369)◀

## Rationale

The transcatheter aortic valve replacement procedures codes 0256T, 0257T, 0258T, and 0259T were moved from Category III status to Category I status, with new guidelines and parenthetical notes established to instruct users on the appropriate reporting of the new codes in the Surgery/Cardiovascular System/Cardiac Valves/Aortic Valve subsection. Category III code 0257T was deleted and replaced with Category III code 0318T for the transapical approach for transcatheter aortic valve placement, because the projected May 17, 2012, FDA-approval had not been received. When peripheral access is inadequate, cardiac procedures involving the placement of an intracardiac prosthesis (ie, stent or valve) can be achieved through transthoracic cardiac exposure via mediastinal, thoracotomy, or subxiphoid approach. The implantation of a prosthetic aortic heart valve through a transthoracic approach can be divided into an approach procedure and a therapeutic (valve implantation) procedure, because two different physicians will often perform different parts of the procedure. Namely, a cardiothoracic surgeon will provide cardiac access, and an interventional cardiologist will manipulate the wire and valve under fluoroscopy.

Therefore, codes 33361-33365, 0318T are used to report transcatheter aortic valve replacement (TAVR) or transcatheter aortic valve implantation (TAVI) procedures. TAVR or TAVI that requires two physician operators and all components of the procedure are reported using modifier 62, *Two Surgeons*. Codes 33361-33365, 0318T include the work, when performed, of percutaneous access, placing the access sheath, balloon aortic valvuloplasty, advancing the valve delivery system into position, repositioning the valve as needed, deploying the valve, temporary pacemaker insertion for rapid pacing (33210), and closure of the arteriotomy, when performed. For additional information regarding the use of codes 33361-33365, 0318T for transcatheter aortic valve replacement (TAVR) or transcatheter aortic valve implantation (TAVI) procedures, see the Rationale for these Category I codes.

**0262T**  Implantation of catheter-delivered prosthetic pulmonary valve, endovascular approach

(0262T includes all congenital cardiac catheterization[s], intraprocedural contrast injection[s], fluoroscopic radiological supervision and interpretation, and imaging guidance performed to complete the pulmonary valve procedure. Do not report 0262T in conjunction with 76000, 76001, 93530, 93563, 93566-93568)

(0262T includes percutaneous balloon angioplasty/valvuloplasty of the pulmonary valve/conduit. Do not report 0262T in conjunction with 92990)

Ⓢ=Modifier 51 Exempt  ⊙=Moderate Sedation  ✚=Add-on Code  𝒩=FDA approval pending

▶(0262T includes stent deployment within the pulmonary conduit. Do not report 37205, 37206, 75960 for stent placement within the pulmonary conduit. Report 37205, 37206, 92928-92944, 75960 separately when cardiovascular stent placement is performed at a site separate from the prosthetic valve delivery site. Report 92997, 92998 separately when pulmonary artery angioplasty is performed at a site separate from the prosthetic valve delivery site)◄

### ✎ Rationale

In support of the percutaneous coronary intervention changes in the Medicine section, the parenthetical note following Category III intravascular procedure code 0262T was revised to reflect the appropriate new percutaneous coronary intervention and catheterization and injection procedure codes.

▶(0276T, 0277T have been deleted. To report, see 31660, 31661)◄

### ✎ Rationale

In conjunction with development of new Category I codes to identify bronchial thermoplasty procedures, codes 0276T and 0277T were deleted. To direct users regarding the correct codes to report for these procedures, a cross-reference was added following code 0277T directing users to new codes (31660 and 31661) for bronchoscopy with bronchial thermoplasty. For more information regarding the intended use for these codes, see the Rationale for these Category I codes.

▶(0279T, 0280T have been deleted. To report, see 86152, 86153)◄

### ✎ Rationale

Category III codes 0279T and 0280T were converted to Category I codes (86152 and 86153) for the reporting of cell enumeration using immunologic selection and identification in fluid specimen. Parenthetical notes directing users to codes 86152 and 86153 for cell enumeration with interpretation and report were added. Parenthetical notes were also added directing users to codes 88184-88189 for flow cytometric immunophenotyping, and codes 86356, 86357, 86359, 86360, 86361, and 86367 for flow cytometric quantitation services.

⊙+●0291T  Intravascular optical coherence tomography (coronary native vessel or graft) during diagnostic evaluation and/or therapeutic intervention, including imaging supervision, interpretation, and report; initial vessel (List separately in addition to primary procedure)

▶(Use 0291T in conjunction with cardiac catheterization codes 92920, 92924, 92928, 92933, 92937, 92941, 92943, 92975, 93454-93461, 93563, 93564)◄

▶(Intravascular optical coherence tomography services include all transducer manipulations and repositioning within the specific vessel being examined, both before and after therapeutic intervention [eg, stent placement])◄

⊙+●0292T  each additional vessel (List separately in addition to primary procedure)

▶(Use 0292T in conjunction with 0291T)◄

▶(For intravascular spectroscopy, use 0205T)◄

### Rationale

Two Category III add-on codes, 0291T for the initial vessel, and 0292T for each additional vessel, were added to report intravascular optical coherence tomography (OCT).

OCT utilizes a near-infrared light from a wavelength swept laser to provide a digital three-dimensional image of the internal structures of the coronary artery, which enables physicians to more precisely assess and treat intravascular lesions with optimal stent and catheter placement. OCT is to be performed during cardiac catheterization or percutaneous coronary intervention (angioplasty, atherectomy, thrombectomy, stent placement).

Add-on codes 0291T and 0292T are to be used in conjunction with cardiac catheterization codes 92920, 92924, 92928, 92933, 92937, 92941, 92943, 93454-93461, 93563, 93564, and 92975. Codes 0291T and 0292T are global procedures, as imaging, supervision, interpretation and report are encompassed in the service descriptors for these codes. Also, as stated in the parenthetical note following code 0291T, all manipulation/repositioning of the transducer within the vessel both before and after the primary procedure (eg, stent or catheterization) are included in the add-on codes. Another parenthetical note following these codes was added to distinguish OCT from another visualization enhancement procedure, intravascular spectroscopy, which should be reported with code 0205T.

### Clinical Example (0291T)

A 65-year-old male with diabetes and peripheral vascular disease presents with unstable angina pectoris. He is admitted, and coronary angiography is ordered. Coronary angiography reveals a long, irregular, severe stenosis in the proximal left anterior descending (LAD) coronary artery and a less severe lesion in the distal LAD artery.

**Description of Procedure (0291T)**

The femoral artery is accessed using standard Seldinger technique and a vascular introducer is placed. Baseline angiography of the left coronary artery is performed. (Note: This preceding work is separately reportable using the applicable diagnostic cardiac catheterization code.) A guide catheter is advanced into the left coronary artery. Under fluoroscopic guidance, a 0.014-in steerable guidewire is advanced through the guiding catheter into the LAD coronary artery, across and distal to the stenotic segment. The physician ensures that accurate patient information is entered into the optical coherence tomography (OCT) console. The OCT imaging catheter is set up, connected to the OCT console, and calibrated. The OCT imaging catheter is back-loaded onto the guidewire and advanced under fluoroscopic guidance distal to the stenotic lesion for the imaging pullback. Similar to performing a diagnostic coronary angiogram, the physician injects contrast through the guiding catheter to temporarily displace blood from the coronary artery for optimal imaging. The contrast injection automatically triggers an OCT imaging acquisition sequence. The physician then reviews the OCT image information and evaluates the information for any abnormalities. The physician further assesses the artery for lesion characteristics (eg, fibrous cap, lipid core, calcium burden), the lumen and stent area, the length of diseased segment, and the presence of thrombus. The OCT imaging catheter is removed from the guiding catheter. The physician determines that stent therapy is required and proceeds with stent deployment into the LAD coronary artery. (Note: Coronary stent placement is reported separately.) After the stent deployment is completed, the OCT imaging catheter is again placed over the guidewire distal to the stented arterial segment. OCT imaging is repeated to confirm stent location, the extent of lesion coverage, whether there is underexpansion or malposition, or whether there is a need for further intervention. After determining that the lesion treatment is complete, the physician removes the catheter(s) and guidewire.

### Clinical Example (0292T)

An 82-year-old morbidly obese male presents with unstable angina pectoris. He is admitted, and coronary angiography is ordered. Coronary angiography reveals two-vessel coronary disease. The proximal segment of the right coronary artery has a long, ulcerated lesion with slow flow (which appears to be the culprit), and a lesion in the left anterior descending (LAD) coronary artery (which involves the bifurcation of the LAD and a large diagonal branch). The procedure is discussed with the patient. The first lesion has been evaluated and treated with optical coherence tomography (OCT), and now the second lesion is evaluated and treated with OCT.

### Description of Procedure (0292T)

The first lesion has been treated and evaluated with OCT. During the same session, the second lesion is evaluated and treated using the same techniques as described in the clinical example for code 0291T. (Note: Additional stenting or angioplasty is reported separately).

⊙●**0293T**  Insertion of left atrial hemodynamic monitor; complete system, includes implanted communication module and pressure sensor lead in left atrium including transseptal access, radiological supervision and interpretation, and associated injection procedures, when performed

▶(Do not report 0293T in conjunction with 93462, 93662)◀

⊙✚●**0294T**  pressure sensor lead at time of insertion of pacing cardioverter-defibrillator pulse generator including radiological supervision and interpretation and associated injection procedures, when performed (List separately in addition to code for primary procedure)

▶(Use 0294T in conjunction with 33230, 33231, 33240, 33262-33264, 33249)◀

▶(Do not report 0294T in conjunction with 93462, 93662)◀

▶(Do not report 0293T or 0294T in conjunction with 33202-33249, 93451-93453 unless performed for separate and distinct clinical indication other than for placement or calibration of left atrial hemodynamic monitoring system)◀

### Rationale

Two Category III codes were established to report the insertion of devices that monitor left atrial pressure (LAP). LAP measurements are used in the early management of congestive heart failure. Code 0293T describes the insertion of a complete left atrial hemodynamic monitor system. The monitor is connected to a hand-held device and communicates the measurements to the device. The patient adjusts his or her medication, based on the physician's changes to the prescription plan that is based on the measurements.

Code 0294T is an add-on code that describes the insertion of a pressure-sensor lead at the time when a pacing cardioverter-defibrillator pulse generator is inserted to allow monitoring of left atrial pressure. It is important to note that pacemaker or pacing cardioverter-defibrillator placement, replacement, and revision procedures are not reported separately, when they are performed only to permit the placement of left atrial hemodynamic monitoring systems or leads.

Codes 0293T and 0294T include radiological supervision and interpretation, as well as any related injection procedures, when performed. Moderate sedation is an inclusive component of this procedure and is not reported separately. The moderate sedation symbol (☉) is listed with codes 0293T and 0294T to indicate this.

 **Clinical Example (0293T)**

A 70-year-old female with a nonischemic cardiomyopathy has a history of multiple hospitalizations for congestive heart failure. The patient is referred by her heart failure managing clinician to undergo implantation of a stand-alone left atrial pressure (LAP) monitoring system.

**Description of Procedure (0293T)**

The procedure is performed under conscious sedation or general anesthesia with the patient in the supine position. The patient is given a dose of intravenous antibiotic prophylaxis and monitored with continuous surface electrocardiography (EKG), pulse oximetry, and noninvasive blood pressure monitoring. The patient is prepped and draped in the standard surgical fashion with surgical sites prepared at the bilateral groins and the left pectoral region. Access is obtained to the left femoral vein and utilized for inserting an intracardiac echocardiography (ICE) probe into the right atrium. The left side of the heart is visualized with ICE to ensure the absence of thrombus, and the interatrial septum (IAS) is examined to assess its thickness and whether there are any anomalies that would complicate the implant procedure. Based on the ICE evaluation, a decision is made to proceed with the implant procedure. Access is obtained to the right femoral vein with a 16-French introducer. A subcutaneous device pocket is created in the left pectoral region and access is obtained to the left axillary vein with a sheath. A purse-string suture is placed around the axillary sheath and hemostasis within the subcutaneous device pocket is achieved. Transseptal puncture is performed from the right groin through the previously placed 16-French introducer across the IAS in the standard fashion using a needle with an 8-French transseptal sheath. Once access is obtained to the left atrium, the patient is administered with intravenous heparin and the LAP is recorded from the transseptal sheath. An activated clotting time (ACT) is obtained to ensure a therapeutic level of anticoagulation. The transseptal sheath is replaced with a 12-French delivery sheath over an exchange guidewire. The LAP is recorded a second time from the delivery sheath. To minimize the risk of an air embolism, care is taken to ensure the absence of an abnormal respiratory pattern and that the LAP waveform does not have negative excursions during inspiration. The LAP implantable sensor lead (ISL) is prepared and loaded into the delivery sheath followed by de-airing the delivery sheath. The ISL is advanced through the delivery sheath and deployed into the left atrium. The delivery sheath is gradually pulled back to the right side of the IAS and a fluoroscopic cineogram with injection of contrast is obtained to define the plane of the IAS. The ISL is gradually pulled back and anchored to the IAS, using gentle tugging under fluoroscopic and ICE guidance. Once the ISL is secured to the IAS, the ISL transfer wire is firmly attached to the connector pin of the ISL. The delivery sheath is removed from the vasculature, while ensuring the ISL has adequate slack. The J-tip end of the ISL transfer wire is inserted back into the vasculature through the 16-French introducer and advanced into the inferior vena cava. A gooseneck snare is inserted from the left pectoral region through the axillary sheath and used to externalize the J-tip end of the ISL transfer wire in the left pectoral region. The ISL transfer wire is pulled superiorly and used for transferring the connector end of the ISL from the groin region to the left pectoral region. The axillary sheath is removed from the vasculature and the ISL transfer wire is detached from the ISL connector pin using a slitter. The slack in the ISL is optimized, and the ISL is secured with a suture sleeve to the subcutaneous tissues within the device pocket. The previously placed purse-string suture is also tied down to ensure the absence of venous back bleeding. The ISL is connected to an implantable communications module (ICM) and calibrated to match the last LAP recorded. ISL function is verified and final position on fluoroscopy is documented. The device pocket is closed in the standard surgical fashion, after a repeat ACT is obtained and hemostasis is achieved. The ICE probe is removed from the vasculature, followed by removal of the groin sheaths once the ACT is normalized. Immediately following the implant, a chest X-ray is obtained to document the absence of any complications, and the patient is started on daily aspirin and clopidogrel. The patient is monitored overnight to ensure stable hemodynamics following transseptal catheterization. A predischarge chest X-ray is obtained to ensure the absence of ISL dislodgement. All wounds and surgical sites are inspected to ensure the absence of any hematomas. A hand-held device is used to communicate with the ISL, and obtain LAP waveform data that are uploaded from the hand-held to a computer and reviewed to ensure proper waveform morphology and device calibration. A set of prescriptions are downloaded into the hand-held, and the patient is instructed on the proper usage of the hand-held and given postprocedure instructions upon discharge to home.

### Clinical Example (0294T)

A 60-year-old male with an ischemic cardiomyopathy has a history of multiple hospitalizations for congestive heart failure despite maximal medical therapy and close monitoring by his heart failure managing physician. The patient was previously implanted with a cardiac resynchronization therapy with defibrillation (CRT-D) device 5 years ago in the left pectoral region. The CRT-D device battery status has recently reached the elective replacement indicator (ERI). The patient is referred by his heart failure managing clinician to undergo an upgrade of his CRT-D device to a CRT-D with left atrial pressure (LAP) monitoring.

**Description of Procedure (0294T)**

The bilateral groins are prepped and draped in the standard surgical fashion. Access is obtained to the left femoral vein and utilized for inserting an intra-cardiac echocardiography (ICE) probe into the right atrium. The left side of the heart is visualized with ICE to ensure the absence of thrombus, and the interatrial septum (IAS) is examined to assess its thickness or whether there are any anomalies that would complicate the implant procedure. Based on the ICE evaluation, a decision is made to proceed with the implant procedure and access is obtained to the right femoral vein with a 16-French introducer. A venogram is obtained to ensure patency of the left subclavian vein. Access is obtained to the left axillary vein with a sheath and a purse-string suture is placed around the axillary sheath. Transseptal puncture is performed from the right groin through the previously placed 16-French introducer across the IAS in the standard fashion using a needle with an 8-French transseptal sheath. Once access is obtained to the left atrium, the patient is administered with intravenous heparin and the LAP is recorded from the transseptal sheath. An activated clotting time (ACT) is obtained to ensure a therapeutic level of anticoagulation. The transseptal sheath is replaced with a 12-French delivery sheath over an exchange guidewire. The LAP is recorded a second time from the delivery sheath. To minimize the risk of an air embolism, care is taken to ensure the absence of an abnormal respiratory pattern and that the LAP waveform does not have negative excursions during inspiration. The LAP implantable sensor lead (ISL) is prepared and loaded into the delivery sheath followed by de-airing of the delivery sheath. The ISL is advanced through the delivery sheath and deployed into the left atrium. The delivery sheath is gradually pulled back to the right side of the IAS, and a fluoroscopic cineogram with injection of contrast is obtained to define the plane of the IAS. The ISL is gradually pulled back and anchored to the IAS using gentle tugging under fluo-roscopic and ICE guidance. Once the ISL is secured to the IAS, the ISL transfer wire is firmly attached to the connector pin of the ISL. The delivery sheath is removed from the vasculature while ensuring the ISL has adequate slack. The J-tip end of the ISL transfer wire is inserted back into the vasculature through the 16-French introducer and advanced into the inferior vena cava. A gooseneck snare is inserted from the left pectoral region through the axillary sheath and used to externalize the J-tip end of the ISL transfer wire in the left pectoral region. The ISL transfer wire is pulled superiorly and used for transferring the connector end of the ISL from the groin region to the left pectoral region. The axillary sheath is removed from the vasculature and the ISL transfer wire is detached from the ISL connector pin using a slitter. The slack in the ISL is optimized, and the ISL is secured with a suture sleeve to the subcutaneous tissues within the device pocket. The previously placed purse-string suture is also tied down to ensure the absence of venous back bleeding. The ISL is connected to the CRT-D with LAP monitor-ing device and calibrated to match the last LAP recorded. ISL function is verified and final position on fluoroscopy is documented. Repeat ACT is obtained prior to closure of the device pocket. The ICE probe is removed from the vasculature followed by removal of the groin sheaths once the ACT is normalized. Prior to discharge, a hand-held device is used to communicate with the ISL, and obtain LAP waveform data that are uploaded from the hand-held to a computer and reviewed to ensure proper waveform morphology and device calibration. A set of prescriptions are downloaded into the hand-held, and the patient is instructed on the proper usage of the hand-held and given postprocedure instructions upon discharge to home.

●**0295T**    External electrocardiographic recording for more than 48 hours up to 21 days by continuous rhythm recording and storage; includes recording, scanning analysis with report, review and interpretation

●**0296T**       recording (includes connection and initial recording)

●**0297T**       scanning analysis with report

●**0298T**       review and interpretation

▶(Do not report 0295T-0298T in conjunction with 93224-93272 for same monitoring period)◀

## 🖎 Rationale

Four Category III codes, 0295T-0298T, were established to report external electrocardiographic recording for more than 48 hours up to 21 days by continuous rhythm recording and storage. These codes differ from existing codes 93224-93227 in that they describe more than 48 hours of recording up to 21 days. Codes 93224-93227 describe up to 48 hours of recording. Recording for more than 48 hours is performed to identify atrial fibrillation recurrence or atrial fibrillation, as a possible cause of stroke. This device employs a single-use patch that adheres to the body for a number of days.

Codes 0295T-0298T are structured similar to codes 93224-93227. Code 0295T includes recording, scanning analysis with report, review, and interpretation. Code 0296T includes only the recording. Code 0297T includes only the scanning analysis and report. Code 0298T includes only the review and interpretation. A cross-reference parenthetical note was added following the 93224-93227 series directing users to codes 0295T-0298T for monitoring of more than 48 hours (see Medicine section of this book).

## 🩺 Clinical Example (0295T)

A 72-year-old female without known structural heart disease and a 10-year history of permanent asymptomatic atrial fibrillation with controlled ventricular response presents to the physician's office with episodes of near-syncope for the past month. The physician elects to proceed with prolonged (ie, greater than 48 hours) external electrocardiographic recording.

### Description of Procedure (0295T)

A decision is reached to place an external electrocardiographic recording monitor for prolonged recording (ie, greater than 48 hours) after the patient is evaluated. The rationale for performance of the diagnostic test and other alternatives are explained to the patient and the patient's family. Teaching regarding the use of the monitoring system is performed, and information is provided on the following: (1) how to connect the device and measures to take to ensure adequate electrode contact to improve diagnostic yield; (2) logging diary entries with accurate time during the recording period; and (3) how to disconnect the device and return the monitoring system. The patient leaves the clinic and the monitoring device records the rhythm during the patient's normal activities. The patient removes the device and returns it. The monitoring system is received. The data is downloaded and a scanning analysis is performed. A technician compiles and prints relevant data and arrhythmias (including logged diary events) to be interpreted by the qualified health care professional or physician. Scanned arrhythmias that meet "immediate notification criteria" are promptly brought to the qualified health care professional's or physician's attention. The compiled report is reviewed and interpreted by the qualified health care professional or physician in a final summary report. Elements of the report requiring a qualified health care professional or physician review and interpretation include: (1) the assessment of heart rate trends (eg, minimum, maximum, and average heart rates); (2) the number of supraventricular premature beats; (3) the presence or absence of supraventricular or ventricular tachycardia; and (4) the presence or absence of significant pauses or bradyarrhythmias. Logged diary entries are also reviewed by the physician or qualified health care professional to determine if a correlative symptomatic arrhythmia exists. The final report and interpretation is also sent to the referring qualified health care professional's or physician's office.

### Clinical Example (0296T)

A 72-year-old female without known structural heart disease and a 10-year history of permanent asymptomatic atrial fibrillation with controlled ventricular response presents to the physician's office with episodes of near-syncope for the past month. The physician elects to proceed with prolonged (ie, greater than 48 hours) external electrocardiographic recording.

#### Description of Procedure (0296T)

Staff apply the device and test the initial recording.

### Clinical Example (0297T)

A 72-year-old female without known structural heart disease and a 10-year history of permanent asymptomatic atrial fibrillation with controlled ventricular response presents to the physician's office with episodes of near-syncope for the past month. The physician elects to proceed with prolonged (ie, greater than 48 hours) external electrocardiographic recording.

#### Description of Procedure (0297T)

The unit is connected to the device that performs a scan or the multiple days of recorded rhythms and generates a report that will be used for review and interpretation. The technician notes key events and, as necessary, notifies the ordering/interpreting clinicians of emergent findings.

### Clinical Example (0298T)

A 72-year-old female without known structural heart disease and a 10-year history of permanent asymptomatic atrial fibrillation with controlled ventricular response presents to the physician's office with episodes of near-syncope for the past month. The physician elects to proceed with prolonged (ie, greater than 48 hours) external electrocardiographic recording.

⦰=Modifier 51 Exempt   ⊙=Moderate Sedation   ✚=Add-on Code   ✗=FDA approval pending

**Description of Procedure (0298T)**

The qualified health care professional or physician reviews the report and symptom log, interprets the findings, and documents an interpretation.

●0299T  Extracorporeal shock wave for integumentary wound healing, high energy, including topical application and dressing care; initial wound

+●0300T      each additional wound (List separately in addition to code for primary procedure)

▶(Use 0300T in conjunction with 0299T)◀

▶(Do not report 0300T in conjunction with 28890, 0101T, 0102T when treating same area)◀

##  Rationale

Two Category III codes 0299T, 0300T were established to report the treatment of extracorporeal shock wave for the integumentary system wound healing, high energy, including topical application and dressing care. Code 0299T is intended to report the initial wound, and code 0300T is an add-on code for each additional wound. This procedure includes a high-energy, noninvasive, biological response activating device utilized by individuals for the repair and regeneration of tissue. Because of its high energy and Class III status, an individual assesses and monitors the patient for any adverse tissue events, such as bleeding, petechiae and hematoma, as well as pain.

To exemplify the intended use for these codes, an instructional parenthetical note was added to indicate that the primary code 0299T is appropriately reported in conjunction with the add-on code 0300T. An exclusionary parenthetical note was also added to preclude the reporting of code 0300T in conjunction with other existing extracorporeal shockwave treatment codes 28890, 0101T and 0102T.

##  Clinical Example (0299T)

A 58-year-old female with a 20-year history of type II diabetes mellitus presents with a stage II ulcer on the plantar aspect of the right foot under the third metatarsal head that shows hyperkeratotic margin with fibrotic borders. Dorsalis pedis and posterior tibial pulses are palpable. The wound was originally documented 36 days prior to this clinician visit, and at that time the patient underwent sharp debridement with home care instruction. The base of the wound is slick in consistency, gray, and presents with some drainage. The ulcer margins are indurated with 1 cm of undermining proximally on 50% of the perimeter. The ulcer measures 3 X 4 X 1 cm.

**Description of Procedure (0299T)**

The patient's history and/or referral for the patient's chronic diabetic foot ulcer are reviewed with the patient. Vitals are checked and concomitant medications and procedures are recorded. The existing dressings are removed and a wound assessment is performed. High-energy extracorporeal shockwave treatment is recommended and discussed with the patient. The procedure room, equipment, and supplies are prepared. The wound is thoroughly cleansed and then photographed. A nylon monofilament is used to test the foot for sensation and to determine the level of neuropathy. The wound is measured for depth and total area and found to measure 3 X 4 X 1 cm. With the use of a wound kit, the physician drapes the high-energy shockwave applicator with a sterile sleeve, and calibrates the device per the patient's diabetic ulcer size, energy setting, number of impulses, and impulse frequency. Sterile conductive gel is applied to the open wound-bed and to the margin of periwound tissue. The sterile gel is also applied to the applicator membrane and sterile sleeve to ensure the integrity of the shockwave impulses delivered into the tissue. The applicator is raised into position with the sterile sleeve in contact with the target ulcer to minimize air bubbles between the wound and sterile sleeve. The patient's protocol settings on the device are rechecked prior to treatment. During treatment, the qualified health care professional glides the active applicator, held perpendicular, over the entire surface of the target ulcer extending 1 cm from the wound perimeter. Posttreatment, the sterile sleeve is removed from the applicator and disposed. The applicator and device is cleaned with a hospital-grade, nonalcohol-based disinfectant. The conductive gel on the diabetic ulcer surface is flushed with normal saline and cleaned. The wound is further assessed for petechiae, bruising, pain, and any other adverse events. Moist dressing is applied to the wound. Home-care instructions are provided regarding appropriate wound care and off-loading procedures. Three additional shockwave treatments over a period of 2 weeks (each reported separately) are coordinated to complete the entire course of treatment.

### Clinical Example (0300T)

A 68-year-old male with a 30-year history of type II diabetes mellitus presents with two ulcers, one on the lateral aspect of the right ankle, and one on the right heel. His medical history includes peripheral vascular disease and hypothyroidism. His surgical history includes a previous amputation of the fourth and fifth toes and portions of the metatarsals of the left foot. The ulcers have shown resistance to multiple treatments, including moist saline dressing and advanced wound therapy. The ulcers present with some drainage and redness. The difficulty in closure is compounded by early treatment delay, venous insufficiency, and peripheral neuropathy. The surrounding tissue is dry, red, and thin. The ankle ulcer measures 5 X 5 X 1 cm and the heel ulcer measures 2 X 2 X 1 cm.

### Description of Procedure (0300T)

The physician reviews the patient's clinical history of two nonhealing chronic diabetic ulcers located on the lateral aspect of the right ankle and right heel. Vitals are checked and concomitant medications are recorded. The patient has a documented history of standard wound and advanced wound treatments with unsuccessful outcomes. Existing dressings are removed and wound assessments are performed. High-energy extracorporeal shockwave treatment is discussed with the patient and a decision is made to move forward with treatment. The procedure room, equipment, and supplies are prepared. The wounds are thoroughly cleansed and then photographed. A nylon monofilament is used to test for sensation and determine the level of neuropathy. The wounds are measured for depth and total area. The ankle ulcer measures 5 X 5 X 1 cm and the heel ulcer measures 2 X 2 X 1 cm. With the use of a wound kit, the physician drapes the high-energy shockwave applicator with a sterile sleeve and calibrates the device per the patient's diabetic ulcer size, energy setting, number of impulses, and impulse frequency.

Ⓢ=Modifier 51 Exempt   ⊙=Moderate Sedation   ✚=Add-on Code   ✗=FDA approval pending

Sterile conductive gel is applied to the open heel wound-bed and to the margin of periwound tissue. The sterile gel is also applied to the applicator membrane and sterile sleeve to ensure the integrity of the shockwave impulses delivered into the tissue. The applicator is raised into position with the sterile sleeve in contact with the target ulcer to minimize air bubbles between the wound and sterile sleeve. The patient's protocol settings on the device are rechecked prior to treatment. During treatment, the qualified health care professional glides the active applicator, held perpendicular, over the entire surface of the target ulcer extending 1 cm from the wound perimeter. Posttreatment, the sterile sleeve is removed from the applicator and disposed. The applicator and device is cleaned with a hospital grade, nonalcohol-based disinfectant. The conductive gel on the diabetic ulcer surface is flushed with normal saline and cleaned. The wound is further assessed for any adverse events such as petechiae, bruising, or pain. Moist dressing is applied to the heel wound. The procedure is repeated for the ankle wound. Home-care instructions are provided regarding appropriate wound care and off-loading procedures. Three additional shockwave treatments for each wound over a period of 2 weeks (each reported separately) are coordinated to complete the entire course of treatment.

⊙●**0301T**  Destruction/reduction of malignant breast tumor with externally applied focused microwave, including interstitial placement of disposable catheter with combined temperature monitoring probe and microwave focusing sensocatheter under ultrasound thermotherapy guidance

▶(Do not report 0301T in conjunction with 76645, 76942, 76998, 77600-77615)◀

### ✎ Rationale

A new Category III code (0301T) was added for reporting focused microwave thermotherapy of the breast involving the use of a new technology. The procedure represented by code 0301T includes interstitial placement of a catheter under ultrasound guidance and adaptive phased array wide-field focused microwave thermotherapy heat treatment for destruction/reduction of a malignant tumor (early stage breast cancer and advanced stage breast cancer). This service currently is only provided nationally during clinical trials for patients receiving preoperative focused microwave thermotherapy, in combination with neoadjuvant chemotherapy for treatment of large breast tumors.

A similar service (0061T) was included in CPT 2004 and was deleted in 2009. Code 0061T was created for the FDA-IDE (Food and Drug Administration-investigational device) exemption approved clinical trials conducted with adaptive phased array wide-field focused microwave thermotherapy technology for heat-alone ablation treatment of early breast cancer and heat, in combination with neoadjuvant chemotherapy for treatment of large breast cancer tumors.

Since then, a larger Phase III randomized clinical trial protocol using adaptive phased array wide-field focused microwave thermotherapy in combination with neoadjuvant chemotherapy for breast cancer patients with large tumors has received FDA-IDE approval. The new code (0301T) was updated to accurately describe current clinical practice. This procedure is only to be used in clinical trials at this time.

Several exclusionary notes were added and revised in the Radiology subsection to preclude reporting code 0301T in conjunction with ultrasound guidance codes 76645, 76942, 76998. A cross-reference note was added following hyperthermia codes 77600-77615 to instruct users to report code 0301T for focused microwave thermotherapy of the breast.

 **Clinical Example (0301T)**

A 59-year-old female presents with primary breast cancer and desires breast conservation treatment. It is elected to treat the cancer with externally applied focused microwave therapy.

**Description of Procedure (0301T)**

The patient undergoes externally applied adaptive phased array wide-field focused microwave thermotherapy to heat and kill the cancerous breast tumor and tumor cells in the margins. Treatment is given in an outpatient, office-based setting on a treatment bed similar to a stereotactic breast needle biopsy table, and the patient is fully awake during the procedure. For early-stage breast tumors, a preoperative heat-alone treatment is used to ablate the cancerous tumor and tumor cells in the margins, which is followed by breast-conserving surgery and standard of care. For patients who are mastectomy candidates with larger breast tumors, the preoperative heat-alone treatment is used in combination with neoadjuvant chemotherapy to provide increased tumor volume reduction, and increase the probability of converting to breast conservation compared to neoadjuvant chemotherapy treatment alone. The patient receives a local anesthetic, and a minimally invasive catheter that contains a temperature probe and a microwave focusing probe is inserted under ultrasound guidance within the tumor to monitor and control the treatment. Wide-field focused microwave thermotherapy treatment lasts 60 minutes or less. The minimally invasive catheter is immediately removed following the thermotherapy treatment, and a thin elastic skin closure is applied at the skin entry site.

⊙●**0302T**    Insertion or removal and replacement of intracardiac ischemia monitoring system including imaging supervision and interpretation when performed and intra-operative interrogation and programming when performed; complete system (includes device and electrode)

⊙●**0303T**        electrode only

⊙●**0304T**        device only

▶(Do not report 0302T-0304T in conjunction with 93000-93010)◀

●**0305T**    Programming device evaluation (in person) of intracardiac ischemia monitoring system with iterative adjustment of programmed values, with analysis, review, and report

▶(Do not report 0305T in conjunction with 93000-93010, 0302T-0304T, 0306T)◀

●**0306T**    Interrogation device evaluation (in person) of intracardiac ischemia monitoring system with analysis, review, and report

▶(Do not report 0306T in conjunction with 93000-93010, 0302T-0305T)◀

▶(Cross Reference 1075008 has been deleted)◀

**Rationale**

An intracardiac ischemic monitoring device system may be used to detect and alert patients during a major ischemic coronary event, such as coronary plaque rupture. The device system includes a generator, adaptor, and transvenous lead to detect an ischemic coronary event in patients, who are at high risk for a repeat ischemic coronary event. These high-risk patients include patients that present (in the past 6 months) with an acute coronary syndrome (unstable angina, ST segment elevation myocardial infarction [STEMI], or non-ST segment elevation myocardial infarction [NSTEMI]), and are scheduled to or have undergone either coronary artery bypass graft or coronary angiography, or a percutaneous coronary intervention, and have other risk factors.

Six new Category III codes have been established describing the procedures related to intracardiac ischemic monitoring.

Codes 0302T-0304T include both insertion or removal and replacement. To further clarify, code 0302T describes insertion of the complete system (device and lead). Code 0303T describes removal and replacement or de novo insertion of only the electrode. Code 0304T describes removal without replacement of only the device—when the patient requires placement of another type of intracardiac device (eg, implantable dual chamber pacemaker).

During de novo insertion or replacement of the intracardiac ischemic monitoring device (IMD), adequate sensing function and data retrieval is established, the IMD is interrogated and electrogram readings are recorded. Therefore, codes 0305T and 0306T are not reported in addition to codes 0302T-0304T. Code 0307T describes removal (without replacement) of the IMD.

**Clinical Example (0302T)**

The patient is a post-menopausal female with prior myocardial infarction, diabetes mellitus, hypertension, and hyperlipidemia, who presents with unstable angina due to a 70% stenosis of the right coronary artery. Medical management is optimized. To manage potential subsequent ischemic events, an intracardiac ischemic monitoring system is implanted.

**Description of Procedure (0302T)**

The patient is transported to the cardiac catheterization laboratory in a fasting state. Moderate sedation is provided. The region of the left deltopectoral groove is prepped and draped. Prior to the incision, the patient undergoes anesthesia. Percutaneous access of the left axillary vein is performed. A guidewire is then advanced into the left axillary vein using fluoroscopy. Following this, a transverse incision is made through the skin and subcutaneous tissue, exposing the pectoral fascia and muscle beneath. A pocket is fashioned in the medial direction. Using the previously placed guidewire, a peel-away sheath is advanced over the guidewire into the vein. The dilator and guidewire are removed. An active pacing lead is then advanced down into the right atrium. The peel-away sheath is removed. The lead is passed across the tricuspid valve and positioned in the apex of the right ventricle. Adequate sensing function is established. The suture sleeve is then advanced to the entry point of the tissue and connected securely to the tissue. The pocket is washed with antibiotic-impregnated saline. An ischemic monitoring device (IMD) is obtained, connected to a lead adaptor, and the lead adaptor is securely connected to the lead. Any excess lead is then coiled within the pocket, and along with the lead adapter, wrapped around the IMD such that the connection between the lead and lead adapter is beside or on top of the IMD. A data retrieval session is initiated using the data retrieval instructions. Upon successful data retrieval, a suture is passed through the holes in the IMD to secure the device, and the device pocket is flushed and closed in layers to reduce dead space. Prior to recovery, the IMD is interrogated and electrogram readings are obtained and recorded. A procedure report is generated.

 **Clinical Example (0303T)**

At the one-year follow-up appointment for a previously placed ischemia monitoring system, it is determined that the patient's transvenous lead is not adequately capturing the intracardiac electrocardiography (ECG) signal. The cardiologist or electrophysiologist determines that this lead requires replacement.

**Description of Procedure (0303T)**

Prior to the incision, the patient undergoes moderate sedation. The device pocket is surgically entered. The device is disconnected from the adaptor and transvenous lead. The lead is extracted. Using a guidewire placed in the axillary vein, a peel-away sheath is advanced over the guidewire into the vein. The dilator and guidewire are removed. An active pacing lead is then advanced into the right atrium. The peel-away sheath is removed. The new lead is passed across the tricuspid valve and positioned in the apex of the right ventricle. Adequate sensing function is established. The new lead is then connected to a new adaptor and reconnected to the existing device. Again, adequate sensing function is verified. Any excess lead is then coiled within the pocket, and along with the lead adapter, wrapped around the ischemic monitoring device (IMD) such that the connection between the lead and lead adapter is beside or on top of the IMD. A data retrieval session is initiated using the data retrieval instructions. Upon successful data retrieval, a suture is passed through the holes in the IMD to secure the device, and the device pocket is flushed and closed in layers. Prior to recovery, the IMD is interrogated, electrogram readings are recorded, and a report is generated.

 **Clinical Example (0304T)**

At the seven-year follow-up appointment for a previously placed ischemia monitoring system, it is determined that the device's battery was depleted and replacement is indicated.

**Description of Procedure (0304T)**

Prior to the incision, the patient undergoes moderate sedation. The indwelling device is detached from the lead adapter and is explanted. The current lead is interrogated to ensure appropriate sensing thresholds. Once this ischemic monitoring device (IMD) has been explanted, a new device is placed either in the same pocket created in the left pectoral tissue dorsal to the skin incision or in an alternate site. The existing lead adaptor is then reconnected to the ischemic intracardiac monitoring device. Any excess lead is then coiled within the pocket with the lead adapter wrapped around the IMD such that the connection between the lead and lead adapter is beside or on top of the IMD. A data retrieval session is initiated using the data retrieval instructions. Upon successful data retrieval, a suture is passed through the holes in the IMD to secure the device, and the incision is flushed and closed in layers to reduce dead space. Prior to recovery, the IMD is interrogated and electrogram readings are recorded. A procedure report is generated.

## Clinical Example (0305T)

A patient with a previously placed intracardiac ischemia monitoring system presents for programming of the device.

### Description of Procedure (0305T)

The ischemic monitoring device (IMD) alarm and alert configuration settings for use by the patient are established by the clinician. The ST thresholds for all subjects are initially set using a feature of the programmer that analyzes ST deviation histogram data. A threshold for myocardial infarction detection is set for the patient's normal heart-rate range with thresholds for demand ischemia set up to four elevated heart-rate ranges. If additional ST data is needed at elevated heart rates, the clinician may have the patient undergo an exercise stress test. (Note: The stress test is reported separately.)

## Clinical Example (0306T)

A patient with a previously placed intracardiac ischemia monitoring system presents at the cardiologist's or electrophysiologist's office for evaluation of the device's status and function.

### Description of Procedure (0306T)

The physician uses an ischemic monitoring device (IMD) interrogation unit to retrieve the ischemia, threshold, and event data from the IMD. The physician then reviews the data and generates a report. The physician also checks the parameter settings and saves any parameter changes based on his or her review, reviews medications taken and records any changes, provides reinforcement training on alarms, and checks the occurrence of any symptomatic adverse experiences. Threshold settings are also updated based on up-to-14 days of ST level data stored in five heart-rate ranges downloaded from the IMD in histogram format. The programmer calculates the appropriate threshold levels for detection of transmural and subendocardial ischemic events, and those thresholds are uploaded to the IMD.

## Clinical Example (0307T)

The patient with an implantable ischemic monitoring system has undergone an intervention that resolves the ischemia. A decision is made to remove the implantable ischemia monitoring device (IMD).

**Description of Procedure (0307T)**

Prior to the incision, the patient undergoes moderate sedation. The device pocket is entered surgically. The indwelling device is detached from the lead adapter, and the device and adaptor are explanted.

⊙⊘●**0308T**    Insertion of ocular telescope prosthesis including removal of crystalline lens

▶(Do not report 0308T in conjunction with 65800-65815, 66020, 66030, 66600-66635, 66761, 66825, 66982-66986, 69990)◀

## ✐ Rationale

A new Category III code (0308T) was established to describe implantation of a prosthetic intraocular telescope for the treatment of central vision loss (bilateral central scotomas) due to end-stage age-related macular degeneration (AMD). Implantation of the telescope is a new surgical procedure that is not described by any current CPT code. The procedure entails physician work that is significantly different from any other corneal or cataract procedure, which involve the removal of the lens of the eye because it includes insertion and implantation of a telescope into the lens capsule. The telescope is a new type of device that is structurally and functionally different from any other device, including all currently available intraocular lens prostheses (IOL), that is inserted into the lens capsule. Two opthalmology procedural codes (66982 and 66984) involve extracapsular removal of a cataract and insertion of an IOL. Neither code describes the telescope implantation procedure in terms of the physician work or the prosthetic telescope that is implanted.

The new Category III code 0308T should not be reported in conjunction with other intraocular lens procedure codes (65800-65815, 66020, 66030, 66600-66635, 66761, 66825, 66982-66986), or operating microscope code 69990. An exclusionary parenthetical note was added following code 0308T to reflect this instruction.

Similarly, cross-reference notes were added in the Eye and Ocular Adnexa subsection following codes 66982 and 66984 to direct users to new code 0308T. A parenthetical note was added following code 66983 to indicate that this code should not be reported in conjunction with code 0308T. Finally, the note following the "Operating Microscope" heading was updated to include Category III code 0308T.

## ☤ Clinical Example (0308T)

A 77-year-old female presents with bilateral central scotomas due to scarred maculas from end-stage dry age-related macular degeneration (AMD). Her visual acuity has deteriorated to 20/300 (ie, severe visual impairment and legal blindness). Retinal fluorescein angiography reveals bilateral nonfoveal sparing geographic atrophy. After assessment, the telescope implant is deemed appropriate for the left eye, and peripheral vision is demonstrated to be adequate for safe orientation and mobility in the right eye. Miniature telescope implantation surgery is scheduled.

**Description of Procedure (0308T)**

Anesthesia is induced by retrobulbar block. A 12- to 13-mm conjunctival incision is made and hemostasis is achieved. The first wound, a biplanar wound, is

---

⊘=Modifier 51 Exempt   ⊙=Moderate Sedation   ✚=Add-on Code   ✎=FDA approval pending

initiated: a 12-mm partial thickness (ie, 50%) vertical groove of at least 12-mm arc length, which can then be used to create a short (eg, 0.5 mm) horizontal plane along the entire length of the groove. Intraocular space for the telescope implant is first created by removal of the lens to accommodate the placement of the telescope in the capsular bag. Lens removal is performed through a second, smaller limbal or clear corneal incisional wound (approximately 3 mm) that is placed approximately 90 degrees from the 12-mm incisional wound created for telescopic implantation, and a 7.0-mm intact anterior capsulorrhexis using the surgeon's preferred phacoemulsification method at lower settings to preserve endothelial cells. After lens removal, the first 12-mm wound is opened to accommodate the dimensions of the rigid and large telescope implant. The device is grasped with forceps on the nonglass portion of the device, across the rigid carrier plate, avoiding grasping or touching the glass windows or cylinder of the telescope. The telescope is coated with dispersive ocular viscoelastic device prior to implantation. Ocular viscoelastic devices are injected prior to and during the telescope implantation, to protect the surrounding intraocular tissue and to establish the required anterior chamber space for telescope maneuvering. This often requires multiple instillations to ensure adequate anterior chamber depth. The incisional wound is opened wide by lifting up the cornea 5 to 6 mm to allow passage of the tall telescope profile under the corneal endothelium, but without corneal touch or tenting of the cornea. A steep entry-angle of 45 degrees is required to place the telescope carrier plate and lead haptic into the capsular bag. With the carrier plate and leading haptic entirely within the anterior chamber, a cyclodialysis spatula is used to help direct the leading haptic downward through the capsulorrhexis and into the bag. (This may require an experienced assistant to lift the cornea.) Bimanual implantation techniques are used to manipulate the telescope through the anterior chamber and into the capsular bag. Forceps are used to compress the trailing haptic superiorly as the telescope is ushered into the capsular bag, while at the same time an inferior hook is placed into the positioning hole in the carrier plate to avoid undue pressure on the inferior capsule and aid in performing this maneuver. Situated in the capsular bag, the anterior window of the device protrudes anteriorly through the iris plane. The telescope is bimanually rotated to the 6 and 12 o'clock positions for maximum stability. Six to 8 sutures are placed using a two-step suturing technique to minimize risk associated with large incisions and to promote healing without inducing postoperative corneal irregularities. Bimanual irrigation and aspiration are performed. A peripheral iridectomy is made. A sub-Tenon's capsule injection of steroid and antibiotic is performed, and topical steroids are applied.

+ ●0309T    Arthrodesis, pre-sacral interbody technique, including disc space preparation, discectomy, with posterior instrumentation, with image guidance, includes bone graft, when performed, lumbar, L4-L5 interspace (List separately in addition to code for primary procedure)

▶(Use 0309T in conjunction with 22586)◀

▶(Do not report 0309T in conjunction with 20930-20938, 22840, 22848, 72275, 77002, 77003, 77011, 77012)◀

## ✎ Rationale

Code 0309T was developed as an add-on code to identify an additional level of pre-sacral interbody fusion performed at the L4-L5 interspace. As an add-on code, this code is intended to be used only in conjunction with code 22586 (which identifies the initial level of pre-sacral interbody fusion), and it includes a parenthetical instructional note that reflects this. There is also an exclusionary cross-reference that restricts the use of fusion (20930-20938), posterior instrumentation (22840-22848), and imaging (72275, 77002, 77003, 77011, 77012) services in conjunction with this code.

For more information regarding the intended use of code 22586, see the Rationale for code 22586.

## ☁ Clinical Example (0309T)

A 45-year-old male presents with a history of low back pain unresponsive to non-operative management for more than one year. Work-up and evaluation show a degenerative disc and/or annular tear at L4/L5 and L5/S1. The patient continues to have limitations to his activities both at home and at work, despite adequate physical therapy and other nonoperative interventions. Examination of the patient is consistent with lumbar annular tear with increased pain with forward bending and or lifting. The patient is a candidate for a level 2 lumbar fusion and desires to proceed with surgery. At the completion of the first level, the second level procedure is performed.

### Description of Procedure (0309T)

After a L5-S1 anterior, pre-sacral discectomy and interbody arthrodesis has been performed, the surgeon performs a L4-5 discectomy and arthrodesis through the same anterior, pre-sacral approach. Bone grafting is performed and the screw across L5-S1 is advanced across the L4-5 disc space. Posterior supplemental instrumentation is performed through a separate incision.

●0310T     Motor function mapping using non-invasive navigated transcranial magnetic stimulation (nTMS) for therapeutic treatment planning, upper and lower extremity

▶(Do not report 0310T in conjunction with 95860-95870, 95928, 95929, 95939)◀

## ✎ Rationale

Category III code 0310T was established to report a new noninvasive technology used in the localization of functional motor cortex for neurosurgical pre-operative planning prior to brain surgery for brain tumors, intractable epilepsy and arterio-venous malformations near or within the motor cortex. Navigated transcranial magnetic stimulation (nTMS) is an integrated system that uses transcranial magnetic stimulation (TMS) and electromyography (EMG) guided by standard magnetic resonance (MR) image data. The nTMS procedure facilitates accurate noninvasive localization of the functional motor cortex to maximize surgery outcomes while minimizing the likelihood of permanent deficits of motor function. An exclusionary parenthetical note was added instructing users not to report code 0310T with codes 95860-95870, 95928, 95929, and 95939. Another parenthentetical note was added following code 90869 directing users to code 0310T for transcranial magnetic stimulation motor function mapping for therapeutic planning other than for repetitive transcranial magnetic stimulation. Modifications to the cross-references following codes 90867 and 90869 were made to clarify the appropriate ranges of codes, including the addition of code 95939 to the list of exclusionary codes that should not be reported in conjunction with codes 90867 and 90869.

## Clinical Example (0310T)

A 59-year-old male presents with a brain tumor located within or close to the assumed location of the primary motor cortex, as well as partial limb paresis. A surgical procedure is considered, but due to unclear neuroanatomy present in the patient's anatomic magnetic resonance imaging (MRI) scan and/or the close proximity of the tumor to the presumed motor cortex, the location of functional motor cortex needs to be verified before a procedure can be planned.

### Description of Procedure (0310T)

A noninvasive, diagnostic, navigated transcranial magnetic stimulation (TMS) procedure is performed to identify the location of the functional primary motor cortex and its relative position to the surgical target on the patient's three-dimensional MRI anatomy to facilitate the planning of a subsequent therapeutic procedure. Initially, the physician checks the safety of the equipment by verifying that there is no damage to the electrical connections and that there is no visible damage to the system. The position of the tracking system unit (infrared camera) is checked to ensure that it will able to visualize all system components are in the correct position. The proper TMS coil that will be used during the session is selected and checked for cleanliness. The patient's MRI scan is uploaded into the system. MRI landmarks are set on the three-dimensional MRI model to register the patient's physical head to the three-dimensional MRI image head-model in the system. The patient is brought in and positioned in the chair. Once the patient is comfortably seated, the position of the tracking-unit camera is adjusted accordingly to view the patient's head. The registration sticker is placed on the patient's forehead to enable verification during the session that the head-trackers have not moved and that the obtained results are valid. Electromyography (EMG) electrodes are placed on the muscles that correspond with the areas of the motor cortex to be mapped. The EMG channels to be used are selected in the software, and the user verifies that the EMG data show no interference. The patient's physical head is registered by placing the digitization tool at the three points (landmarks) on the scalp marked in the magnetic resonance images. Nine additional points on the patient's head are touched with the digitization tool for advanced registration, after which the user verifies that the software indicates that the registration was accurate. A further verification of the successful registration is done by placing the digitization tool at three preset locations on the registration sticker. The physician places the coil on the patient's head and presses a foot pedal that triggers the system and the TMS coil to stimulate the cortex to locate the motor functions. Multiple stimulations are performed to locate the motor functions. Once the motor function hotspot is located, TMS is used to determine the patient's motor threshold. The stimulator output is set to optimal mapping intensity (110% of motor threshold), and is used to determine the locations eliciting motor evoked potentials (MEPs) from the target muscles with high spatial resolution for accurate mapping of the motor cortex. As the coil is moved over the patient's head, the physician can see in real time the electronic field location, strength, and direction in the three-dimensional intracranial rendering. After the mapping is completed, the EMG electrodes and the head-tracker are removed from the patient. Postprocessing is performed by analyzing the EMG responses and reviewing the mapping results. A digital imaging and communications in medicine (DICOM) export of the results can be created so that the results can be used in the operating room or in other third-party software. Color-coded maps of the MEP response strengths can be viewed at any intracranial depth. The physician performing subsequent therapeutic procedures can view the results. The results and their implications can also be immediately discussed with the patient with results presented on software.

●**0311T**   Non-invasive calculation and analysis of central arterial pressure waveforms with interpretation and report

### Rationale

A Category III code 0311T was established to report noninvasive calculation and analysis of central arterial pressure waveforms with interpretation and report. Code 0311T is intended to describe collection and interpretation of pressure waveform data through a high-fidelity pressure transducer.

The printed report includes peripheral and central waveforms, multiple indices of the blood pressure waveform, and systemic arterial stiffness (eg, peripheral and central systolic, diastolic and pulse pressures, as well as normal values and ranges). This information is not available and cannot be inferred from standard cuff blood-pressure measurements.

The individual thus makes hypertension management decisions incorporating additional data available from central blood-pressure and waveform analysis.

### Clinical Example (0311T)

A 58-year-old male with difficult-to-control hypertension has a central blood pressure determination to help manage his hypertension.

#### Description of Procedure (0311T)

A trained operator (generally office staff) performs the test as follows: The patient's sitting blood pressure is measured by brachial cuff sphygmomanometry according to guidelines (ie, the cuff blood pressure is used to calibrate the noninvasive central pressure measurement). Patient information is entered into the device or computer controlling the device. A peripheral blood pressure waveform is acquired noninvasively (eg, from arterial tonometry at the radial artery). The quality of the waveform is then assessed and a printed report is generated. The printed report includes peripheral and central waveforms, multiple indices of the blood pressure waveform, and systemic arterial stiffness. The physician assesses these measurements for validity and generates an interpretation.

●**0312T** Vagus nerve blocking therapy (morbid obesity); laparoscopic implantation of neurostimulator electrode array, anterior and posterior vagal trunks adjacent to esophagogastric junction (EGJ), with implantation of pulse generator, includes programming

●**0313T** laparoscopic revision or replacement of vagal trunk neurostimulator electrode array, including connection to existing pulse generator

●**0314T** laparoscopic removal of vagal trunk neurostimulator electrode array and pulse generator

●**0315T** removal of pulse generator

●**0316T** replacement of pulse generator

▶(Do not report 0315T in conjunction with 0316T)◀

●**0317T** neurostimulator pulse generator electronic analysis, includes reprogramming when performed

▶(For implantation, revision, replacement, and/or removal of vagus [cranial] nerve neurostimulator electrode array and/or pulse generator for vagus nerve stimulation performed other than at the EGJ [eg, epilepsy], see 64568-64570)◀

▶(For analysis and/or [re]programming for vagus nerve stimulator, see 95970, 95974, 95975)◀

### 🖎 Rationale

Category III codes 0312T-0317T are used to report laparoscopic vagus nerve blocking therapy for treatment of obesity. The services identified by the use of these codes includes: (1) laparoscopic implantation of the neurostimulator electrode array (0312T); (2) revision or replacement of the neurostimulator array (0313T); (3) removal of the neurostimulator electrode array and pulse generator (together) (0314T); and (4) removal of the pulse generator independent of the electrode array (0315T), replacement of the pulse generator (0316T), and electronic analysis of the pulse generator (along with reprogramming when performed) (0317T). To indicate the intended use of these codes, a number of parenthetical notes were placed in this section as well as other sections to identify exclusions that exist, and to provide instruction regarding the use of these codes versus the use of other codes that identify neurostimulator implantation/removal, analysis, and/or reprogramming (43647 series for laparoscopic gastric neurostimulator placement, 64568 series for open procedures regarding implant, revision, and/or removal of cranial nerve neurostimulators [such as vagus nerve], and 95980 series for programming of implants). For more information regarding the intent of the parenthetical notes that follows these codes, see the Rationale for these codes.

The new codes for laparascopic vagal blocking therapy procedures identify intermittent intra-abdominal vagal blocking to treat obesity using high-frequency electrical currents. The electrodes are positioned laparoscopically on the anterior and posterior vagal trunks near the esophagogastric junction (EGJ), without anatomic modification or tissue compression of the alimentary tract. The procedures utilize high-frequency electrical currents that demonstrate reversible inhibition of the propagation of vagus and sciatic nerve compound action potentials in both A$\delta$ and C fibers of the nerves, as well as reversible inhibition of pancreatic exocrine secretion and gastric contractions. This is all accomplished while preserving neural anatomy, histology, and function.

## 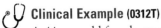 Clinical Example (0312T)

A 44-year-old female presents with a body mass index (BMI) of 45 kg/m², hypertension, and poorly controlled diabetes. She has failed nonoperative obesity interventions. She is a single mother and is fearful of the operative complications of bands, sleeves, and bypasses. She is interested in vagal nerve blocking therapy.

### Description of Procedure (0312T)

The vagal blocking therapy induces intermittent intra-abdominal vagal blocking to treat obesity using high-frequency electrical currents. The electrodes are positioned laparoscopically around the anterior and posterior vagal trunks near the esophagogastric junction (EGJ), without anatomic modification or tissue compression of the alimentary tract. The device consists of two electrodes (one for each vagal trunk), a neuroregulator placed subcutaneously, and an external mobile charger attached to a transmit coil to recharge the device. The electrode itself has an active surface area of 10 mm² and is "C"-shaped to partially encircle the nerve. The procedure for placement is as follows: After general anesthesia and the customary abdominal sterile prepping and draping, the abdominal cavity is accessed for laparoscopic surgery and an angled laparoscope is inserted along with three to four working ports that are either 5 or 10 mm. Two leads (electrodes) of the vagal blocking system are inserted into the abdomen thorough a 10-mm trocar. The left lateral segment of the liver is retracted anteriorly and the gastroesophageal junction is identified. The gastrohepatic ligament is dissected to expose the EGJ, and the stomach is retracted downward and laterally to keep slight tension on the EGJ. To locate the posterior vagal trunk, the right diaphragmatic crus is identified and separated from its esophageal attachments. The anterior vagal trunk is identified by locating it as it courses through the diaphragmatic hiatus. After both vagal trunks have been identified, a right angle grasper is used to dissect a 5-mm window underneath the posterior vagal trunk. The electrode is then placed by positioning a right-angle grasper through the window that had been created under the vagal nerve. The electrode's distal suture tab is then grasped, and the electrode is pulled into place, seating the nerve within the electrode cup. The same steps are repeated to place a second electrode around the anterior vagal trunk. Finally, each electrode is secured in position using a single suture placed through each electrode's distal suture tab and affixed to the outer layers of the esophagus. Care is taken to assure that the nerve is comfortably and completely in the electrode cup and that the nerve is neither stretched nor kinked. The leads are further secured by suturing the proximal suture sleeve to the gastrohepatic ligament or to the lesser curvature of the stomach. The proximal ends of the leads are then pulled out of the abdominal cavity through the 10-mm trocar and connected to the neuroregulator. After successful device interrogation, the neuroregulator is implanted in a subcutaneous pocket on the lateral upper abdomen of the lower chest wall. At implantation, proper electrode placement can then be determined in two different ways. First, correct anatomic electrode and nerve alignment can be verified visually. Second, effective electrical contact can be verified using impedance measurements intraoperatively (and at frequent intervals thereafter). After recovery from the surgery, a mobile charger connected to a transmit coil is used to recharge the implanted neuroregulator transdermally. The neuroregulator is programmed for frequency, amplitude, and duty cycle using a computer programmer. The therapeutic frequency selected to block neural impulses on the vagal trunks is 5,000 Hz, based on animal studies of vagal inhibition of pancreatic exocrine secretion. Amplitudes utilized range from 1 mA to 8 mA. However, in almost all instances, the amplitude is 6 mA. The device is usually activated in the morning and turned off before sleep. The protocol specified an algorithm of 5 minutes of blocking, alternating with 5 minutes without blocking, for approximately 12 hours of therapy per day. Effective electrical contact is verified using impedance measurements at frequent intervals postoperatively.

 **Clinical Example (0313T)**

A 40-year-old male had a vagal nerve blocking therapy device implanted 2 months earlier. Unfortunately, on interrogation, the system demonstrates very high impedance levels. It is thought that there is a lead malfunction. The patient wishes to continue therapy and requests lead replacement.

**Description of Procedure (0313T)**

The vagal nerve blocking therapy device is interrogated and deactivated. The patient is placed in the supine, lithotomy, or legs spread position depending on the surgeon's preference. Antibiotics and thromboprophylaxis are administered. The abdomen and left lower chest are prepped with an antiseptic solution, and the patient is draped sterilely. Standard abdominal cavity access is performed and a pneumoperitoneum is created. Port placement is also according to the surgeon's preference. An angled laparoscope is inserted. The liver is elevated anteriorly and superiorly off of the stomach. The leads are located. Adhesions are taken down as needed to free the liver and the leads. The leads are traced back to the gastroesophageal junction (EGJ). Careful dissection is employed to locate the distal suture tabs. When freed, the sutures of the distal suture tabs are cut and the leads are carefully pulled off of the vagus nerves. The leads are then moved away from the EGJ. The proximal suture sleeves are located and detached from the stomach wall by cutting their sutures. New leads are carefully placed into the abdominal cavity. The electrode cup is passed around each vagus nerve through the plain created by the removal of the old leads. The new leads are secured in a similar fashion as the old ones by suturing the distal suture tab to the esophageal wall and the proximal suture sleeves to the anterior gastric wall or gastrohepatic ligament. The proximal ends of both the old and new leads are brought out of the abdominal cavity via a left upper-quadrant trocar. At this point, the laparoscopic portion of the procedure is completed. The pocket overlying the neuroregulator is opened through the old incision, and the neuroregulator is freed by cutting adhesions, the fibrous capsule, and the tacking sutures. The neuroregulator is pulled out of its pocket. The old leads are disconnected by loosening the setscrews. The old leads are then discarded. The new leads are pushed into the neuroregulator connectors and the setscrews are tightened. The system is then interrogated. If function is normal, the neuroregulator is replaced back in the pocket and secured with sutures. The wounds are then closed per the surgeon's usual routine. The patient recovers, and is discharged when stable.

### Clinical Example (0314T)

A 50-year-old female had a vagal nerve blocking therapy device implanted one year earlier. Unfortunately, her results did not meet her expectations, and she requested that the device be explanted.

#### Description of Procedure (0314T)

The vagal nerve blocking therapy device is interrogated and deactivated. The patient is placed in the supine, lithotomy, or legs spread position depending on the surgeon's preference. Antibiotics and thromboprophylaxis are administered. The abdomen and left lower chest are prepped with an antiseptic solution, and the patient is draped sterilely. Standard laparoscopic abdominal cavity access is performed and a pneumoperitoneum is created. Port placement is also according to the surgeon's preference. An angled laparoscope is inserted. The liver is elevated anteriorly and superiorly off of the stomach. The leads are located. Adhesions are taken down as needed to free up the proximal stomach and the leads. The leads are traced back to the gastroesophageal junction (EGJ). Careful dissection is employed to locate the distal suture tabs. When freed, the sutures of the distal suture tabs are cut and the leads are carefully pulled off of the vagus nerves. The leads are then moved away from the EGJ. The proximal suture sleeves are located and detached from the stomach wall by cutting their sutures. The leads are cut and the proximal ends of both leads are brought out of the abdominal cavity via a left upper-quadrant trocar. At this point the laparoscopic portion of the procedure is completed. The pocket overlying the neuroregulator is opened through the old incision, and the neuroregulator is freed by cutting adhesions, the fibrous capsule, and the tacking sutures. The neuroregulator is pulled out of its pocket. The neuroregulator and the distal leads can then be explanted and discarded. The wounds are then closed per the surgeon's usual routine. The patient recovers, and is discharged when stable.

### Clinical Example (0315T)

A 45-year-old male patient had the vagal nerve blocking therapy device implanted 2 years earlier and has achieved his weight-loss goal. The patient requested that the pulse generator be removed due to its prominence as a result of successful weight loss. The patient wishes to have the option to continue therapy at a later time if he regains weight, and therefore, requests that the leads be left in place for potential future use.

#### Description of Procedure (0315T)

The patient is placed in the supine position depending on the surgeon's preference. Antibiotics and thromboprophylaxis are administered. The abdomen and left lower chest are prepped with an antiseptic solution, and the patient is draped sterilely. The pocket overlying the neuroregulator is opened through the old incision, and the neuroregulator is freed by cutting adhesions, the fibrous capsule, and the tacking sutures. The neuroregulator is pulled out of its pocket. The leads are disconnected by loosening the setscrews. The old neuroregulator is discarded. The leads are secured within the pocket to be attached to a new neuroregulator at a later point. The wound is then closed per the surgeon's usual routine. The patient recovers, and is discharged when stable.

⃠=Modifier 51 Exempt   ⨀=Moderate Sedation   ✚=Add-on Code   ⅄=FDA approval pending

## Clinical Example (0316T)

A 40-year-old female had the vagal nerve blocking therapy device implanted 5 years earlier. Unfortunately, on interrogation, the system demonstrates that the pulse generator battery is no longer viable. The patient wishes to continue therapy and requests a pulse generator replacement.

### Description of Procedure (0316T)

The patient is placed in the supine or lithotomy position depending on the surgeon's preference. Antibiotics and thromboprophylaxis are administered. The abdomen and left lower chest are prepped with an antiseptic solution, and the patient is draped sterilely. The pocket overlying the neuroregulator is opened through the old incision, and the neuroregulator is freed by cutting adhesions, the fibrous capsule, and the tacking sutures. The neuroregulator is pulled out of its pocket. The leads are disconnected by loosening the setscrews. The old neuroregulator is discarded. A new neuroregulator is brought into the surgical field. The leads are pushed into the new neuroregulator connectors and the setscrews are tightened. The system is then interrogated. If function is normal, the neuroregulator is replaced back in the pocket and secured with sutures. The wound is then closed per the surgeon's usual routine. The patient recovers, and is discharged when stable.

## Clinical Example (0317T)

A 36-year-old female with a body mass index (BMI) of 46 kg/m², hypertension, gastroesophageal reflux, dypsnea, and stress urinary incontinence has undergone placement of the vagal nerve blocking therapy device with initial weight loss success over the first 4 months after implant. However, over the next 2 months, her weight loss plateaued and she has had some increase in appetite.

### Description of Procedure (0317T)

The neuroregulator is programmed for frequency, amplitude, and duty cycle using a computer programmer. The therapeutic frequency selected to block neural impulses on the vagal trunks is 5,000 Hz, based on animal studies of vagal inhibition of pancreatic exocrine secretion. Amplitudes utilized range from 1 mA to 8 mA. However, in almost all instances, the amplitude is 6 mA. The device is usually activated in the morning and turned off before sleep. The protocol specified an algorithm of 5 minutes of blocking, alternating with 5 minutes without blocking, for approximately 12 hours of therapy per day. Effective electrical contact is verified using impedance measurements at frequent intervals postoperatively. The patient is assessed for possible contraindications. The nature of the procedure, why it is being performed, and possible complications are discussed with the patient. The transmit coil is placed over the subcutaneous neuroregulator on the thoracic sidewall and connected to the mobile charger, which is then connected to the computer programmer. Interrogation and measurement of impedance, current amplitude, block on/off time, ramp-up time, battery-charge status, lead status, therapy delivery, therapy schedule and parameters, and patient compliance are completed. The patient is determined to be set at an amplitude of 6 mA. Her clinician decides to reprogram the device to a higher amplitude. The results of the analysis are communicated to the patient. The clinician increases the amplitude to 6.5 mA using the computer programmer amplitude features. The patient is observed for 15 minutes using the "live test" feature at the changed level of amplitude to determine acceptability of the change. When reprogramming is successful, and the device is delivering the desired mA of current, the procedure is terminated and the patient is disconnected from the computer programmer. All adjustments made to the blocking parameters are documented in the patient's medical record. The patient is sent home.

●0318T  Implantation of catheter-delivered prosthetic aortic heart valve, open thoracic approach, (eg, transapical, other than transaortic)

▶(For percutaneous femoral artery, open femoral artery, open axillary artery, open iliac artery, or transaortic approach, see 33361-33365)◀

▶(To report cardiopulmonary bypass in conjunction with 0318T, see 33367, 33368, or 33369)◀

### ✍ Rationale

In conjunction with the new transcatheter aortic valve replacement (TAVR) codes 33361-33364 and 33367-33369, Category III code 0318T was established to represent the transapical approach for transcatheter aortic valve placement. When peripheral access is inadequate, cardiac procedures involving the placement of an intracardiac prosthesis (ie, stent or valve) can be achieved through transthoracic cardiac exposure via mediastinal, thoracotomy, or subxiphoid approach. The implantation of a prosthetic aortic heart valve through a transthoracic approach can be divided into an approach procedure and a therapeutic (valve implantation) procedure, because two different physicians will often perform different parts of the procedure.

### ☤ Clinical Example (0318T)

An 83-year-old male presents with aortic stenosis, coronary artery disease, and Class III-IV heart failure. The aortic stenosis is life-limiting and severely symptomatic, and is characterized as critical with a documented aortic valve orifice area of 0.6 cm². He has multiple additional co-morbidities that make his risk of mortality with conventional open heart aortic valve replacement greater than 10% by objective predictive criteria. He is evaluated by the valve-team comprised of a cardiac surgeon and an interventional cardiologist, who agree that the operative risks outweigh the benefit. The team, therefore, recommends transcatheter aortic valve replacement. Because of severe peripheral vascular disease, including severe aortoiliac, femoral axillary artery disease, and the presence of a porcelain aorta, a transapical approach is recommended.

**Description of Procedure (0318T)**

A temporary transvenous pacemaker electrode is advanced into the apex of the right ventricle and tested for proper electrical capture. Arterial access (eg, femoral, radial, or brachial) for the reference pigtail catheter is obtained by needle puncture (Seldinger technique), followed by passage of a standard guidewire and pigtail angiographic catheter. The catheter is positioned within the aortic root using fluoroscopy. A root aortogram(s) is obtained using power contrast injection and cine angiography to determine the optimal angiographic angle relative to the native

⊘=Modifier 51 Exempt   ⊙=Moderate Sedation   ✚=Add-on Code   𝒩=FDA approval pending

aortic valve. The heart is exposed through a left anterior thoracotomy in the fifth or sixth intercostal space. Single lung ventilation is initiated, and the left lung is collapsed. A pericardiotomy is performed, and pacing wires are affixed to the ventricular muscle. Two circumferential pledgeted purse-string sutures are placed in the apex of the left ventricle. Anticoagulant therapy is administered to achieve therapeutic anticoagulation levels. A sheath is introduced into the left ventricle, and a pigtail catheter is advanced over a guidewire into the ascending aorta using fluoroscopy. A root aortogram(s) is obtained using power contrast injection and cine angiography to determine the optimal angiographic angle relative to the native aortic valve. Typically, several aortograms in different angles are required.

Under fluoroscopic guidance, access across the native aortic valve is obtained using a guidewire and catheter of the physician's choice. This typically requires multiple attempts and multiple angiographic views due to the severe aortic valve stenosis. Once the guidewire is across the aortic valve and positioned in the aorta, a small catheter is advanced over the guidewire, and the guidewire is exchanged for a stiff guidewire. A large balloon catheter is passed over the guidewire and positioned within the native aortic valve. Rapid pacing is initiated to minimize balloon movement and balloon aortic valvuloplasty is performed: the balloon is inflated by one physician, while another physician continuously adjusts the balloon catheter position to minimize any potential movement and resultant left ventricular trauma/perforation. Typically, this results in hypotension and ventricular ectopy. The balloon is then rapidly deflated and the patient is monitored for hemodynamic recovery. Supravalvular aortography is performed to assess the aorta and ventricle for trauma and to assess for aortic insufficiency. Concurrently, the prosthetic valve is loaded into or onto the delivery catheter. Correct orientation of the valve on the delivery catheter is confirmed by the physician before inserting the valve-delivery catheter system into the introducer sheath. The valvuloplasty catheter is exchanged for the prosthetic delivery catheter over the previously positioned stiff guidewire, while maintaining access across the native aortic valve. The delivery catheter is advanced across the native aortic valve annulus to the aortic root and positioned under fluoroscopic guidance. In addition, transesophageal echocardiography (TEE) may be used to position the prosthesis within the aortic annulus. (If performed, TEE is reported separately.) Multiple supravalvular aortograms may be performed to facilitate placement, before a satisfactory valve position is chosen. The prosthesis is then deployed within the native aortic valve, typically during rapid ventricular pacing.

After confirming satisfactory position and function of the valve, as well as assessing the degree of any paravalvular regurgitation or presence of mechanical complications that might require open, urgent surgical intervention or coronary compromise requiring percutaneous coronary intervention, the delivery catheter and guidewire are removed from the patient. The left ventricular apical sheath is removed and the purse-string sutures are tied. Hemostasis is assured. Protamine is given to reverse the heparin. Chest tube(s) is placed. Double lung ventilation is resumed. The incision is closed in layers, and dressings are placed.

# Appendixes

## Appendix A

For CPT 2013, Appendix A has been updated in tandem with the CPT nomenclature reporting neutrality, which is discussed in the CPT Nomenclature Reporting Neutrality section beginning on page 1 of this book.

Appendix A was also updated with a revision to modifier 62.

## Appendix I

The Genetic Testing Code Modifiers (formerly Appendix I) has been removed from the CPT code set.

## Appendix J

Appendix J has been revised to reflect the deletion of codes 95900-95904 and the addition of codes 95907-95913.

## Appendix O

The CPT code set contains a new administrative code list (Appendix O) with 3 new administrative and 9 new Category I, multianalyte assays with algorithmic analyses (MAAA) codes.

# Appendix A

For CPT 2013, Appendix A was updated in tandem with the CPT nomenclature reporting neutrality, which is discussed in the CPT Nomenclature Reporting Neutrality section beginning on page 1 of this book.

Appendix A was also updated with a revision to modifier 62. Language in modifier 62 was revised to more accurately represent the role of each surgeon. This revision is intended to assist in discerning when to append either CPT modifier 62, *Two Surgeons*, CPT modifier 80, *Assistant Surgeon*, or CPT modifier 82, *Assistant Surgeon (when qualified resident surgeon not available)*, as appropriate, to each code reported. The revision to modifier 62 also offers clarification in the event additional procedure(s) [including add-on procedure(s)] are performed during the same surgical session, those separate code(s) may also be reported with modifier 62 appended. Furthermore, if the co-surgeon acts as an assistant in the performance of additional procedure(s) during the same surgical session, those services may also be reported by that physician using the appropriate procedure code(s) with either modifier 80 or modifier 82 appended.

# Appendix I

## Genetic Testing Code Modifiers

The Genetic Testing Code Modifiers (formerly Appendix I) has been removed from the CPT codebook.

The addition of more than 100 molecular pathology codes to the 2012 code set and still more codes to the 2013 CPT code set has resulted in the deletion of the molecular laboratory procedures related to genetic testing. The genetic testing code modifiers applied to those codes, and therefore, the modifiers are no longer applicable to the 2013 code set.

# Appendix J

## Electrodiagnostic Medicine Listing of Sensory, Motor, and Mixed Nerves

This summary assigns each sensory, motor, and mixed nerve with its appropriate nerve conduction study code in order to enhance accurate reporting of codes 95907-95913. Each nerve constitutes one unit of service.

## Motor Nerves Assigned to Codes 95900 and 95907-95913

Upper extremity, cervical plexus, and brachial plexus motor nerves.

## Sensory and Mixed Nerves Assigned to Codes 95907-95913

Upper extremity sensory and mixed nerves.

## Type of Study/Maximum Number of Studies

| Indication | Limbs Studied by Needle EMG (95860-95864, 95867-95870, 95885-95887) | Nerve Conduction Studies (Total nerves studied, 95907-95913 | Neuromuscular Junction Testing (Repetitive Stimulation, 95937) |
|---|---|---|---|
| Carpal Tunnel (Unilateral) | 1 | 7 | — |
| Carpal Tunnel (Bilateral) | 2 | 10 | — |
| Radiculopathy | 2 | 7 | — |
| Mononeuropathy | 1 | 8 | — |
| Polyneuropathy/Mononeuropathy Multiplex | 3 | 10 | — |
| Myopathy | 2 | 4 | 2 |
| Motor Neuronopathy (eg, ALS) | 4 | 6 | 2 |
| Plexopathy | 2 | 12 | — |
| Neuromuscular Junction | 2 | 4 | 3 |
| Tarsal Tunnel Syndrome (Unilateral) | 1 | 8 | — |
| Tarsal Tunnel Syndrome (Bilateral) | 2 | 11 | — |
| Weakness, Fatigue, Cramps, or Twitching (Focal) | 2 | 7 | 2 |
| Weakness, Fatigue, Cramps, or Twitching (General) | 4 | 8 | 2 |
| Pain, Numbness, or Tingling (Unilateral) | 1 | 9 | — |
| Pain, Numbness, or Tingling (Bilateral) | 2 | 12 | — |

### Rationale

In support of the changes to the Nerve Conduction Tests section, Appendix J was revised to reflect the deletion of codes 95900-95904 and the addition of codes 95907-95913.

⊘=Modifier 51 Exempt   ☉=Moderate Sedation   ✚=Add-on Code   ⟋=FDA approval pending

# Appendix O

## Multianalyte Assays with Algorithmic Analyses

The 2013 CPT code set contains a new Administrative Code List (Appendix O). Appendix O contains 3 new Administrative and 9 new Category I Multianalyte Assays with Algorithmic Analyses (MAAA) codes. Also included are introductory guidelines that provide specific guidance on how to accurately report or assign codes and the specific requirements for inclusion in the Administrative Code List or as a Category I code. Codes 81508 and 81599 were inadvertently left out of Appendix O. This correction will be included in the 2013 CPT errata document and posted on the AMA CPT Web site (www.ama-assn.org/ama/pub/physician-resources/solutions-managing-your-practice/coding-billing-insurance/cpt/about-cpt/errata.page).

# Tabular Review of the Changes

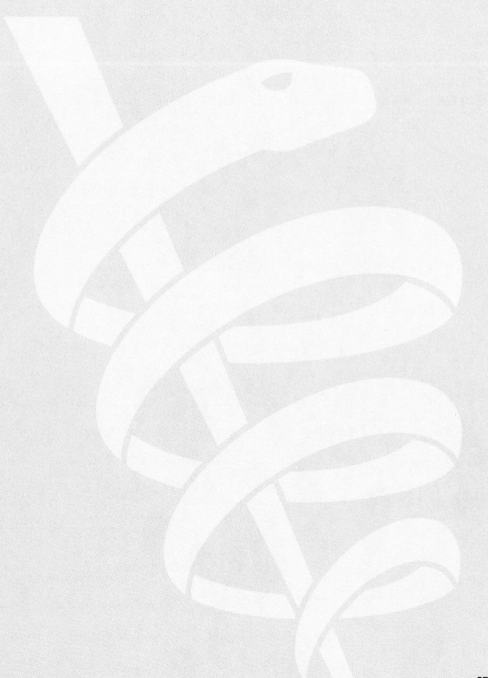

## Evaluation and Management

### Office or Other Outpatient Services

#### New Patient

| Section/Code | Added | Deleted | Revised | Grammatical Revision | Cross-reference |
|---|---|---|---|---|---|
| 99201 | | | X | | X |
| 99202 | | | X | | |
| 99203 | | | X | | |
| 99204 | | | X | | X |
| 99205 | | | X | | |

#### Established Patient

| Section/Code | Added | Deleted | Revised | Grammatical Revision | Cross-reference |
|---|---|---|---|---|---|
| 99211 | | | X | | X |
| 99212 | | | X | | |
| 99213 | | | X | | |
| 99214 | | | X | | |
| 99215 | | | X | | X |

### Hospital Observation Services

#### Observation Care Discharge Services

| Section/Code | Added | Deleted | Revised | Grammatical Revision | Cross-reference |
|---|---|---|---|---|---|
| 99217 | | | X | | X |

#### Initial Observation Care

New or Established Patient

| Section/Code | Added | Deleted | Revised | Grammatical Revision | Cross-reference |
|---|---|---|---|---|---|
| 99218 | | | X | | X |
| 99219 | | | X | | |
| 99220 | | | X | | X |

#### Subsequent Observation Care

| Section/Code | Added | Deleted | Revised | Grammatical Revision | Cross-reference |
|---|---|---|---|---|---|
| 99224 | | | X | | X |
| 99225 | | | X | | |
| 99226 | | | X | | X |

| Section/Code | Added | Deleted | Revised | Grammatical Revision | Cross-reference |
|---|---|---|---|---|---|

**Hospital Inpatient Services**

Initial Hospital Care

New or Established Patient

| Section/Code | Added | Deleted | Revised | Grammatical Revision | Cross-reference |
|---|---|---|---|---|---|
| 99221 | | | X | | X |
| 99222 | | | X | | |
| 99223 | | | X | | X |

Subsequent Hospital Care

| Section/Code | Added | Deleted | Revised | Grammatical Revision | Cross-reference |
|---|---|---|---|---|---|
| 99231 | | | X | | X |
| 99232 | | | X | | |
| 99233 | | | X | | X |

Observation or Inpatient Care Services (Including Admission and Discharge Services)

| Section/Code | Added | Deleted | Revised | Grammatical Revision | Cross-reference |
|---|---|---|---|---|---|
| 99234 | | | X | | X |
| 99235 | | | X | | |
| 99236 | | | X | | X |

**Consultations**

Office or Other Outpatient Consultations

New or Established Patient

| Section/Code | Added | Deleted | Revised | Grammatical Revision | Cross-reference |
|---|---|---|---|---|---|
| 99241 | | | X | | X |
| 99242 | | | X | | |
| 99243 | | | X | | |
| 99244 | | | X | | |
| 99245 | | | X | | X |

Inpatient Consultations

New or Established Patient

| Section/Code | Added | Deleted | Revised | Grammatical Revision | Cross-reference |
|---|---|---|---|---|---|
| 99251 | | | X | | X |
| 99252 | | | X | | |
| 99253 | | | X | | |
| 99254 | | | X | | |
| 99255 | | | X | | X |

⊘=Modifier 51 Exempt  ⊙=Moderate Sedation  ✚=Add-on Code  ⁄V=FDA approval pending

| Section/Code | Added | Deleted | Revised | Grammatical Revision | Cross-reference |
|---|---|---|---|---|---|

**Emergency Department Services**

New or Established Patient

| Section/Code | Added | Deleted | Revised | Grammatical Revision | Cross-reference |
|---|---|---|---|---|---|
| 99281 | | | X | | X |
| 99282 | | | X | | |
| 99283 | | | X | | |
| 99284 | | | X | | |
| 99285 | | | X | | X |

Other Emergency Services

| Section/Code | Added | Deleted | Revised | Grammatical Revision | Cross-reference |
|---|---|---|---|---|---|
| 99288 | | | X | | X |

**Nursing Facility Services**

Initial Nursing Facility Care

New or Established Patient

| Section/Code | Added | Deleted | Revised | Grammatical Revision | Cross-reference |
|---|---|---|---|---|---|
| 99304 | | | X | | X |
| 99305 | | | X | | |
| 99306 | | | X | | |

Subsequent Nursing Facility Care

| Section/Code | Added | Deleted | Revised | Grammatical Revision | Cross-reference |
|---|---|---|---|---|---|
| 99307 | | | X | | X |
| 99308 | | | X | | |
| 99309 | | | X | | |
| 99310 | | | X | | X |

Other Nursing Facility Services

| Section/Code | Added | Deleted | Revised | Grammatical Revision | Cross-reference |
|---|---|---|---|---|---|
| 99318 | | | X | | X |

**Domiciliary, Rest Home (eg, Boarding Home), or Custodial Care Services**

New Patient

| Section/Code | Added | Deleted | Revised | Grammatical Revision | Cross-reference |
|---|---|---|---|---|---|
| 99324 | | | X | | X |
| 99325 | | | X | | |
| 99326 | | | X | | |
| 99327 | | | X | | |
| 99328 | | | X | | |

| Section/Code | Added | Deleted | Revised | Grammatical Revision | Cross-reference |
|---|---|---|---|---|---|
| **Established Patient** | | | | | |
| 99334 | | | X | | X |
| 99335 | | | X | | |
| 99336 | | | X | | |
| 99337 | | | X | | X |
| **Home Services** | | | | | |
| **New Patient** | | | | | |
| 99341 | | | X | | X |
| 99342 | | | X | | |
| 99343 | | | X | | |
| 99344 | | | X | | |
| 99345 | | | X | | |
| **Established Patient** | | | | | |
| 99347 | | | X | | X |
| 99348 | | | X | | |
| 99349 | | | X | | |
| 99350 | | | X | | X |
| **Prolonged Services** | | | | | |
| **Standby Services** | | | | | |
| 99360 | | | X | | X |
| **Care Plan Oversight Services** | | | | | |
| 99374 | | | X | | X |
| 99375 | | | X | | X |
| 99377 | | | X | | X |
| 99378 | | | X | | X |
| 99379 | | | X | | |
| 99380 | | | X | | X |

⊘=Modifier 51 Exempt   ⊙=Moderate Sedation   ✚=Add-on Code   ⫫=FDA approval pending

| Section/Code | Added | Deleted | Revised | Grammatical Revision | Cross-reference |
|---|---|---|---|---|---|

**Non-Face-to-Face Services**

Telephone Services

| Section/Code | Added | Deleted | Revised | Grammatical Revision | Cross-reference |
|---|---|---|---|---|---|
| 99441 | | | X | | X |
| 99442 | | | X | | |
| 99443 | | | X | | X |

On-Line Medical Evaluation

| Section/Code | Added | Deleted | Revised | Grammatical Revision | Cross-reference |
|---|---|---|---|---|---|
| 99444 | | | X | | X |

**Newborn Care Services**

Delivery/Birthing Room Attendance and Resuscitation Services

| Section/Code | Added | Deleted | Revised | Grammatical Revision | Cross-reference |
|---|---|---|---|---|---|
| 99464 | | | X | | X |

**Inpatient Neonatal Intensive Care Services and Pediatric and Neonatal Critical Care Services**

Pediatric Critical Care Patient Transport

| Section/Code | Added | Deleted | Revised | Grammatical Revision | Cross-reference |
|---|---|---|---|---|---|
| 99466 | | | X | | X |
| 99467 | | | X | | X |
| 99485 | X | | | | |
| 99486 | X | | | | X |

**Complex Chronic Care Coordination Services**

| Section/Code | Added | Deleted | Revised | Grammatical Revision | Cross-reference |
|---|---|---|---|---|---|
| 99487 | X | | | | |
| 99488 | X | | | | |
| 99489 | X | | | | |

**Transitional Care Management Services**

| Section/Code | Added | Deleted | Revised | Grammatical Revision | Cross-reference |
|---|---|---|---|---|---|
| 99495 | X | | | | |
| 99496 | X | | | | |

| Section/Code | Added | Deleted | Revised | Grammatical Revision | Cross-reference |
|---|---|---|---|---|---|

## Anesthesia

**Other Procedures**

| Section/Code | Added | Deleted | Revised | Grammatical Revision | Cross-reference |
|---|---|---|---|---|---|
| 01991 | | | X | | |
| 01992 | | | X | | |

## Surgery

**Integumentary System**

Repair (Closure)

Other Flaps and Grafts

| | | | | | |
|---|---|---|---|---|---|
| 15740 | | | X | | X |

**Musculoskeletal System**

General

Introduction or Removal

| | | | | | |
|---|---|---|---|---|---|
| 20665 | | | X | | X |

Spine (Vertebral Column)

Vertebral Body, Embolization or Injection

| | | | | | |
|---|---|---|---|---|---|
| 22522 | | | X | | X |

Arthrodesis

| | | | | | |
|---|---|---|---|---|---|
| 22586 | X | | | | X |

Shoulder

Repair, Revision, and/or Reconstruction

| | | | | | |
|---|---|---|---|---|---|
| 23473 | X | | | | X |
| 23474 | X | | | | X |

Humerus (Upper Arm) and Elbow

Repair, Revision, and/or Reconstruction

| | | | | | |
|---|---|---|---|---|---|
| 24370 | X | | | | X |
| 24371 | X | | | | X |

⊘=Modifier 51 Exempt   ⊙=Moderate Sedation   ✚=Add-on Code   ⊿=FDA approval pending

| Section/Code | Added | Deleted | Revised | Grammatical Revision | Cross-reference |
|---|---|---|---|---|---|
| **Foot and Toes** | | | | | |
| Other Procedures | | | | | |
| 28890 | | | X | | X |
| **Application of Casts and Strapping** | | | | | |
| Lower Extremity | | | | | |
| 29590 | | X | | | X |
| **Respiratory System** | | | | | |
| **Trachea and Bronchi** | | | | | |
| Endoscopy | | | | | |
| 31647 | X | | | | X |
| 31648 | X | | | | X |
| 31649 | X | | | | X |
| 31651 | X | | | | X |
| 31656 | | X | | | X |
| Bronchial Thermoplasty | | | | | |
| 31660 | X | | | | |
| 31661 | X | | | | |
| Introduction | | | | | |
| 31715 | | X | | | X |
| **Lungs and Pleura** | | | | | |
| Removal | | | | | |
| 32420 | | X | | | X |
| 32421 | | X | | | X |
| 32422 | | X | | | X |
| Introduction and Removal | | | | | |
| 32551 | | | X | | X |
| 32554 | X | | | | X |
| 32555 | X | | | | X |

| Section/Code | Added | Deleted | Revised | Grammatical Revision | Cross-reference |
|---|---|---|---|---|---|
| 32556 | X | | | | X |
| 32557 | X | | | | X |
| Stereoatic Radiation Therapy | | | | | |
| 32701 | X | | | | X |

## Cardiovascular System

### Heart and Pericardium

| Pacemaker or Pacing Cardioverter-Defibrillator | | | | | |
|---|---|---|---|---|---|
| 33225 | | | X | | X |
| Cardiac Valves | | | | | |
| 33361 | X | | | | X |
| 33362 | X | | | | X |
| 33363 | X | | | | X |
| 33364 | X | | | | X |
| 33365 | X | | | | X |
| 33367 | X | | | | X |
| 33368 | X | | | | X |
| 33369 | X | | | | X |
| Cardiac Assist | | | | | |
| 33990 | X | | | | X |
| 33991 | X | | | | X |
| 33992 | X | | | | X |
| 33993 | X | | | | X |

### Arteries and Veins

| Vascular Injection Procedures | | | | | |
|---|---|---|---|---|---|
| 36010 | | | X | | |
| 36140 | | | X | | X |
| 36221 | X | | | | X |
| 36222 | X | | | | X |

⊘=Modifier 51 Exempt   ⊙=Moderate Sedation   ✚=Add-on Code   ⩘=FDA approval pending

| Section/Code | Added | Deleted | Revised | Grammatical Revision | Cross-reference |
|---|---|---|---|---|---|
| 36223 | X | | | | X |
| 36224 | X | | | | X |
| 36225 | X | | | | X |
| 36226 | X | | | | X |
| 36227 | X | | | | X |
| 36228 | X | | | | X |
| 36400 | | | X | | X |
| 36405 | | | X | | X |
| 36406 | | | X | | X |
| 36410 | | | X | | X |

Transcatheter Procedures

| Section/Code | Added | Deleted | Revised | Grammatical Revision | Cross-reference |
|---|---|---|---|---|---|
| 37197 | X | | | | |
| 37201 | | X | | | |
| 37203 | | X | | | X |
| 37209 | | X | | | X |
| 37211 | X | | | | X |
| 37212 | X | | | | X |
| 37213 | X | | | | X |
| 37214 | X | | | | X |

## Hemic and Lymphatic Systems

Transplantation and Post-Transplantation Cellular Infusions

| Section/Code | Added | Deleted | Revised | Grammatical Revision | Cross-reference |
|---|---|---|---|---|---|
| 38240 | | | X | | X |
| 38241 | | | X | | X |
| 38242 | | | X | | X |
| 38243 | X | | | | |

| Section/Code | Added | Deleted | Revised | Grammatical Revision | Cross-reference |
|---|---|---|---|---|---|
| **Digestive System** | | | | | |
| Esophagus | | | | | |
| Endoscopy | | | | | |
| 43206 | X | | | | X |
| 43234 | | X | | | X |
| 43252 | X | | | | X |
| Intestines (Except Rectum) | | | | | |
| Other Procedures | | | | | |
| 44705 | X | | | | X |
| **Urinary System** | | | | | |
| Bladder | | | | | |
| Transurethral Surgery | | | | | |
| 52287 | X | | | | |
| **Maternity Care and Delivery** | | | | | |
| Repair | | | | | |
| 59300 | | | X | | |
| **Nervous System** | | | | | |
| Spine and Spinal Cord | | | | | |
| Reservoir/Pump Implantation | | | | | |
| 62370 | | | X | | X |
| Extracranial Nerves, Peripheral Nerves, and Autonomic Nervous System | | | | | |
| Neurostimulators (Peripheral Nerve) | | | | | |
| 64561 | | | X | | |
| Destruction by Neurolytic Agent (eg, Chemical, Thermal, Electrical or Radiofrequency), Chemodenervation | | | | | |
| 64612 | | | X | | X |
| 64614 | | | X | | X |
| 64615 | X | | | | X |

⃠=Modifier 51 Exempt  ⊙=Moderate Sedation  ✚=Add-on Code  𝒩=FDA approval pending

| Section/Code | Added | Deleted | Revised | Grammatical Revision | Cross-reference |
|---|---|---|---|---|---|

## Eye and Ocular Adnexa

### Anterior Segment

#### Anterior Chamber

| Section/Code | Added | Deleted | Revised | Grammatical Revision | Cross-reference |
|---|---|---|---|---|---|
| 65800 | | | X | | X |
| 65805 | | X | | | X |

### Ocular Adnexa

#### Eyelids

| Section/Code | Added | Deleted | Revised | Grammatical Revision | Cross-reference |
|---|---|---|---|---|---|
| 67810 | | | X | | X |

# Radiology

## Diagnostic Radiology (Diagnostic Imaging)

### Chest

| Section/Code | Added | Deleted | Revised | Grammatical Revision | Cross-reference |
|---|---|---|---|---|---|
| 71040 | | X | | | X |
| 71060 | | X | | | X |

### Spine and Pelvis

| Section/Code | Added | Deleted | Revised | Grammatical Revision | Cross-reference |
|---|---|---|---|---|---|
| 72040 | | | X | | |
| 72050 | | | X | | |
| 72052 | | | X | | |

### Vascular Procedures

#### Aorta and Arteries

| Section/Code | Added | Deleted | Revised | Grammatical Revision | Cross-reference |
|---|---|---|---|---|---|
| 75650 | | X | | | X |
| 75660 | | X | | | X |
| 75662 | | X | | | X |
| 75665 | | X | | | X |
| 75671 | | X | | | X |
| 75676 | | X | | | X |
| 75680 | | X | | | X |
| 75685 | | X | | | X |

 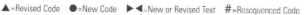

| Section/Code | Added | Deleted | Revised | Grammatical Revision | Cross-reference |
|---|---|---|---|---|---|
| Transcatheter Procedures | | | | | |
| 75896 | | | X | | X |
| 75898 | | | X | | X |
| 75900 | | X | | | X |
| 75961 | | X | | | X |
| **Other Procedures** | | | | | |
| 76000 | | | X | | X |
| 76001 | | | X | | X |
| 76376 | | | X | | X |
| 76377 | | | X | | X |
| **Diagnostic Ultrasound** | | | | | |
| Extremities | | | | | |
| 76885 | | | X | | |
| 76886 | | | X | | |
| **Breast, Mammography** | | | | | |
| 77051 | | | X | | |
| 77052 | | | X | | |
| **Bone/Joint Studies** | | | | | |
| 77071 | | | X | | |
| **Nuclear Medicine** | | | | | |
| Diagnostic | | | | | |
| Endocrine System | | | | | |
| 78000 | | X | | | X |
| 78001 | | X | | | X |
| 78003 | | X | | | X |
| 78006 | | X | | | X |
| 78007 | | X | | | X |

⊘=Modifier 51 Exempt   ⊙=Moderate Sedation   ✚=Add-on Code   ✓=FDA approval pending

| Section/Code | Added | Deleted | Revised | Grammatical Revision | Cross-reference |
|---|---|---|---|---|---|
| 78010 | | X | | | X |
| 78011 | | X | | | X |
| 78012 | X | | | | X |
| 78013 | X | | | | X |
| 78014 | X | | | | X |
| 78070 | | | X | | X |
| 78071 | X | | | | X |
| 78072 | X | | | | X |

## Pathology and Laboratory

**Molecular Pathology**

Tier 1 Molecular Pathology Procedures

| | Added | Deleted | Revised | Grammatical Revision | Cross-reference |
|---|---|---|---|---|---|
| 81201 | X | | | | |
| 81202 | X | | | | |
| 81203 | X | | | | |
| 81235 | X | | | | |
| 81252 | X | | | | |
| 81253 | X | | | | |
| 81254 | X | | | | |
| 81321 | X | | | | |
| 81322 | X | | | | |
| 81323 | X | | | | |
| 81324 | X | | | | |
| 81325 | X | | | | |
| 81326 | X | | | | |

Tier 2 Molecular Pathology Procedures

| | Added | Deleted | Revised | Grammatical Revision | Cross-reference |
|---|---|---|---|---|---|
| 81400 | | | X | | X |
| 81401 | | | X | | |
| 81402 | | | X | | X |

| Section/Code | Added | Deleted | Revised | Grammatical Revision | Cross-reference |
|---|---|---|---|---|---|
| 81403 | | | X | | |
| 81404 | | | X | | |
| 81405 | | | X | | |
| 81406 | | | X | | |
| 81407 | | | X | | |
| 81408 | | | X | | X |
| 81479 | X | | | | X |

**Multianalyte Assays with Algorithmic Analyses**

| | | | | | |
|---|---|---|---|---|---|
| 81500 | X | | | | |
| 81503 | X | | | | |
| 81506 | X | | | | |
| 81508 | X | | | | |
| 81509 | X | | | | |
| 81510 | X | | | | |
| 81511 | X | | | | |
| 81512 | X | | | | |
| 81599 | X | | | | |

**Chemistry**

| | | | | | |
|---|---|---|---|---|---|
| 82009 | | | X | | |
| 82010 | | | X | | |
| 82777 | X | | | | |
| 83890 | | X | | | X |
| 83891 | | X | | | X |
| 83892 | | X | | | X |
| 83893 | | X | | | X |
| 83894 | | X | | | X |
| 83896 | | X | | | X |
| 83897 | | X | | | X |

⊘=Modifier 51 Exempt ⊙=Moderate Sedation ✚=Add-on Code ⃥=FDA approval pending

| Section/Code | Added | Deleted | Revised | Grammatical Revision | Cross-reference |
|---|---|---|---|---|---|
| 83898 | | X | | | X |
| 83900 | | X | | | X |
| 83901 | | X | | | X |
| 83902 | | X | | | X |
| 83903 | | X | | | X |
| 83904 | | X | | | X |
| 83905 | | X | | | X |
| 83906 | | X | | | X |
| 83907 | | X | | | X |
| 83908 | | X | | | X |
| 83909 | | X | | | X |
| 83912 | | X | | | X |
| 83913 | | X | | | X |
| 83914 | | X | | | X |

## Immunology

| Section/Code | Added | Deleted | Revised | Grammatical Revision | Cross-reference |
|---|---|---|---|---|---|
| 86152 | X | | | | X |
| 86153 | X | | | | X |
| 86711 | X | | | | |

## Tissue Typing

| Section/Code | Added | Deleted | Revised | Grammatical Revision | Cross-reference |
|---|---|---|---|---|---|
| 86828 | X | | | | X |
| 86829 | X | | | | X |
| 86830 | X | | | | X |
| 86831 | X | | | | X |
| 86832 | X | | | | X |
| 86833 | X | | | | X |
| 86834 | X | | | | |
| 86835 | X | | | | |

| Section/Code | Added | Deleted | Revised | Grammatical Revision | Cross-reference |
|---|---|---|---|---|---|
| **Microbiology** | | | | | |
| 87498 | | | X | | |
| 87521 | | | X | | |
| 87522 | | | X | | |
| 87535 | | | X | | |
| 87536 | | | X | | |
| 87538 | | | X | | |
| 87539 | | | X | | |
| 87631 | X | | | | X |
| 87632 | X | | | | X |
| 87633 | X | | | | X |
| 87901 | | | X | | |
| 87910 | X | | | | |
| 87912 | X | | | | |
| **Surgical Pathology** | | | | | |
| 88375 | X | | | | X |
| 88384 | | X | | | X |
| 88385 | | X | | | X |
| 88386 | | X | | | X |

# Medicine

**Vaccines, Toxoids**

| Section/Code | Added | Deleted | Revised | Grammatical Revision | Cross-reference |
|---|---|---|---|---|---|
| 90653 | X | | | | |
| 90655 | | | X | | |
| 90656 | | | X | | |
| 90657 | | | X | | |
| 90658 | | | X | | |
| 90660 | | | X | | |
| 90665 | | X | | | X |

⊘=Modifier 51 Exempt  ⊙=Moderate Sedation  ✚=Add-on Code  ⁄⁄=FDA approval pending

| Section/Code | Added | Deleted | Revised | Grammatical Revision | Cross-reference |
|---|---|---|---|---|---|
| 90672 | X | | | | |
| 90701 | | X | | | X |
| 90718 | | X | | | X |
| 90739 | X | | | | |
| 90746 | | | X | | |

**Psychiatry**

Interactive Complexity

| | | | | | |
|---|---|---|---|---|---|
| 90785 | X | | | | |

Psychiatric Diagnostic Procedures

| | | | | | |
|---|---|---|---|---|---|
| 90791 | X | | | | |
| 90792 | X | | | | |
| 90801 | | X | | | X |
| 90802 | | X | | | X |
| 90804 | | X | | | X |
| 90805 | | X | | | X |
| 90806 | | X | | | X |
| 90807 | | X | | | X |
| 90808 | | X | | | X |
| 90809 | | X | | | X |
| 90810 | | X | | | X |
| 90811 | | X | | | X |
| 90812 | | X | | | X |
| 90813 | | X | | | X |
| 90814 | | X | | | X |
| 90815 | | X | | | X |
| 90816 | | X | | | X |
| 90817 | | X | | | X |
| 90818 | | X | | | X |

| Section/Code | Added | Deleted | Revised | Grammatical Revision | Cross-reference |
|---|---|---|---|---|---|
| 90819 | | X | | | X |
| 90821 | | X | | | X |
| 90822 | | X | | | X |
| 90823 | | X | | | X |
| 90824 | | X | | | X |
| 90826 | | X | | | X |
| 90827 | | X | | | X |
| 90828 | | X | | | X |
| 90829 | | X | | | X |

Psychotherapy

| Section/Code | Added | Deleted | Revised | Grammatical Revision | Cross-reference |
|---|---|---|---|---|---|
| 90832 | X | | | | X |
| 90833 | X | | | | X |
| 90834 | X | | | | X |
| 90836 | X | | | | X |
| 90837 | X | | | | X |
| 90838 | X | | | | X |

Other Psychotherapy

| Section/Code | Added | Deleted | Revised | Grammatical Revision | Cross-reference |
|---|---|---|---|---|---|
| 90839 | X | | | | X |
| 90840 | X | | | | X |
| 90857 | | X | | | X |

## Psychiatric Therapeutic Procedures

Other Psychiatric Services or Procedures

| Section/Code | Added | Deleted | Revised | Grammatical Revision | Cross-reference |
|---|---|---|---|---|---|
| 90862 | | X | | | |
| 90863 | X | | | | X |
| 90875 | | | X | | |
| 90876 | | | X | | |
| 90889 | | | X | | |

⃠=Modifier 51 Exempt  ⊙=Moderate Sedation  ✚=Add-on Code  ✗=FDA approval pending

| Section/Code | Added | Deleted | Revised | Grammatical Revision | Cross-reference |
|---|---|---|---|---|---|
| **Dialysis** | | | | | |
| Hemodialysis | | | | | |
| 90935 | | | X | | X |
| Miscellaneous Dialysis Procedures | | | | | |
| 90945 | | | X | | X |
| 90947 | | | X | | X |
| End-Stage Renal Disease Services | | | | | |
| 90951 | | | X | | X |
| 90952 | | | X | | |
| 90953 | | | X | | |
| 90954 | | | X | | |
| 90955 | | | X | | |
| 90956 | | | X | | |
| 90957 | | | X | | |
| 90958 | | | X | | |
| 90959 | | | X | | |
| 90960 | | | X | | |
| 90961 | | | X | | X |
| 90962 | | | X | | X |
| **Gastroenterology** | | | | | |
| 91110 | | | X | | X |
| 91111 | | | X | | X |
| 91112 | X | | | | X |
| **Ophthalmology** | | | | | |
| Special Ophthalmological Services | | | | | |
| Other Specialized Services | | | | | |
| 92286 | | | X | | X |
| 92287 | | | X | | |

| Section/Code | Added | Deleted | Revised | Grammatical Revision | Cross-reference |
|---|---|---|---|---|---|
| **Special Otorhinolaryngologic Services** | | | | | |
| Evaluative and Therapeutic Services | | | | | |
| 92613 | | | X | | |
| 92615 | | | X | | |
| 92617 | | | X | | |
| **Cardiovascular** | | | | | |
| Therapeutic Services and Procedures | | | | | |
| Other Therapeutic Services and Procedures | | | | | |
| 92920 | X | | | | X |
| 92921 | X | | | | X |
| 92924 | X | | | | X |
| 92925 | X | | | | X |
| 92928 | X | | | | X |
| 92929 | X | | | | X |
| 92933 | X | | | | X |
| 92934 | X | | | | X |
| 92937 | X | | | | X |
| 92938 | X | | | | X |
| 92941 | X | | | | X |
| 92943 | X | | | | X |
| 92944 | X | | | | X |
| 92973 | | | X | | X |
| 92980 | | X | | | X |
| 92981 | | X | | | X |
| 92982 | | X | | | X |
| 92984 | | X | | | X |
| 92995 | | X | | | X |
| 92996 | | X | | | X |

⊘=Modifier 51 Exempt   ⊙=Moderate Sedation   ✚=Add-on Code   ✎=FDA approval pending

| Section/Code | Added | Deleted | Revised | Grammatical Revision | Cross-reference |
|---|---|---|---|---|---|
| **Cardiography** | | | | | |
| 93015 | | | X | | X |
| 93016 | | | X | | X |
| **Cardiovascular Monitoring Services** | | | | | |
| 93224 | | | X | | X |
| 93227 | | | X | | X |
| 93228 | | | X | | X |
| 93229 | | | X | | X |
| 93268 | | | X | | X |
| 93272 | | | X | | X |
| **Implantable and Wearable Cardiac Device Evaluations** | | | | | |
| 93279 | | | X | | X |
| 93280 | | | X | | X |
| 93281 | | | X | | X |
| 93282 | | | X | | X |
| 93283 | | | X | | X |
| 93284 | | | X | | X |
| 93285 | | | X | | X |
| 93286 | | | X | | X |
| 93287 | | | X | | X |
| 93288 | | | X | | X |
| 93289 | | | X | | X |
| 93290 | | | X | | |
| 93291 | | | X | | X |
| 93292 | | | X | | X |
| 93293 | | | X | | X |
| 93294 | | | X | | X |
| 93295 | | | X | | X |
| 93297 | | | X | | X |
| 93298 | | | X | | X |

| Section/Code | Added | Deleted | Revised | Grammatical Revision | Cross-reference |
|---|---|---|---|---|---|
| **Echocardiography** | | | | | |
| 93351 | | | X | | X |
| **Intracardiac Electrophysiological Procedures/Studies** | | | | | |
| 93651 | | X | | | X |
| 93652 | | X | | | X |
| 93653 | X | | | | X |
| 93654 | X | | | | X |
| 93655 | X | | | | X |
| 93656 | X | | | | X |
| 93657 | X | | | | X |
| **Noninvasive Physiologic Studies and Procedures** | | | | | |
| 93745 | | | X | | X |
| 93750 | | | X | | |
| 93790 | | | X | | |
| **Other Procedures** | | | | | |
| 93797 | | | X | | |
| 93798 | | | X | | |
| **Pulmonary** | | | | | |
| **Pulmonary Diagnostic Testing and Therapies** | | | | | |
| 94014 | | | X | | |
| 94016 | | | X | | |
| 94452 | | | X | | X |
| 94453 | | | X | | X |
| 94610 | | | X | | X |
| 94774 | | | X | | X |
| 94777 | | | X | | X |

⊘=Modifier 51 Exempt  ⊙=Moderate Sedation  ✚=Add-on Code  ⩍=FDA approval pending

| Section/Code | Added | Deleted | Revised | Grammatical Revision | Cross-reference |
|---|---|---|---|---|---|
| **Allergy and Clinical Immunology** | | | | | |
| *Allergy Testing* | | | | | |
| 95004 | | | X | | X |
| 95010 | | X | | | X |
| 95015 | | X | | | X |
| 95017 | X | | | | |
| 95018 | X | | | | |
| 95024 | | | X | | |
| 95027 | | | X | | |
| 95075 | | X | | | X |
| *Ingestion Challenge Testing* | | | | | |
| 95076 | X | | | | X |
| 95079 | X | | | | X |
| *Allergen Immunotherapy* | | | | | |
| 95120 | | | X | | |
| 95125 | | | X | | |
| 95130 | | | X | | |
| 95131 | | | X | | |
| 95132 | | | X | | |
| 95133 | | | X | | |
| 95134 | | | X | | |
| **Neurology and Neuromuscular Procedures** | | | | | |
| *Sleep Medicine Testing* | | | | | |
| 95808 | | | X | | |
| 95810 | | | X | | X |
| 95811 | | | X | | X |
| 95782 | X | | | | |
| 95783 | X | | | | X |

| Section/Code | Added | Deleted | Revised | Grammatical Revision | Cross-reference |
|---|---|---|---|---|---|
| **Routine Electroencephalography (EEG)** | | | | | |
| 95830 | | | X | | |
| **Nerve Conduction Tests** | | | | | |
| 95900 | | X | | | X |
| 95903 | | X | | | X |
| 95904 | | X | | | X |
| 95907 | X | | | | |
| 95908 | X | | | | |
| 95909 | X | | | | |
| 95910 | X | | | | |
| 95911 | X | | | | |
| 95912 | X | | | | |
| 95913 | X | | | | |
| **Intraoperative Neurophysiology** | | | | | |
| 95920 | | X | | | X |
| 95940 | X | | | | |
| 95941 | X | | | | |
| **Autonomic Function Tests** | | | | | |
| 95924 | X | | | | X |
| 95943 | X | | | | X |
| **Evoked Potentials and Reflex Tests** | | | | | |
| 95934 | | X | | | X |
| 95936 | | X | | | X |
| **Special EEG Tests** | | | | | |
| 95954 | | | X | | |
| 95961 | | | X | | X |
| 95962 | | | X | | X |
| **Other Procedures** | | | | | |
| 95991 | | | X | | X |

⊘=Modifier 51 Exempt  ⊙=Moderate Sedation  ✚=Add-on Code  ⑅=FDA approval pending

| Section/Code | Added | Deleted | Revised | Grammatical Revision | Cross-reference |
|---|---|---|---|---|---|
| **Motion Analysis** | | | | | |
| 96004 | | | X | | X |
| **Functional Brain Mapping** | | | | | |
| 96020 | | | X | | |

### Physical Medicine and Rehabilitation

| Section/Code | Added | Deleted | Revised | Grammatical Revision | Cross-reference |
|---|---|---|---|---|---|
| **Therapeutic Procedures** | | | | | |
| 97530 | | | X | | |
| 97532 | | | X | | |
| 97533 | | | X | | |
| 97535 | | | X | | |
| 97537 | | | X | | |
| **Tests and Measurements** | | | | | |
| 97755 | | | X | | X |

### Non-Face-to-Face Nonphysician Services

| Section/Code | Added | Deleted | Revised | Grammatical Revision | Cross-reference |
|---|---|---|---|---|---|
| **On-line Medical Evaluation** | | | | | |
| 98969 | | | X | | X |

### Special Services, Procedures and Reports

| Section/Code | Added | Deleted | Revised | Grammatical Revision | Cross-reference |
|---|---|---|---|---|---|
| **Miscellaneous Services** | | | | | |
| 99000 | | | X | | X |
| 99001 | | | X | | |
| 99002 | | | X | | |
| 99070 | | | X | | X |
| 99071 | | | X | | X |
| 99078 | | | X | | X |
| 99091 | | | X | | X |

| Section/Code | Added | Deleted | Revised | Grammatical Revision | Cross-reference |
|---|---|---|---|---|---|

**Moderate (Conscious) Sedation**

| Section/Code | Added | Deleted | Revised | Grammatical Revision | Cross-reference |
|---|---|---|---|---|---|
| 99143 | | | X | | X |
| 99144 | | | X | | X |
| 99145 | | | X | | X |
| 99148 | | | X | | X |
| 99149 | | | X | | X |
| 99150 | | | X | | X |

**Other Services and Procedures**

| Section/Code | Added | Deleted | Revised | Grammatical Revision | Cross-reference |
|---|---|---|---|---|---|
| 99174 | | | X | | X |
| 99183 | | | X | | |

## Category II Codes

**Patient History**

| Section/Code | Added | Deleted | Revised | Grammatical Revision | Cross-reference |
|---|---|---|---|---|---|
| 1005F | | | X | | |
| 1052F | X | | | | |

**Physical Examination**

| Section/Code | Added | Deleted | Revised | Grammatical Revision | Cross-reference |
|---|---|---|---|---|---|
| 2060F | | | X | | |

**Diagnostic/Screening Processes or Results**

| Section/Code | Added | Deleted | Revised | Grammatical Revision | Cross-reference |
|---|---|---|---|---|---|
| 3517F | X | | | | |
| 3520F | X | | | | |
| 3750F | X | | | | |

**Therapeutic, Preventive, or Other Interventions**

| Section/Code | Added | Deleted | Revised | Grammatical Revision | Cross-reference |
|---|---|---|---|---|---|
| 4069F | X | | | | |
| 4142F | X | | | | |
| 4240F | | | X | | |

⊘=Modifier 51 Exempt ⊙=Moderate Sedation ✚=Add-on Code ◢=FDA approval pending

| Section/Code | Added | Deleted | Revised | Grammatical Revision | Cross-reference |
|---|---|---|---|---|---|

**Follow-up or Other Outcomes**

| Section/Code | Added | Deleted | Revised | Grammatical Revision | Cross-reference |
|---|---|---|---|---|---|
| 5010F | | | X | | |
| 5020F | | | X | | |
| 5100F | | | X | | |

**Patient Safety**

| Section/Code | Added | Deleted | Revised | Grammatical Revision | Cross-reference |
|---|---|---|---|---|---|
| 6150F | X | | | | |

# Category III Codes

| Section/Code | Added | Deleted | Revised | Grammatical Revision | Cross-reference |
|---|---|---|---|---|---|
| 0030T | | X | | | X |
| 0048T | | X | | | X |
| 0050T | | X | | | X |
| 0173T | | X | | | X |
| 0195T | | | X | | X |
| 0196T | | | X | | X |
| 0206T | | | X | | X |
| 0242T | | X | | | X |
| 0250T | | X | | | X |
| 0251T | | X | | | X |
| 0252T | | X | | | X |
| 0256T | | X | | | X |
| 0257T | | X | | | X |
| 0258T | | X | | | X |
| 0259T | | X | | | X |
| 0276T | | X | | | X |
| 0277T | | X | | | X |
| 0279T | | X | | | X |
| 0280T | | X | | | X |
| 0291T | X | | | | X |
| 0292T | X | | | | X |

| Section/Code | Added | Deleted | Revised | Grammatical Revision | Cross-reference |
|---|---|---|---|---|---|
| 0293T | X | | | | X |
| 0294T | X | | | | X |
| 0295T | X | | | | X |
| 0296T | X | | | | X |
| 0297T | X | | | | X |
| 0298T | X | | | | X |
| 0299T | X | | | | X |
| 0300T | X | | | | X |
| 0301T | X | | | | X |
| 0302T | X | | | | X |
| 0303T | X | | | | X |
| 0304T | X | | | | X |
| 0305T | X | | | | X |
| 0306T | X | | | | X |
| 0307T | X | | | | |
| 0308T | X | | | | X |
| 0309T | X | | | | X |
| 0310T | X | | | | X |
| 0311T | X | | | | |
| 0312T | X | | | | |
| 0313T | X | | | | |
| 0314T | X | | | | |
| 0315T | X | | | | X |
| 0316T | X | | | | |
| 0317T | X | | | | |
| 0318T | X | | | | X |

⊘=Modifier 51 Exempt ⊙=Moderate Sedation ✚=Add-on Code ⟋=FDA approval pending

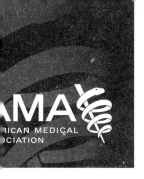

# When you think December, think learning with the AMA.

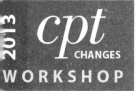

## CPT® Changes 2013 Workshops

A unique one-day, straight-from-the source CPT Changes Workshop educates you on the process, rationale, and application for numerous changes to the CPT code set. Expert instructors provide a hands-on, practical explanation of the changes to the 2013 code set along with some deeper insight into the subject and examples for better understanding.

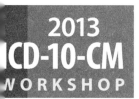

## ICD-10-CM Workshops

Now is the time to increase your awareness of one of the biggest changes to hit health care—the transition from ICD-9-CM to ICD-10-CM. Learn, implement, and code in a one-day ICD-10-CM workshop where subject experts will explain the details and how-to of ICD-10-CM coding.

| CPT Changes | ICD-10-CM | Location |
| --- | --- | --- |
| Mon., Dec. 3 | Tues., Dec. 4 | Baltimore |
| Mon., Dec. 3 | Tues., Dec. 4 | New Brunswick, NJ |
| Wed., Dec. 5 | Thurs, Dec. 6 | Irving, TX |
| Mon., Dec. 10 | Tues., Dec. 11 | Las Vegas |
| Thurs., Dec. 13 | Fri., Dec. 14 | Atlanta |

**Sign up for both and make it a two-day learning retreat.**

For more information on dates and locations and to register, visit **ama-assn.org/gocptchangesworkshops** or **ama-assn.org/go/icd10workshops** or call **(800) 621-8335**.

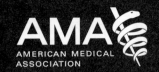

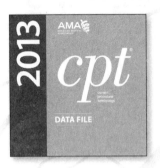

2013
cpt
DATA FILE

# New Descriptors Added to the CPT® 2013 Data File

Purchasers of the *CPT® 2013 Data File* will now have access to two new sets of code descriptors: **CPT® Consumer Friendly Descriptors** and **CPT® Clinician Descriptors**. This is the first time that the American Medical Association has made these descriptors available with the *CPT Data File*.

**Consumer friendly descriptors** translate each code descriptor from the official CPT code set into language that is easily understood by the average patient and/or his or her caregiver.

Consumer friendly descriptors have the potential to be used within electronic health record patient portals, discharge summaries, and explanation of benefits forms.

**Clinician descriptors** describe clearly and specifically the procedure or service performed by a physician or qualified health care provider at the point of care.

Clinician descriptors have the potential to be used for defining a subset of medical procedures and services within an electronic health record, documenting medical procedures and services, conducting research, and reporting clinical and statistical data.

Learn more and order at **ama-assn.org/go/CPTdatafile** or by calling **(800) 621-8335**. For pricing and to license this content for more than 10 users, please send an email message to **Intellectual. Property.Services@ama-assn.org** or call **(312) 464-5022**.

### Interested in licensing additional data files from the AMA?

The AMA also makes available for licensing purposes the *CPT® Enhanced Data File* and the *CPT® Developer's Toolkit*.

The *CPT Enhanced Data File* includes the same content as the *CPT 2013 Data File* but with numeric concept identifiers, machine-readable and computable elements, and additional content for application development and maintenance. It is available in XML and ASCII tab-delimited formats.

*The CPT Developer's Toolkit*, also known as CPT DTK, augments the *CPT 2013 Data File* and the *CPT Enhanced Data File* with the following three main files: type, property, and relationship. In addition to a change history file, the CPT DTK also includes a history file and deleted file. The CPT DTK introduces attributes and relationships based on CPT code characteristics (e.g., anatomic site, method, and device) and also includes enhanced guidelines.

For more information visit **ama-assn.org/go/CPTenhancedfile** and **ama-assn.org/go/CPTDTK**. For pricing and licensing information, please send an email message to **Intellectual.Property. Services@ama-assn.org** or call **(312) 464-5022**.